Praise for *Psychedelic Revival*

"Prepare to embark on a fascinating journey that transcends conventional boundaries. *Psychedelic Revival* offers a groundbreaking exploration into the transformative power of psychedelics and their potential to usher in a new era of healing and the collective evolution of consciousness. Sean Lawlor encourages us to consider the broader implications of their integration into Western culture, acknowledging the benefits, the drawbacks, and the need for responsible and ethical use and for drug policy reform. Whether you are a seasoned enthusiast, a curious skeptic, or someone seeking a deeper understanding of the psychedelic experience, this book is a must-read."

Rick Doblin, PhD
founder (in 1986) and president of MAPS

"If you only buy one book about psychedelics, make it this one. Sean writes with clarity and humility, a truly balanced and trustworthy voice."

Rosalind Watts, PhD
clinical psychologist, founder of ACER Integration, and developer of the ACE model and the Watts Connectedness Scale for measuring outcomes of psychedelic therapy

"If you'd like to understand the full landscape of the psychedelic revival—the good, the not so good, the absurd, and the wonderful—you could not find a better guide and a better guidebook. Separating the myths and the mistakes from the miracles is no easy job. Fortunately, Lawlor is a seasoned astronaut, a fine investigative journalist, and a wonderful storyteller. I don't know a better guide through yesterday's history and today's labyrinth."

James Fadiman, PhD
author of *The Psychedelic Explorer's Guide* and (with Jordan Gruber) *All About Microdosing*

T0322222

"An exceptionally well-written and comprehensive description of the rich history and great potential of psychedelic medicines in psychotherapy. Bursting with vivid quotes, fascinating anecdotes, and engaging references to popular culture, this is a must-read resource for professionals or laypersons seeking to use psychedelic catalysts in their own or their clients' healing journeys. This inspired, compassionate, and grounded book is sure to be an invaluable contribution to the psychedelic renaissance."

Stanislav Grof, MD, PhD
author of *The Way of the Psychonaut* and *LSD Psychotherapy*
and cofounder of the Grof® Legacy Training

Renn Butler, PhD
author of *Pathways to Wholeness* and
director of Grof Studies Graduate Programs

PSYCHEDELIC
REVIVAL

PSYCHEDELIC
REVIVAL

Toward a New Paradigm
of Healing

SEAN LAWLOR

RIDER

Rider, an imprint of Ebury Publishing
20 Vauxhall Bridge Road
London SW1V 2SA

Rider is part of the Penguin Random House group of companies whose
addresses can be found at global.penguinrandomhouse.com

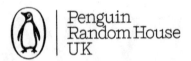

First published in Great Britain by Rider in 2024
First published in the United States by Sounds True in 2024

www.penguin.co.uk

The information in this book is not a substitute for and is not to be
relied on for medical or healthcare professional advice. Please consult your
GP before changing, stopping or starting any medical treatment. So far as the
author is aware the information given is correct and up to date as at 6 June 2024.
The author and publishers disclaim, as far as the law allows, any liability arising
directly or indirectly from the use or misuse of the information contained in this book.

A CIP catalogue record for this book is available from the British Library

ISBN 9781846048449

Printed and bound in Great Britain by Clays Ltd, Elcograf S.p.A.

The authorised representative in the EEA is Penguin Random House Ireland,
Morrison Chambers, 32 Nassau Street, Dublin D02 YH68

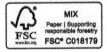

Penguin Random House is committed to a sustainable
future for our business, our readers and our planet.
This book is made from Forest Stewardship
Council® certified paper.

"The further one goes, the less one knows."

—Lao Tzu, *Tao Te Ching*

Contents

Introduction

"Increasingly, the authority of traditional medical science, with
its firm separation between mind and body, is becoming
suspect, and people are seeking more holistic alternatives."

—Stanislav Grof, foreword to *LSD: My Problem Child*

The more we try to define something, the more it eludes our grasp.
Applying strict categories and parameters to concepts, individuals, and
physical things establishes limited viewpoints that wall off inherent complexities. Rather than aiming my longbow of writerly intention at some clever
but narrow synthesis of the variety of substances called *psychedelics*, I set my
sights on considering numerous perspectives to evoke the multitudes of phenomena stirred up by these powerful, polarizing substances.

My psychedelic initiation occurred during a college semester abroad in
Australia, when seven friends and I took "magic" mushrooms one overcast
afternoon and ventured to the sculpture park on campus where I'd spent
countless hours reading philosophy beneath a weeping willow. Fifteen years
have passed since that day, and when I remember the laughter, exploration,
and tender love we shared, I recognize a turning point in my life—a realization there was more happening in the present moment than I had been
taught to believe. Although I had suspected as much through my burgeoning
interest in Zen Buddhism and mysticism, the mushrooms allowed me to
experience it, and every supposition strengthens when immediate perception
grounds it. That afternoon in the sculpture park, I revived vibrant parts of
myself I hadn't realized I'd lost, and my reconnection with the earth, wind,
and sky nourished my body, mind, and spirit. The thought of passing it off
as a mere "high" was absurd.

If there is anything consistent in the infinite expanse of potential effects of psychedelics, it may be their propensity for shaking up one's sense of reality and revealing the limitations of one's dogmas, if not obliterating them completely. Psychedelics consistently reveal that despite our greatest efforts to fit the world into clever models of predictability, life remains infused with mystery, and the truth is never as simple as it seems. To begin answering the question "What are psychedelics?" is to illuminate the vast physical, intellectual, emotional, and spiritual territory upon which their effects shed light.

Since the third millennium CE got rolling, Western society's regard for psychedelics has pivoted from dismissive judgment to widespread interest in their healing potential. By 2013, this shift in zeitgeist had become dramatic enough to require a nickname, and U.K.-based psychiatrist Ben Sessa stepped up to the plate and called it a "psychedelic renaissance." As I write these words ten years later, Sessa's term remains in widespread use. After decades of Federal prohibition of scientific and personal inquiry into these mysterious molecules, psychiatric research has opened Western blockades by demonstrating that psychedelics, when used in specific contexts, are profound medicines capable of healing a seemingly endless array of conditions. From depression to Lyme disease, PTSD to Parkinson's, and anxiety to addiction, it seems no diagnosis is exempt from psychedelic science's inquiry, leading scientists and laypersons alike to regard this renaissance as the foundation of a new paradigm of Western healing, particularly when it comes to mental health.

The abstract, otherworldly, and oftentimes spiritual dimensions of psychedelic-assisted healing present a stark contrast to the biomedical model upon which Western medicine is built. Biomedicine focuses on physical solutions to ailments. As these solutions can be explained via biological mechanisms, the body is regarded as a complex machine whose health is characterized by lack of immediate symptoms. If a pharmaceutical medication represses symptoms to a manageable level without too many side effects, it is considered effective, whether or not the underlying cause gets addressed.

As much as scientists attempt to explain psychedelic-assisted healing through physiological models, these substances' medicinal properties continue to defy medical reductionism. More than any contemporary Western medicine, it seems the *experiences* that psychedelics catalyze are of prevailing significance, as their subjective qualities can either heighten or negate the boons to which the physiological effects grant access. As such, psychedelic science has called for the creation of abstract models to accompany biomedical explanations. This amplifies a tension inherent in confronting mysteries whose solutions elude the reaches of established frameworks.

Mystery has energized the history of science and religion, fueling centuries of contrasting responses vying for supremacy. Science accuses religion of medieval superstition, and religion accuses science of material reductionism antithetical to apprehending the sacred. The unfolding resurgence of Western psychedelic interest has magnified this battle: while many laypersons attribute religious qualities to psychedelic visions, many scientists dismiss such explanations as unscientific, calling instead for research grounded in quantifiable data.

The many important advancements of medical science have yielded increased longevity, improved quality of life, and healing for millions of people. Less frequently acknowledged are biomedicine's limitations, which have become particularly apparent in the field of psychiatry. Following the introduction of psychiatric medication into mental health treatment in the mid-1900s, psychiatry has perpetuated the myth that just as medications can help the body, they can likewise heal the physiological imbalances underpinning mental health ailments. Despite the breakthrough invention of Prozac hitting the market to widespread enthusiasm in 1988, for example, depression continues to afflict 300 million people across the world. While antidepressants undoubtedly help many people, studies have shown they are no more effective than a placebo for up to 85% of users.[1]

Now, in the third millennium CE, psychedelics are generating enthusiasm in medicine and psychiatry, suggesting forms of healing that reach well beyond biomedicine's limits. Since the medical establishment has been slow to adopt these molecules, countless people suffering from a wide range of physical, mental, and emotional illnesses now travel to non-Western communities in such regions as West Africa and the Amazon basin in search of healing through psychoactive plants and fungi that have been used ceremonially for centuries, if not millennia. This trend, which shows no signs of slowing, expresses a Western yearning for a type of healing most hospitals and psychiatric facilities cannot offer. Beneath this yearning is a pervasive sense that something of immense importance is missing in the West, and psychedelic plants and molecules may hold the key to recovering it.

The viewpoint that psychedelics are medicines of remarkable healing potential contrasts significantly with their longstanding reputation in the West. For over five decades, psychedelics have been generally associated with the 1960s hippie counterculture. The hippies' free and open use of psychedelics like LSD was tagged as a prime mover of their anti-Vietnam, anti-authoritarian ethos aimed at manifesting a revolutionary utopia to challenge the uber-capitalistic American Dream their Greatest Generation and Silent Generation parents had instilled after World War II. The threat this antiestablishment mentality posed to the nationalistic status quo prompted US Presidents Lyndon B. Johnson and Richard Nixon to mobilize Federal forces to stomp out its spread. Politically motivated media coverage of psychedelics focused on depravity, promoting propaganda-fueled messages that a single hit of LSD would render its user permanently insane. The anti-psychedelic agenda reached its zenith when the media capitalized on the Charles Manson trial in 1969, pointing its cameras at the cult leader's LSD-guzzling followers carving X's into their foreheads outside the Los Angeles courthouse while expressing no remorse for the grisly Tate-LaBianca murders that had sent tsunamis of fear across the nation. Nixon faced little resistance passing the Controlled Substances Act in 1970, thereby relegating all psychedelics to the new classification of Schedule I.

Schedule I rendered psychedelic production, sale, use, and possession a felony. Stubborn hippies found in possession of LSD could land in prison. A blow of equal proportion was dealt through the act's fine print, which established that Schedule I drugs have a high potential for abuse and no accepted medical use. As a result, the US government effectively blocked all research into the therapeutic and medicinal potential of psychedelics. These blockades remained shatterproof for decades.

Significant as this government-versus-hippie story is, decades of excessive focus on its myriad dramatizations edited an important chapter of psychedelic history out of collective awareness. This lesser-known chronicle is more relevant to the chapter of psychedelic history currently being written than stories of anti-war rallies and peace signs. Before the hippies started taking LSD in the mid-sixties, researchers around the world published promising results on its therapeutic potential. Dozens of studies dating to the early 1950s examined LSD's efficacy for treating addiction, depression, and end-of-life anxiety in people facing terminal cancer diagnoses. Other "classic psychedelics" like mescaline and psilocybin sparked similar enthusiasm, prompting Czech psychiatrist Stanislav "Stan" Grof, perhaps the most prolific "first-wave" researcher, to assert, "Psychedelics, used responsibly and with proper caution, would be for psychiatry what the microscope is for biology and medicine or the telescope is for astronomy. These tools make it possible to study important processes that under normal circumstances are not available for direct observation."[2]

To convince the population that psychedelics had no medicinal value, the US government ignored numerous scientific discoveries, essentially erasing them from public awareness. The government's intended erasure, however, amounted merely to a lengthy suppression for first-wave discoveries came back into the spotlight through "second-wave" research built on the first wave's foundation. Jim Fadiman, one of the few individuals bridging current research with the first wave due to his involvement in both, told me that while the unfolding surge in Western interest is commonly labeled a renaissance, it's really a psychedelic *revival*. While the renaissance has its roots in the West, the revival's origins extend back far before the twentieth century.

Human consumption of psychedelics for healing purposes dates to periods of history where primary records were kept through paintings on cave walls. Several psychoactive "plant medicines" have been consumed by Indigenous cultures around the world for thousands of years. In its many colonial exploits, the Judeo-Christian West has traditionally met such practices with hostility. Colonists and conquistadors have been keener to associate plant medicine use with paganism and devil worship than to take interest in its value. In this sense, Western psychedelic research can be viewed as a revival of healing practices more fundamental to human history than observing molecules through a microscope.

This book is about the second wave of psychedelic research, including many of the histories it implicitly and explicitly revives. It covers foolish chapters in Western history, critiquing the reductive mindset woven into culture while paying homage to the wisdom and bravery of those who maintained steadfast allegiance to meaningful practices in the face of enormous oppression. My hope is to instill an attitude of reverence and humility toward these powerful molecules, eroding the ill-informed pomposity that erroneously declares psychedelic healing a Western discovery. Humility paves the road to allowing these molecules' intrinsic mystery to illuminate aspects of life that defy clear explanation. Such illumination can revive the spirit, even for those lost in a pale void of oversaturated cultural values that fail to imbue their lives with significance.

No attempt of science, mathematics, or philosophy can grasp the entirety of existence, and psychedelics consistently reveal how much remains to be explored and discovered. A web of infinite mystery lies beyond the material immediacy of the present moment. While this web can entangle those who travel into its depths, it can also animate life with a renewed sense of possibility, especially for those whose sense of wonder has been buried beneath heartache and pain. Perhaps this animation provides an antidote to more modern afflictions than we realize.

Can psychedelics shed light on the incorporeal layers of illness Western medicine ignores, linking physical symptoms with nonphysical causes? Might these molecules meet the emptiness so many people face with forms of healing the Western world has seldom known—or, perhaps more accurately, has long forgotten?

Psychedelic advocates are often eager to make such claims. This mentality, however, can devolve into "Psychedelics will save the world!" sensationalism, which damaged the substances' reputation in the 1960s when folks like psychologist-turned-hippie-guru Timothy Leary proselytized about LSD's capacity to awaken the masses to political repression and heal a broken culture. "Turn on, tune in, and drop out," Leary instructed a crowd of around 30,000 at San Francisco's Golden Gate Park in 1967. As his words evolved into a countercultural mantra for detaching from social conventions through psychedelic use, their orator attracted the ire of Johnson and Nixon, resulting in Leary's imprisonment after a string of arrests for marijuana possession. One of the many lessons Leary and the hippie counterculture taught us is that claiming widespread psychedelic use will yield a utopia accomplishes little apart from crafting a naïve dreamworld. Like many worlds envisioned in dreams, the psychedelic utopia crumbles beneath reality's boots.

It's easy to get excited about psychedelics, especially amid increased mainstream recognition of their potential. However, research repeatedly demonstrates the healing they induce is more complicated than taking a drug. Psychedelics will not in and of themselves recover the elusive pieces missing from Western medicine. What they can do is open access to inner and outer realities more expansive than physical symptoms, and specific contexts, models, and techniques implemented by trained, ethically guided professionals can profoundly enhance these realities' potential to catalyze behavioral and psychological transformation. Transformation comes through intentionally engaging with the content the psychedelic evokes—memories, emotions, visions, and so on—especially when the content is challenging to behold. That's a radically different approach from taking LSD to soar through the starry Woodstock sky on currents of Janis Joplin's wailing vibrations.*

The mysterious nature of psychedelic medicine gives rise to one of this book's core questions: What does it mean to *heal*? It wasn't until diving into the subject that I recognized how complex and nuanced healing can be. Physical healing tends to be obvious: broken bones heal when they mend, and colds heal when our immune system prevails. When it comes to mental and emotional wounds, the process is less precise.

Psychedelics may infuse the world with a sense of magic, but they are not magical cure-alls. The healing process requires active engagement, with or without psychedelics. The length and form an individual's process assumes are impossible to quantify objectively. Nevertheless, human beings, in their limitless curiosity, continue to create theories and protocols that bring consistency to the unpredictable subjectivity of psychedelic-assisted healing.

---

*   This is not to suggest that watching a Janis Joplin performance on LSD would be anything short of amazing, nor is it to declare that I wouldn't pay a hefty sum for the time machine I'd need to make it happen.

Rather than over-glorifying psychedelics as a prophesied panacea, I draw from extensive research and over fifty interviews with subject matter experts to encourage an increasingly psychedelic-positive society to incorporate these compounds into its systems with wisdom, care, and respect. Of the many things psychedelic research has demonstrated, an essential tenet is that when certain conditions are accounted for, these mysterious, consciousness-altering agents can yield relatively predictable and positive outcomes. This book synthesizes numerous patterns, trends, and lessons from the swirling mass of psychedelic strangeness in hope of offering guidance for clinicians, clients, and every curious cat among us looking to kickstart their life in a new direction.

Perhaps there is an inherent order to the inner life. Perhaps we can revive that order in the face of life's chaos through patience, trust, and courage. For those embarking upon or deep in the throes of a healing journey, I hope this book serves you as an ally, helping you relate to your circumstances with compassion and equanimity. If nothing else, I hope these words reveal what mushrooms showed me in that sculpture park in Australia many years ago: no matter how certain we feel about life, there is always more to discover.

I

PSYCHEDELICS
IN THE WEST

1

Setting the Stage

"To fathom hell or soar angelic, just take a pinch of psychedelic."

—Humphry Osmond, in a letter to Aldous Huxley

The word "psychedelic" first appeared in 1956, when psychiatrist Humphry Osmond proposed the term in a letter to esteemed scholar, philosopher, and *Brave New World* author Aldous Huxley. Seeking to describe the strange and powerful substances that had recently garnered Western interest, Osmond combined the Greek words *psyché*—translated as "soul" or "mind"—and *dêlos*—translated as "manifest"—into psychedelic, which translates to "mind-" or "soul-manifesting." Huxley raised no objections, for he agreed with Osmond's assessment that these drugs expanded the reaches of consciousness, granting access to heightened capacities of human perception. Despite the blowback these mind-manifesting molecules attracted in the decades that followed Osmond's letter, his term endured, and it remains the most common appellation for these drugs today.

A subclass of psychoactive drugs known to the medical world as "hallucinogens," psychedelics evoke powerful "non-ordinary" states of consciousness that carry the potential to catalyze inner transformation. The variety of purposes for which people take these drugs include psychological and emotional healing, self-exploration, cognitive enhancement, interpersonal bonding, spiritual growth, connection with nature, and deepening bonds with loved ones. Their range of effects includes visual distortions, increased empathy, existential and spiritual insight, reliving of memories, spatiotemporal distortion, out-of-body and near-death experiences, closed-eye visions of geometrical patterns, and a sense of connection to life's fundamental processes. On the flipside, psychedelics can induce anxiety, confusion, nausea, disconnection from reality, and terror of a profundity that cannot be adequately described.

Given this vast spectrum, no theorist can concisely capture everything psychedelics do. Stan Grof, however, came pretty darn close. Based on decades of LSD research, Grof defined psychedelics as "nonspecific amplifiers of the unconscious."[1] With these words, he evoked psychedelics' capacity to shine conscious light on unconscious content. The nonspecific nature of what this light illuminates means anything is fair game, from traumatic memories to repressed desires to visions of spiritual beings and parallel dimensions. Psychedelics don't create an experience in a vacuum; they take what's inside a person, plug it into a multisensory PA system, and crank up the overdrive.[*]

As helpful as definitions and metaphors are for understanding psychedelics, discussing them in a general sense obscures important differences between the numerous compounds assembled beneath this categorical umbrella. People mistakenly believe that all psychedelics are essentially the same and that the benefits science demonstrates for one molecule can be drawn from the others. This inaccurate perception can get people into trouble, as certain psychedelics are significantly more powerful than those receiving positive mainstream press. If each psychedelic is individually mind-manifesting, then the mind they collectively manifest is stranger than we can possibly comprehend.

Unless I discover the technology to create some ever-updating encyclopedia like *The Hitchhiker's Guide to the Galaxy*, it will remain impossible to elucidate every psychedelic in a single book. I've thus restricted my focus to eight substances, each of which continues to play a significant role in the Western revival:

- Psilocybin
- LSD
- MDMA
- Ketamine

- Mescaline
- Ibogaine
- 5-MeO-DMT
- DMT

---

[*] For the *Spinal Tap* fans out there, the psychedelic amps definitely go to eleven.

This list constitutes a drop in the psychedelic ocean. For proof, one needn't look further than the books *PIHKAL: A Chemical Love Story* and *TIHKAL: The Continuation*. Written by psychedelic pioneers Alexander (better known as "Sasha") and Ann Shulgin, *PIHKAL* (an acronym for "Phenethylamines I Have Known and Loved") and *TIHKAL* (an acronym for "Tryptamines I Have Known and Loved") are filled with more than two hundred recipes for various psychoactive compounds, many of which Sasha, a widely respected chemist, created. The majority of these compounds could fit into today's psychedelic categorical boundaries, for their edges have proven more permeable than those established in the 20th century.

Classic Psychedelics and New Additions

Several compounds that have historically belonged to separate classes of drugs have been adopted as psychedelics. Their properties tend to differ significantly from the "classic psychedelics." The four classic psychedelics— LSD, psilocybin, mescaline, and DMT—elicit non-ordinary states of consciousness characterized by visual distortions, vivid mental imagery, and dramatic shifts in emotion and cognition.[2] Researchers have correlated their hallucinogenic effects with action on receptor sites for serotonin, the complex neurotransmitter that modulates numerous processes including mood, cognition, learning, and memory.

The two most significant adoptees in second-wave psychedelic categorization are MDMA and ketamine, both of which have made waves in mental health research when combined with therapy. MDMA—better known as "ecstasy"—belongs to the "empathogen" class of drugs, for its heart-opening properties yield an increased sense of empathy and emotional connection. These empathogenic effects have been correlated with a release of oxytocin, the hormone associated with love and interpersonal bonding. MDMA also modulates release of serotonin, dopamine (connected to motivation and reward), and norepinephrine (connected to alertness and adrenaline). The cumulative effect replaces the visual distortions of classic psychedelics with increased focus and embodiment.

Ketamine, on the other hand, is a "dissociative anesthetic" used primarily for conking out people preparing to undergo surgery and instantaneously numbing agonizing pain. While MDMA intensifies the immediacy of the physical world, ketamine rapidly dissolves it into oblivion. After taking "sub-anesthetic" doses, however, ketamine users maintain awareness as they travel through nonphysical spaces of dark textures, trippy imagery, or a combination of the two. Although serotonin plays no role in its glutamate-driven effects, ketamine's visionary and antidepressant properties have afforded it a seat at the psychedelic table.

You need neither to understand nor care about neurotransmitters to get a sense of the differences between each psychedelic. Even the classic psychedelics catalyze a wide range of effects, with DMT being notorious for swiftly inducing otherworldly visions of a parallel realm that may or may not house humanoid alien entities. I explore each substance in depth in its corresponding chapter, but if you find yourself jonesing for a trip as soon as possible, take care to research your chosen psychedelic and recognize what you're getting into. Otherwise, you might think DMT will bliss you out like MDMA and find yourself blasted out of an intergalactic cannon toward a destination you weren't prepared to visit.

Plant Medicines

Like psychedelics, the range of plants and fungi belonging to the category of hallucinogenic "plant medicines" is too extensive to detail exhaustively. My focus thus centers on five primary plant medicines* that have attracted significant attention since they entered Western awareness:

- Psilocybin-containing mushrooms
- *Amanita muscaria* mushrooms

- Iboga
- Ayahuasca
- Peyote

---

* Some of these medicines belong to the Fungi kingdom, which is taxonomically distinct from the kingdom Plantae. Nevertheless, these fungi are typically included in the plant medicine category. For simplicity's sake, I will maintain this inclusion.

Many psychedelic compounds are derived from these and other plant medicines. Psilocybin was first isolated from the *Psilocybe mexicana* mushroom, ibogaine was derived from the African *Tabernanthe iboga* shrub, and mescaline was synthesized from *Lophophora williamsii*, the peyote cactus. This does not mean that the isolated chemicals and their organic hosts are the same.

Plant Medicines as a Separate Category

Issues stemming from assuming all psychedelics are the same grow exponentially when plant medicines are included in the category. For starters, plant medicines are not synthesized molecules delivered through a pill, powder, or syringe. Their psychoactive properties result from natural alkaloids found in fungi, cacti, vines, leaves, flowers, roots, bark, and other organic materials.

Unlike the cultural neutrality of psychedelics, plant medicines are inextricable from their cultural context. They are traditionally consumed in ceremonial rituals of cultures indigenous to the specific regions where the given plant or fungi grows. The structures of these ceremonies develop through generations of navigating and understanding the medicine's effects. Often, the plant medicine is so essential to a culture that the culture's mythology and value system is woven into the fabric of their healing rituals. When a Western seeker thus consumes a plant medicine because they heard about psychedelics on CNN, they may find themselves beholding a reality as foreign to them as the culture that holds the medicine as sacred.

A few years ago, a US Army veteran seeking psychedelic treatment contacted me after reading an article I wrote on the therapeutic use of LSD. He'd seen the 2018 documentary *From Shock to Awe*, which follows veterans Matt Kahl and Mike Cooley's use of the Amazonian plant medicine ayahuasca to heal their treatment-resistant PTSD alongside veteran Brooke Cooley's therapeutic use of MDMA for the same reason. The documentary gives the impression that ayahuasca and MDMA are similar in their induction of a non-ordinary state that catalyzes healing from combat-related trauma. In reality, they are not similar at all.

While both can potentially help heal complex PTSD, MDMA was synthesized in a lab, and ayahuasca comes from brewing a leaf and a vine native to the Amazon jungle. MDMA has been used therapeutically for about fifty years, while ayahuasca has been consumed ceremonially by Amazonian tribes for centuries, if not millennia.* If you want to get nerdy, DMT, the primary psychoactive alkaloid of ayahuasca, belongs to the tryptamine class of compounds, while MDMA is of the phenethylamine class. Each chemical interacts with different parts of the brain—ayahuasca's DMT is an agonist of 5HT2A receptors, mimicking serotonin through molecular similarity, while MDMA, as you'll recall, prompts a large release of serotonin, norepinephrine, dopamine, and oxytocin.

Just because two substances can help the same condition does not mean those two substances are the same. Taking part in a ceremony in the Amazon is fundamentally different from taking MDMA in a Western therapeutic context. If this veteran had continued assuming MDMA and ayahuasca were essentially identical, he could have found himself in the grip of an overwhelming journey through ayahuasca's otherworldly depths. Due to differences in histories, syntheses, cultural contexts, and effects, psychedelics and plant medicines are best regarded as separate categories.

A Unique Class of Compounds

A paradigm of scientific materialism operates at the core of the biomedical model. This model dominates Western health care, including mental health treatment. Diagnosis is the name of the game, prompting psychiatrists to prescribe antidepressants, antipsychotics, anxiolytics, and a plethora of other symptom-reducing drugs targeting the molecular manifestations of the condition. Though therapists are not MDs like psychiatrists, counseling master's programs train them to employ "evidence-based therapies" that have weathered the scientific method to receive the mighty stamp of approval from "peer reviewers," the gatekeepers of academia.

Such therapeutic approaches are wonderful, but since a modality must become evidence-based in order for insurance companies to cover treatment, data-driven methods are venerated over experimental or alternative therapies.

---

* This ambiguity is not due to lack of research. It's because nobody knows for certain when ayahuasca was first consumed. It's generally assumed ayahuasca has been used for thousands of years, but some scholars, such as anthropologist Bernd Brabec de Mori, claim the plant medicine could be less than five hundred years old.

Measurable, linear models reign over nonlinear approaches, and strict therapeutic procedures with verifiable checkpoints gain priority over open exploration of the vast domains of consciousness. "If you can't prove it with numbers and figures, it isn't worth considering," say the Scientific Overlords.

Following Nixon's Controlled Substances Act of 1970, the scientific mainstream rejected psychedelic research as buffoonery. Scientists who expressed interest essentially committed career suicide, for the experiences psychedelics evoked were as nonmaterial as they come. To change the narrative, second-wave researchers dusted off their creativity specs and established elegant methods to usher psychedelics through the gauntlet of scientific materialism. It's largely due to their success that the revival has reached its current mainstream status in the West.

In the early 2000s, leading institutions like Johns Hopkins University and the Multidisciplinary Association for Psychedelic Studies (MAPS) developed rigorous, placebo-controlled protocols for administering psilocybin and MDMA in therapeutic settings to participants with specific diagnoses. They communicated the effectiveness of psychedelic treatments through the esoteric data and technical verbiage required to satisfy the peer reviewers and the US government, prompting Uncle Sam to relax his long-standing, unwilling-to-budge embargo. The data demonstrated that specific protocols of psychedelic administration in the context of therapy were not only safe, but more effective than leading evidence-based treatments for pervasive conditions like treatment-resistant depression and post-traumatic stress disorder. That's because unlike other psychiatric medicines, psychedelics help people dig into root causes of their conditions. In the words of American Buddhist teacher Jack Kornfield, psychedelic-assisted healing arises through "the power of bringing into consciousness that which has been below the threshold of awareness."[3] For someone suffering from depression, a selective serotonin reuptake inhibitor (SSRI) like Prozac may dull emotional pain and help them function in everyday life, but it will not reveal *why* they are depressed. Unlike SSRIs, psychedelics expand the lens of consciousness, allowing one to observe emotions, memories, and unmet needs underpinning their depressive patterns. Regardless of the cause, broadened awareness opens the opportunity to recognize and shift the habits that unconsciously lock the doors of depression's dungeons.

Grof's definition of psychedelics as "nonspecific ampliers of the unconscious" means they can reveal an infinite array of possible causes. Sometimes, those causes are imprecise. Perhaps a dose of psilocybin connects a depressed individual to a spiritual reality, prompting them to pinpoint a lack of recognition of the sacred as the foundation of their suffering. While most prescription drugs have predictable effects—opiates reduce pain, benzodiazepines calm anxiety—psychedelics take people on unpredictable inner journeys whose content arises from their personal lives. The quotient of variability between psychedelic experiences far outweighs that of modern pharmaceuticals.

Psychedelic healing is not as simple as taking a drug, because psychedelics respond to *intention*. Approaching them with respect, humility, and hope to gain insight is more likely to yield a beneficial outcome than taking them because you're bored. Given their unpredictability, intentions of openness and trust help pave the road to personal transformation.

Case Study: A Navy SEAL Battles Alcoholism with Psychedelics

Before diving into theories on how psychedelic healing works, I'll share a story of a retired Navy SEAL I had the pleasure of interviewing. I'll refer to him as Sam. When Sam was discharged in 2016, he rapidly lost his sense of purpose.

"Two years ago, I was a point man in Afghanistan, getting shot at, planning operations, doing interesting things," he said. "All of a sudden, I'm working for a bank, answering phone calls eight hours a day, thinking, 'What the fuck *am* I?'"

To cope with his confusion, Sam turned to alcohol. Soon, he was drinking around the clock. After getting a DUI, he quit his job. When he informed his girlfriend, whom he'd planned on marrying, she broke up with him, told him not to contact her, and blocked his number. Sam went into a tailspin.

"Fifth of whiskey, every single day, and usually some beers afterward," he recalled. "I would wake up and drink whiskey. If I didn't have any left, I'd panic because I had to wait until ten a.m. when the liquor store opened. It snowballed out of control."

Sam knew he needed help. When he told psychiatrists he was a SEAL, they diagnosed PTSD and prescribed pharmaceuticals. He knew combat trauma wasn't the problem, and the drugs didn't work. Alcoholics Anonymous helped, but not enough, and things went from bad to worse.

When Sam left the SEALs, he weighed 215 pounds, a healthy weight for his 6'2" frame. Now, he weighed 163 pounds. He was "at death's door" when he heard from a close friend he'd served with in Afghanistan. After discharge, his friend had become addicted to alcohol and methamphetamine. He told Sam a nonprofit foundation had arranged for him to travel to a psychedelic retreat center in Mexico. There, he'd taken ibogaine and 5-MeO-DMT with other veterans, and he'd been sober ever since.

"Honestly, lying down blindfolded in a room full of strangers doing psychedelics sounded like the stupidest shit I'd ever heard of," Sam recalled. "But I was out of options, so I said, 'Fuck it. I'll give it a try, and I'll go into it with an open mind.'"

He contacted a similar foundation that funds veterans' trips to psychedelic retreat centers. The next opening in Mexico was two months away, but a clinic in Texas that offered mushrooms instead of ibogaine had an opening in four days. In the midst of an attempt to cut the booze cold turkey, Sam was so sick from withdrawals that he wasn't sure he could physically make it to the airport. He found the strength to persevere, and four days later, he was imbibing mushrooms alongside other veterans and first responders in a group ceremony.

At first it was excruciating. "I'm blindfolded, seeing kaleidoscope shit. I'm throwing up, gagging, spitting into the bowl next to me, thinking, 'This fucking sucks.' Eventually, I just went into it."

Once he'd surrendered, the mushrooms brought up a repressed memory, a concept Sam had previously thought was bullshit. The memory had nothing to do with his time overseas.

"When I was five and living in Florida, I was playing around at a park one day, and there was a bathroom nearby. I ran in, and a dude molested me. I didn't do anything. I just stood there. It just *happened*."

On mushrooms, he didn't simply observe the memory—he relived it, realizing it had profoundly affected his life. "From the time I was five, I never wanted to feel weak, helpless, or scared like that again. That manifested in bad ways. I was starting fights in fifth grade. At the same time, I was super shy and quiet."

His challenges compounded as his family moved from city to city. Always the new kid, he needed to prove he was tough. If anyone ridiculed him or got on his nerves, he'd punch them in the jaw. "My mom told me that when I was in kindergarten, I threatened my teacher that I would go to my grandpa's house, get his gun, and shoot her in the head. I don't remember that, but I'm not surprised. I was constantly pissed off at the world."

Reliving the memories, Sam felt associated emotions of anger, shame, helplessness, fear. He hadn't cried in decades, but he found himself sobbing uncontrollably. "I was finally able to *feel* and be okay with feeling. That comes from being vulnerable, and vulnerability isn't a strong suit for SEALs."

As his insights deepened, Sam recognized the patterns he developed after being molested led him to join the SEALs. "By becoming a SEAL, no one can question whether or not you're tough. I thought, 'If I can do this, I've proven I'm a badass, and all those feelings will go away. I won't need to deal with that shit anymore, because I'll have proven myself through doing this impossible thing.' Then, you become a SEAL, you go to war, and when it's over, you realize, 'I don't feel any different than I did before. None of it is solved.'"

After Sam had moved through the painful memories, the mushrooms directed his mind's eye toward alcohol. He had a vision of his younger cousins, who looked up to him, observing his body at his funeral after drinking had killed him. "The psilocybin showed me, 'If you keep going, you're going to end up in an early grave, and you'll be an embarrassment.' Your cousins will remember, 'He was a hero to the three of us, and then we didn't hear from him again until he showed up dead because he drank himself to death.'"

In another vision, Sam saw himself standing at the altar with his ex-girlfriend, and he saw the family they could have had. "It was like, 'Look at all this stuff that could have been that you fucked up.'"

Unpleasant as it was to endure, Sam didn't resist. He stayed with the unpleasantness, and eventually, the tone shifted. "By the end, it was like, 'There's so much more out there. You're still young. That's over with. Where you go from here is up to you.'" He saw that amid all the anger, rage, and struggle to maintain control, he had developed tremendous passion and drive. "The psilocybin was like, 'There's another way forward. You can use the positive stuff that came from the negative, and you can funnel it a different way. But you have to leave drinking behind.'"

As the effects dwindled, Sam felt like he'd "run two marathons." In his exhaustion, he noticed something extraordinary: for the first time in recent memory, he felt at peace. "I felt so much gratitude to be where I was. I thought, 'Thank God for that experience. Thank God people cared enough about me to reach out and get me here.' It was so profound."

It didn't take long for him to realize his relationship to the past had shifted. "When I thought back on those memories, I didn't feel anger or sadness or shame. The psilocybin allowed me to leave it in the past. I confronted that shit head-on and got through it, and I got a second chance at life. It was like, 'Day one of part two of your life starts now. Go.' It was exciting, man."

In part two of his life, the anger Sam had felt since early childhood transformed. "If some random guy walked up to me right now and said, 'Hey, dude, *fuck you*,' I'd say, 'All right, man. Have a good day.' If you did that to me seven months ago, I was going to try to put you in the hospital. Now, I think, 'Poor guy's having a bad day.' I can be more empathetic. I'm not going to indulge those temptations to get pissed off, because you don't know what other people are going through. It's not worth spending your time on Earth locked in fucking combat all the time. There are better ways to live."

One element of Sam's better way of living is to feel challenging emotions without allowing them to grip him. "The psilocybin enabled me to feel things like sadness and anger and react appropriately. I cry now. I let it out. That's done wonders for me. I've been able to let so much of that anger and hatred inside of me go."

His newfound gratitude permeated our conversation, and it came as little surprise when he said he reminds himself of his blessings every day. "I've got a great job, and I'm doing well at it. I've got friends. I've damaged relationships with people in the past, and I've repaired them. Things have gotten so much better."

There's one more way his life has improved: since his journey, he hasn't had a drink of alcohol. "I don't know why, but I haven't felt tempted to get a bottle of whiskey and get fucked up," he said. "A few times, I've been watching a baseball game and thought, 'A beer would be pretty good right now.'

But I think back on what I experienced, and I'm like, 'Fuck that. Let's watch the game without a beer. I'm good.'"

Sam's story exemplifies numerous aspects of the psychedelic healing process. Although his ceremony transpired outside legal boundaries, his inner journey and transformation exemplify the aspirations of the primary model of psychedelic healing in the West. That model, which lies at the foundation of the psychedelic research that has attracted widespread enthusiasm, is psychedelic-assisted therapy.

2

Foundations of
Psychedelic-Assisted Therapy

"What I have learned in the last five years is that the greatest threat to
a healthy psychedelic future is the fetishizing of just the drug alone."

—Rosalind Watts,
"It's Time to Start Studying the Downside of Psychedelics"[1]

Psychedelic-assisted therapy, or *psychedelic therapy*, is more similar to traditional therapy than often gets recognized. In the majority of sessions,
clients are sober as they meet with a therapist. They process fears, explore
traumatic memories, define treatment goals, and expand their capacity to
regulate their nervous system amid challenging emotions. Adding a psychedelic to the mix can accelerate the therapeutic process, giving the client and
therapist a trove of rich material to work with.

Psychedelic therapy is less of an independent modality than a framework within which numerous modalities can be implemented. Applicable
approaches appear to be limitless, and new synergistic methods continue
to emerge as practitioners explore the psychedelic frontier. Nevertheless,
certain psychological schools and methods have provided a general foundation for psychedelic therapy since it emerged in the 1950s. First-and
second-wave researchers alike have found that these models of the psyche
relate symbiotically to the non-ordinary states psychedelics catalyze.

Psychoanalysis and the Unconscious

The founder of psychoanalysis has perhaps the most widely recognized name in the history of Western psychology. Known to pop culture's beloved consciousness voyagers Bill and Ted as "The Frood Dude," this cigar-loving provocateur is Sigmund Freud. While Freud certainly snorted his fair share of cocaine in the late 1800s, his work predated psychedelics' arrival in the West by several decades. Still, he inadvertently influenced psychedelic therapy through his conceptualization of the unconscious mind and its defense mechanisms.

Freud and his followers regarded the psyche as an iceberg: what we see on the surface (consciousness) amounts to a minute percentage of the whole, while the most powerful layers (the unconscious) lurk in unseen depths. Consciousness does not give rise to the unconscious; it's the other way around. The conscious "ego" is more like a vessel controlled by unconscious forces than a domain of free thinking.

The unconscious houses an individual's desires, fantasies, fears, and defense mechanisms. According to Freud, an unconscious war wages between one's aggressive, sexual, and primal instincts—the "id"—and one's internalized moral compass dictating how to behave—the "superego." Drawing on implicit and explicit messages from the individual's education, family system, religion, and culture, the superego develops through childhood and adolescence to repress the id's primitive, chaotic energy. But the id fights against this control, and the resultant neurosis expresses as the tangled mess of the ego. (Though Freud continues to draw accusations of chauvinism, dogmatism, and penile obsession, he's rarely been accused of optimism.*)

Freud's psychoanalytic approach is commonly understood as a method of *making the unconscious conscious.* This is the path to establishing internal balance and learning to express desires in healthy ways. Psychoanalysis

---

* He was, after all, heavily influenced by German philosopher Arthur Schopenhauer, whose 19th-century work exemplified "philosophical pessimism." Given Schopenhauer's over-the-top misogyny, it's little surprise that Freud frequently attracts chauvinist accusations, especially given his delineation of a female's development as "penis envy," which means exactly what it suggests. Coincidentally, one of the most potent strains of psilocybin-containing mushrooms carries the name "penis envy" due to their uncanny—another Freudian term!—resemblance to phalli.

derives insight into the unconscious through dream interpretation, hypnosis, and free association—a technique wherein an analyst says a word or phrase and the client responds with whatever leaps to mind. Freud's controversial interest in cocaine shared a core commonality with later psychoanalysts' interest in psychedelics: both theorized their drug of interest relaxed defense mechanisms, opening access to the unconscious.

Unlike cocaine, psychedelics didn't seem to have negative long-term side effects when mid-twentieth century psychoanalysts administered them in supportive environments. LSD, psilocybin, and mescaline appeared to ease defensive strategies that habitually sealed off traumatic memories and shame-ridden impulses, creating opportunities to recognize how such unconscious conflicts affected one's day-to-day functioning. More than dreams or free association, psychedelics appeared to accelerate the process of making the unconscious conscious.

Freud's interest in symbols as an unconscious language also lent itself to making meaning of the dreamlike imagery common to psychedelic experiences. One of his downfalls, however, was dogmatism. Freud positioned the psychoanalyst as the expert who held the Rosetta Stone for deciphering unconscious imagery. By extension, the client relied on the analyst's interpretive power—which, for Freud, usually led to sex—to make sense of things. Psychedelic therapists have abandoned Freud's dogmatism when it comes to interpreting clients' visions, drawing instead from a school of psychology that developed in response to the cognitive, emotionally neutral stance of the psychoanalyst. Psychoanalysis informed the intellectual development of psychedelic therapy, but its heart developed through the person-centered approach of humanistic psychology.

Humanistic Psychology

The humanistic approach to psychotherapy aimed to reduce the hierarchical power differential between client and therapist. Early humanistic thought leaders like Carl Rogers and Abraham Maslow theorized that excessive insistence on interpretation and diagnosis actually *thwarted* the healing process. To Rogers in particular, the most important factor in client healing was the immediacy and quality of the therapeutic relationship.

Healing didn't come through hypnotizing someone or interpreting their freely associated thoughts on words like "cigar" and "anus"; it came through being with another person and following the lead of a compassionate heart. Humanistic therapists aimed to ensure their clients felt understood, cared for, and empowered in their unique human expression.

Humanistic therapists don't conceive of themselves as the "expert in the room." The expert is the *client*, whose inner world contains intuitive wisdom of what they need to heal. The therapist reflects and affirms the client's words, meeting their testimony with three primary qualities that Rogers called "necessary and sufficient conditions" for healing.[2] Rogers maintained that when therapists embody these conditions, "the process of constructive personality change will follow."[3]

1. Genuineness—*realness, congruence,* and *authenticity* as a fellow human

2. Accurate Empathy—*caring* for the client and entering their experience *as if* it's the therapist's own

3. Unconditional Positive Regard—affirming the validity of the client's subjectivity rather than interpreting, casting judgment, or projecting a personal value system

The humanistic approach grounds psychedelic therapy. Psychedelic therapists are trained to resist the urge to interpret a client's experience or offer advice. Instead, they focus on following the client's inner process, emphasizing the validity of the client's thoughts and emotions, and maintaining empathetic, authentic presence. When the client feels safe in the room with the therapist, the substance can facilitate an organic healing process, for the client can relax enough to allow their natural inclination toward self-actualization to guide them.

In this sense, psychedelic therapy can be seen as enhanced humanistic therapy, for the establishment of trust in an authentic therapeutic relationship is essential for inner transformation. No matter how far out the psychedelic blasts one's consciousness, psychedelic sessions are always, at their core, human beings relating to one another in a room.

Somatic Therapy

A more recent therapeutic development from which psychedelic therapy draws influence is somatic therapy. The term "somatic" comes from the Greek word *sôma*, which translates to "body." Whereas psychotherapy focuses on thoughts, memories, and emotions, somatic—or "body-based"—therapy concerns itself with the client's embodied experience in the present.

Sensorimotor Psychotherapy and Somatic Experiencing, two prevailing body-based approaches, were developed specifically to treat trauma. Pat Ogden created the former in the 1970s when she recognized a link between clients' traumatic memories and their nervous systems' patterns, such as the tendency to dissociate into a detached, ungrounded state. In teaching clients to become aware of their autonomic responses, Ogden helped them reestablish trust in their bodies. Doing so allowed their nervous systems to express through movements that were truncated in the traumatic event.[4] If, for example, someone felt disempowered while being bullied as a teenager, a sensorimotor therapist might help them locate their body's thwarted desire to scream in anger. Once the desire has been located, the therapist encourages its expression to "complete" the interrupted process.

Somatic Experiencing focuses even less on discussing thoughts or traumatic memories. Peter Levine began developing the approach in the 1970s after observing that prey animals, after escaping predatorial attacks, tended to shake, spasm, and convulse—and then resume their lives as if nothing had happened. Levine theorized that human bodies, like those of other mammals, have a physiological need to discharge stress through autonomic processes. Whether due to social conventions or legitimate threats to safety, people often block their bodies from releasing the energy of stress. As a result, they accumulate and "store" that energy in the nervous system. When the blocked energy overwhelms the system, the body enters a dissociated state of hypoarousal—a freeze response common to survivors of trauma. Levine and thousands of therapists trained in Somatic Experiencing encourage mindfulness to help clients titrate into the "stuck" energy, learn to feel it without becoming overwhelmed, and allow their bodies to discharge it naturally. The client's body may shake and spasm, punch and kick, or even move as if running away from the traumatic incident as it desired when the onset of hypoarousal locked the limbs in stasis. In the safety of the therapeutic space, the nervous system can recognize the threat is no longer present and complete its natural cycle of release.*

Western psychology has been slow to embrace somatic therapy, but that has not thwarted its popularity. I suppose people realize how much sense it makes. When my skepticism arises around far-out terms like "stuck energy," I think about the car crash I experienced when I was eighteen. I remember seeing the sedan's brake lights as we barreled toward it. Our driver swerved, to dodge the sedan, and the brake lights became the headlights of a pickup truck. We collided head-on, and both vehicles were destroyed. Somehow, everyone made it out alive.

To this day, when I'm a passenger and see brake lights flash ahead, my body stiffens, my breath constricts, and I brace for impact. It's an "irrational" response, but some piece of the helplessness I felt in that situation remains stuck in my nervous system and automatically responds to associated stimuli. People who have experienced more severe trauma often have more severe responses to phenomena that evoke the painful past, and unless they find a way to release the stuck somatic energy, those phenomena will continue to trigger them into dysregulated states. Amid such overwhelm, many turn to coping strategies such as drug abuse, binge eating, and any number of chronic behaviors bringing short-term reprieve and long-term harm.

As psychedelics amplify thoughts and emotions, they likewise magnify bodily sensations, including blocked somatic charges. A significant dose can intensify such charges to a degree that feels nearly impossible to endure. When this level of intensity takes hold, talking about it seldom helps—in fact, it might even reinforce the trauma by encouraging the client to flee their embodied experience by means of a distracting story. Many psychedelic therapists thus incorporate somatic techniques to help clients connect to a calm,

---

*   Although these two somatic approaches were developed in the 1970s, their seeds were planted far earlier. Somatic therapy is often traced back to Wilhelm Reich, who, in the early 1900s, presented an innovative theory that repressed psychosexual energy manifested as "body armor." These physical blocks were stored in the muscles and organs and prevented a natural flow of energy until they were released. And wouldn't you know it that Reich was an Austrian psychoanalyst who apprenticed under none other than Sigmund Freud. The Frood Dude strikes again!

regulated state from which they can "pendulate" into the pain and return when necessary. Over time, clients build emotional resilience, widening their "window of tolerance" and expanding their capacity to remain calm in difficult situations both inside and outside of the psychedelic journey.

It's common for psychedelic therapy sessions to involve tensing, relaxing, hyperventilating, screaming, and weeping, each of which could facilitate somatic discharge. It's also common for clients to quake, shiver, and convulse. Therapists informed on the neurophysiology of trauma, as conceptualized by such innovators as Ogden and Levine, can distinguish such energetic releases from alarming reactions like epileptic seizures, saving paramedics a pointless trip and encouraging an organic healing process. When therapists provide proper psychological and physical support, somatic discharge can help restore a client's sense of being at home in their bodies, where they can now rest to a degree they had forgotten was possible.

Transpersonal Psychology

Unlike the first three therapeutic frameworks, the fourth arose in tandem with psychedelic therapy. Among its earliest developers were first-wave researchers like Stan Grof and Jim Fadiman, who found psychoanalysis, behaviorism, and humanism failed to describe and appreciate the value of psychedelic states and other "peak experiences" that defied rational explanation. Reluctant to use the word "spiritual" in fear of academic backlash, these 1960s practitioners named their framework "transpersonal psychology," for its lens focused beyond the personal layers of the inner world.

The psyche's personal layers are composed of memories, fears, fantasies, hopes, traumas, and other phenomena related to autobiographical identity that begins at birth and ends at death. Transpersonal phenomena cannot be reduced to individualistic narratives. Examples include near-death experiences, extrasensory perception (ESP), visions of other dimensions, regression into "past lives," communication with the deceased, and profound spiritual connection to the Cosmos. Many of these dissolve the dichotomy between the inner and outer world that's been cemented into Western thought since René Descartes distinguished the mind from the body in the 17th century. The resulting "oneness" may give rise to a mystical vision of life's sacredness, or it could manifest as *flow state*—a state of consciousness familiar to many artists and athletes wherein their analytical thoughts recede and their bodies move in perfect attunement to the moment, as if prescient about the movements required for optimal performance.[*]

Rather than reinforcing Western trends of pathologizing such phenomena, transpersonal psychologists recognize their importance and help clients integrate them into meaningful shifts in behavior and perspective. The same applies to psychedelic states, which can give rise to any of the aforementioned experiences. In the spirit of the humanistic approach from which their framework emerged, transpersonal psychologists eschew the application of interpretive corsets, opting instead to follow clients into "irrational" realms while honoring their subjective truth.

Psychedelic therapists trained in transpersonal psychology equip themselves to meet the vast array of psychedelic effects with curiosity instead of diagnostic pathology. If a client on ketamine is flooded with visions of Egyptian hieroglyphs or Mesoamerican temples, the transpersonal psychologist explores these images with the client rather than labeling them "delusional hallucinations." In this sense, transpersonal psychology became the first major development of Western psychology that looked beyond the limits of scientific materialism, replacing neurobiological distillation with intrigue and respect for the mysterious, infinite reaches of consciousness.

The Tripartite Structure of Psychedelic Therapy

These four psychological frameworks clarify foundational elements of psychedelic therapy's philosophy and approach, but they do not comprise a complete list of approaches that synergize with non-ordinary states. Many others have been applied, and more will gain popularity, for psychedelics seem to amplify the benefits of most therapies if sessions are facilitated with skill, care, and understanding of the molecules' manifold effects.

---

[*]   For fellow cinephiles out there, a great example occurs at the climax of *The Matrix*. Having just risen from the dead, Keanu Reeves stops bullets with ease, exerts kung fu dominance over Agent Smith, and Superman-dives into Agent Smith's chest to explode him from the inside. When Reeves flexes his pipes and exhales, the world warbles around him. He triumphs not through struggle but through the ease of a flow state, the natural disposition of "The One." That movie will never not be awesome.

While these four psychological schools provide important scaffolding, psychedelic therapy proceeds according to a unique map, the structural protocol of which consistently follows a tripartite sequence.

1. Preparation session(s)

2. Psychedelic ("dosing" or "medicine") session(s)

3. Integration session(s)

In short, preparation sessions prime clients for journeys, psychedelic sessions are the journeys, and integration sessions help clients make meaning out of journeys and apply insights to their lives. Practitioners routinely emphasize the essential importance of each session type; when they are skillfully facilitated, the likelihood of a healing outcome increases dramatically. Though dosing sessions attract the most widespread interest and attention, psychedelic therapists often say that the journey begins with preparation, which starts the moment one decides to take a psychedelic.

Set and Setting

Timothy Leary's most enduring contribution to psychedelic therapy was his popularization of *set* and *setting* as the key factors in determining a trip's quality and outcome. One of the most important goals of preparation sessions is establishing optimal manifestations of these two conditions.

"Set" refers to the mindset and inner state of the individual embarking on the psychedelic voyage. It includes emotions, beliefs, intentions, expectations, and attitudes toward the drug. When one imbibes a psychedelic while fear grips their heart, fear will likely factor into—if not dominate—the trip. If the therapist helps the client approach the trip calmly, serenity may structure the journey, even if the client's mind kicks up bizarre and freaky visions.

"Setting" refers to the external environment where the trip transpires. This includes the physical surroundings—office décor, cleanliness, choice of music, etc.—as well as the cultural environment. If a psychedelic witch hunt is taking place in your town, the cultural setting of paranoia may seep into the space, no matter how much sage is burned.

Perhaps the most important setting consideration is safety. If a client feels unsafe, healing is less likely to transpire, and the possibility of psychological harm increases. Practitioners can enhance safety by paying careful attention to feng shui. For instance, well-positioned portraits of serene landscapes and water flowing over smooth rocks will enhance well-being more consistently than paintings of red-eyed dragons breathing fire on the Pentagon or a ten-foot print of Edvard Munch's *The Scream*. As participants in shady, Cold-War-era, CIA-funded psychedelic research had the displeasure of discovering, tripping in a windowless, fluorescent-lit room under the observant eyes of emotionless agents can lead to a very bad time.[*]

You can see how setting influences set: if the office is fashioned after the lair of Edward Scissorhands (minus the beautiful topiaries), fear and apprehension would be legitimate responses (unless, of course, you're a Tim Burton devotee). It's ideal to establish cohesion between set and setting, where the décor promotes a mindset of ease, and the client finds comfort and safety wherever they look. In a sense, the setting is the external expression of the mindset one intends to carry through the psychedelic session.

Safety is not all about ambiance. A therapist can create a sanctuary, but their clients may still feel unsafe if there's something "off" about the therapist's vibe. People can sense inauthenticity, and the sensory expansion psychedelics catalyze can broaden one's ability to sniff out BS. If a therapist tells a client, "I hear how challenging things are with your job," while thinking, "Get over it, ya whiner!" chances are the psychedelic-influenced client will sense something screwy afoot.

That's not to say therapists should be upfront about such thoughts with clients; doing so could destroy trust and erode the session's potential. Therapists instead need to be skilled at tracking their own inner experience, honestly reckoning with it, and healing their personal wounds so the client's pain doesn't trigger "countertransference," the phenomenon in which a therapist projects their own "stuff" onto the client. The incongruence of feeling one thing and saying another can rupture trust in the therapeutic alliance.

---

[*] I explain the point of reference in chapter 4. For now, consider this reference an ominous foreshadowing of a sketchy episode of Western psychedelic history.

It should also be noted that even when a therapist *is* trustworthy, buried unconscious content can arise in clients and evoke profound terror. Psychedelics can prompt clients to project their terror onto the therapist, whose prior trustworthiness will be no match for the client's sudden, all-encompassing perception that their therapist is the reincarnation of Hannibal Lecter.

If trust hasn't been established, it will be difficult for the therapist to help the client return to reality amid such perceptual distortions. This will yield a traumatizing trip if the unprocessed terror remains stuck in the client's nervous system. Trust equips clients to deepen into their journeys, no matter how challenging they are. As memories, fantasies, and shadowed impulses come to light, they feel safe to speak truthfully without fear of judgment or misunderstanding, and the sheer act of voicing what is happening within can reveal influences underpinning one's subjective reality. Without trust, the client will likely keep things hidden, which can snowball into an avalanche of panic and shame. Shame festers in silence like a poison; expressing shame to a compassionate person provides an antidote, allowing one to experience unconditional acceptance in the eyes of another.

Clear Intention with Minimal Expectation

Psychedelic therapists and researchers agree that approaching psychedelics with clear intention benefits the therapeutic outcome. It's so widely agreed upon, in fact, that people rarely question what intention really means.

Simply stated, intention centers on what an individual hopes to get from the trip. The problem is, when this becomes too specific, the individual attaches unrealistic desires to the non-ordinary state, and if the journey goes in a different direction, they may think it was all for naught.

An *expectation* brings a specific agenda to the psychedelic session. It's like taking mushrooms and thinking, "I will process my pain around Chaz Barkley humiliating me in grade 7, and that will cure my addiction problems." Expectation narrows the focus, whereas a good *intention* expands the focus to meet whatever arises. We may think we know what we need, but an amazing thing about psychedelics is their capacity to reveal what we *actually* need.

Imagine a client we'll call Gary. Convinced his anxiety stems from his contentious relationship with his mother as a child, Gary intends to dive into his painful memories on LSD to gain closure. Three hours into the session, Gary discovers thoughts related to his mother are as murky as the Pleiades on a cloudy night. As he forces himself to remember arguing with his mother after school, his discomfort increases, and the memories come no closer. If Gary continues this struggle, he will emerge from the experience feeling worse and decide the session was a failure and this whole psychedelic therapy thing is bogus.

In a parallel universe, Gary releases his expectation. He notices his discomfort, and he recognizes the familiarity of the mental pressure that accompanies his attempts to coerce his emotional experience into something other than what it is. A realization emerges that this inclination to change his present reality operates at the core of Gary's struggle to feel calm. By deepening into his emotions and releasing his preoccupation with changing them, the pressure in his head recedes. He notices a sense of calmness emerging, the calmness that stems from accepting things exactly as they are without needing to change them. Amid such grounded peace, Gary is flooded with memories of his mother reading his favorite book to him after tucking him in at night, and he watches his bitterness drift away.

Intention concerns how one orients toward what arises. For Sam—the retired Navy SEAL—intention manifested as openness to everything the mushrooms evoked. He hoped to heal a pattern, and he did so by releasing preconceived notions of what he needed, reckoning instead with the murky underground that surfaced.

Taking all this into consideration, a more accurate understanding of intention, as conceptualized by *VICE* writer Suzannah Weiss, can provide ". . . a guiding, girding idea for you to come back to if you start to feel adrift in a trip, or provide you with a safe thought to return to if you start feeling scared or spiral-y."[5] Like a mantra, intention is a mooring that anchors you when you find yourself at the whim of a stormy sea.

Specificity is not necessarily bad. An intention to feel your way into a specific painful memory could facilitate processing the memory. To mitigate the potentially detrimental consequences of excessive specificity, one must simply recognize it as an expectation and accept the possibility of things not playing out as desired. A reminder to "hold expectations lightly" will help one bring hopes to the medicine without fixating on the necessity of their fulfillment. If the journey goes in an unexpected direction, the traveler will be equipped to surf the waves instead of struggling to change their direction.

The Greek myth of Hercules and the Hydra illustrates these ideas. Each time Hercules cut off the monstrous Hydra's head, three heads grew in its place. The more furiously Hercules tried to defeat his foe through force, the more powerful she became. The client's most Herculean efforts will be fruitless if they try to assert dominance over the multi-headed Hydra of the psychedelic journey, inadvertently increasing the likelihood of emerging from the session feeling stuck. If the client replaces the struggle with compassionate surrender, the Hydra will transform into possibilities the battle had rendered impossible to envision.

Therapeutic Presence

How interactive should therapists be during a psychedelic session? Are they responsible for more than crisis management, or are they merely "trip sitters" for their clients' psychonautical adventures?

As clients lie down during psychedelic sessions, therapists often appear to do very little. They may even appear to do nothing—which can be exactly what the client needs. Doing nothing, however, is different from getting lost in one's thoughts or daydreaming about Mai Tais in Maui. Doing nothing is being as present as possible. While this may sound simple, it takes discipline and skill to remain engaged for hours on end, especially when the client remains silent.

As psychedelic research pioneer Rick Doblin said when we spoke in 2020, "In an eight-hour session with MDMA, around half the time, the therapists are just sitting there while the patient has their eyes closed, listening to music, going through all sorts of stuff. The therapists kind of need to be in a meditative state."[6]

If therapists become too *directive*, perhaps telling a client what to think about or how to interpret a vision, they risk interrupting the client's healing process by projecting a personal agenda. Directiveness is typically discouraged in psychedelic therapy and sometimes regarded as an ethical violation. How can someone know what another person needs? The therapist's thoughts are informed by their own belief system and biases, which may not line up with the needs of the client.

Psychedelic therapists are taught to respond to clients rather than prompt them. If a client says they're having a difficult time, the therapist offers support and, if necessary, guidance, such as a breathing exercise. Therapists must be attuned to their clients, for important matters are sometimes communicated nonverbally.

Imagine a therapist we'll call Joanna is facilitating her client Kendra's low-dose ketamine session. Kendra isn't saying anything, but Joanna notices her anguished expression as she squirms on the couch. During their preparation sessions, Joanna learned Kendra has difficulty asking for help—her parents considered it weak to rely on others and encouraged her to navigate her struggles alone. Joanna recognizes this dynamic could be playing out in the session—but Kenda's anguish could also be something else. Rather than assuming, Joanna says, "It looks like you have something coming up. I'm wondering if you'd like to talk about it or if you'd like some support." Kendra now has the power to validate Joanna's intuition or tell her, "I'm doing fine. I'll let you know if I need anything."

The last thing you want in a psychedelic session is for the client to feel responsible for the therapist's well-being. Psychedelic therapists must check their egos at the door. If they come in thinking, "I have the power to heal this person," they've already made the client's healing about themselves. If the client doesn't ask for support, the therapist's ego may feel bruised, negatively affecting their capacity to embody open-hearted presence.

Deb Dana, renowned clinician and trauma expert, told me, "If I'm in the therapist role, my responsibility is to be anchored in regulated energy, which means that I am open, engaged, safe, and sending safety cues to my client's nervous system through *neuroception*—the unconscious way nervous systems communicate. If I move out of that, my responsibility is to return to that anchored state." A therapist's calm and consistent attentiveness nonverbally communicates, "I'm here with you," encouraging the client to release control to whatever is unfolding.

Time to Move On, Time to Get Going

As much as these models and approaches elucidate what psychedelic therapy looks like, they only begin to answer questions related to why and how it works. So far, you've had to take me at my word that it's efficacious, and I know modern folks tend to reserve their trust for claims backed by scientific evidence.

Though psychedelic science is a relatively recent addition to the Western narrative, results published in numerous international journals demonstrate that psychedelic-assisted therapy can be more beneficial than traditional therapy, psychiatric medication, or their combination. Many psychedelics have emerged into the forefront of Western interest, but one in particular was central in reviving interest in the first place. This compound, which bridged traditional plant medicine healing with psychedelic science when it emerged into Western focus in the 1950s, is *psilocybin*, the psychoactive alkaloid of "magic" mushrooms.

3

Psilocybin: The Bridge Between Science and Mysticism

"The mushrooms give me the power of universal contemplation. I can see from the origin. I can arrive where the world is born."

—*María Sabina: Her Life and Chants*

Psilocybin occurs naturally in hundreds of species of mushrooms spanning several genera. The most notable of these genera, *Psilocybe*, accounts for more than a hundred "magic" mushroom species. Archaeological evidence suggests the Mazatec people of southern Mexico have ceremonially imbibed the psilocybin-containing mushrooms endemic to their region for hundreds of years. Further evidence, garnered through pictographs and other relics displaying carvings of humans and mushrooms in harmonious relationship, points to Mesoamerican use of *Psilocybe* among the Aztecs. They called it *teonanácatl*, commonly translated as "flesh of the gods."

With the exception of Antarctica, psilocybin-containing mushrooms grow on all continents.[1] Although origins of human consumption remain ambiguous, speculation traces their use back to the Stone Age, drawing from Mesolithic-Neolithic rock art found in Africa and Europe depicting humanoid figures with *Psilocybe*-appearing mushrooms growing out of their heads, torsos, and limbs.[2] It wasn't until the 1950s, however, that Western culture became aware of these fantastic fungi and their ritual use in sacred ceremonies.

The Grandmother of the Magic Mushroom

The Western origin story follows amateur mycologists R. Gordon and Valentina P. Wasson on a series of journeys from America to Mexico to "seek the magic mushroom." The Wassons had read a journal article containing a quote from Harvard University professor Richard Evans Schultes—often considered the "father" of ethnobotany, a research field concerned with traditional uses of regional plants—referencing the contemporary survival of a visionary mushroom ritual dating to sixteenth-century Mesoamerica. Drawing inspiration from anthropologist Jean Bassett Johnson's 1930s journey to Mexico's Sierra Mazateca region, where he'd reportedly witnessed the sacred mushroom ritual, the Wassons packed up their goods and headed south in 1953. It was their first of several excursions to the Mazatec village of Huautla de Jiménez, and it yielded a fateful meeting with María Sabina.

Sabina was a Mazatec *curandera*, a Spanish term for a "medicine woman" who administers plant-based medicines to heal a variety of physical, mental, emotional, and spiritual conditions. Among the many remedies she offered, Sabina facilitated traditional mushroom ceremonies called *veladas*, ushering people of her community into the visionary, healing world the mushrooms opened. The mushrooms contained psilocybin, but she did not use that word, for it had not been invented. For Sabina, the mushrooms were Los Niños Santos, "the holy children."

In his book *Singing to the Plants*, explorer Stephan V. Beyer wrote, "When Sabina ingested the mushrooms, the mushroom spirits would show her the cause of the sickness—for example, through soul loss, malevolent spirits, or human sorcerers." Beyer quoted Sabina's explanation: "'The sickness comes out if the sick vomit. They vomit the sickness. They vomit because the mushrooms want them to. If the sick don't vomit, I vomit. I vomit for them and in that way the malady is expelled.'" Beyer added that Sabina "would then be able to cure the patient through the power of her singing."[3]

In 1955, Sabina allowed Gordon Wasson, along with photographer Allan Richardson, to participate in one of her ceremonies, permitting them to become, in Wasson's boastful words, "the first white men in recorded history to eat the divine mushrooms." Two years later, Wasson unlatched Pandora's box when *Life* magazine, then the leading news magazine in the US, featured his photo essay, titled "Seeking the Magic Mushroom," on its front page.[4] His protection of Sabina's identity—he called her "Eva Mendez" in the article—was short-lived, for soon after, he and Valentina included details of Sabina and her village in *Mushrooms, Russia, and History: Volume II.*

Starting in the early 1960s, hordes of Western hippies, scientists, and curiosity seekers flocked to Sabina's small village in search of the magic mushroom.* Sabina was keenly aware their motivations did not align with the Mazatec ways. The White people did not seek healing; they desired an experience where, if they were lucky, they would find God.

The story took a tragic turn when Mexican Federales became suspicious of the influx of Westerners. Their ensuing involvement in the Mazatec community threatened to destroy the mushroom custom. Sabina's community turned on her, blaming her for allowing the outside world to enter their sacred ceremony. During the years of the Wassons' visits, Sabina's house and store were burned to the ground, forcing her to move into the woods. Even more devastating was the unprompted murder of Aurelio Carreras, her nineteen-year-old son-in-law, an occurrence about which Sabina had been forewarned during harrowing mushroom-induced visions.

"They were warnings of the pain that was approaching," Sabina remembered. In her visions, she saw a man dressed as a Mazatec who said, "I'm the one . . . With this one it will be five I've murdered." When the man from her vision entered her store, Sabina recognized him, and minutes later, he shot and killed Aurelio.

She did not know why these events occurred. Given their concurrence with Wasson's visit, she acknowledged, "Some people thought it was because I had revealed the ancestral secret of our native medicine to foreigners." She was aware that before Wasson, "nobody spoke so openly about the *children.*"[5] By the end of her life in 1985, Sabina had come to regret giving mushrooms to Wasson.

---

* Rumored seekers who visited Sabina include Bob Dylan, Mick Jagger, and John Lennon, though none have been corroborated as fact. See Paul Roberts, "Huautla de Jiménez: in the footsteps of María Sabina and John Lennon," *livingandworkinginmexico* (blog), August 28, 2010, livingandworkinginmexico.wordpress.com/2010/08/28/huautla-de-jimenez-in-the -footsteps-of-maria-sabina/.

After Wasson's article appeared, he sent samples of *Psilocybe mexicana* to Albert Hofmann, the brilliant chemist who had synthesized LSD almost twenty years prior, in Switzerland. In 1958, Hofmann isolated psilocybin from the mushrooms and, recognizing its similarity to LSD, presented it as the primary psychoactive alkaloid. Four years later, Wasson and Hofmann visited Sabina and offered her several pills of isolated psilocybin. In a 1984 interview with Stan Grof, Hofmann recalled, "María Sabina told us that these tablets really contained the spirit of the mushrooms."[6]

Sabina remains widely respected in the psychedelic world. Her story reflects an important tension in the Western history of plant medicines: in revealing the mushrooms' healing power to the Western world, she, an Indigenous woman, suffered great loss as a result. Her sacrifice was enormous, and the revival's headline-making psilocybin research should be contextualized through recognition of her exploitation. None of the developments that comprise the remainder of this chapter would have been possible without María Sabina.

Psilocybin-Assisted Therapy

Journalist Michael Pollan helped open the revival's floodgates with his widely influential 2018 book, *How to Change Your Mind*. Early in the book, Pollan suggested the revival, which he called the "renaissance," began with three events in 2006, the most significant of which was Johns Hopkins University's publication of a research paper in the esteemed scientific journal *Psychopharmacology*. The lead author of the paper (which was titled "Psilocybin can occasion mystical-type experiences having substantial and sustained personal meaning and spiritual significance") was Roland Griffiths, who'd gained prominence in the field of psychopharmacology through decades of researching behavioral and subjective effects of mood-altering drugs like sedative-hypnotics and caffeine. Griffiths didn't approach psychedelics until 1999, when he launched the first of many Johns Hopkins psilocybin studies to come.

Rather than focusing on therapeutic applications, Griffiths investigated psilocybin's potential to induce a "mystical experience," a profound state of consciousness central to stories of spiritual initiation and conversion. With a double-blind, placebo-controlled approach applied to thirty-six volunteers, Griffiths and his team discovered psilocybin "occasioned" a "complete mystical experience" in more than 60% of participants. Additionally, the team found these mystical experiences appeared to have long-term positive effects of therapeutic significance.

According to the *Psychopharmacology* publication, "67% of the volunteers rated the experience with psilocybin to be either the single most meaningful experience of his or her life or among the top five most meaningful experiences of his or her life."[7] That's worth repeating: two-thirds of participants considered their psilocybin journey one of the five most meaningful experiences *of their entire lives.* In comparison, 8% of participants who'd received a placebo of methylphenidate, the stimulant sold under the brand name Ritalin, ascribed a comparable degree of significance.*

After the publication, Johns Hopkins became one of the world's leading psychedelic research hubs. The majority of the institution's ensuing investigations into psilocybin have aimed to demonstrate that a psilocybin-induced mystical experience catalyzes mental health benefits up to and including psychospiritual transformation, a fancy way of saying "improving your life in every way."

Johns Hopkins' studies have primarily focused on psilocybin-assisted therapy. After a series of preparation sessions, psilocybin is administered, and co-therapists support the participant through an eight-hour journey. During dosing sessions, participants are encouraged to wear eyeshades as they listen to curated playlists of evocative music. They then stay the night in the medically equipped facility in case of an adverse response. Therapists return in the morning for the first of several integration sessions, helping participants translate their psilocybin experiences into insight and healing.

In the research world, participants don't eat mushrooms. They consume capsules of synthetic psilocybin, like those Hofmann gave to Sabina. The dose has traditionally been determined based on the individual's weight, following a conversion of 30 mg for each 70 kg of body weight; however, the

---

*   It's noteworthy in itself that 8% of participants who took Ritalin reported life-changing mystical experiences. You don't tend to hear this with Ritalin. Perhaps the "placebo effect" was at play, and participants' expectations created the desired reality. Perhaps the serene setting Johns Hopkins created helped facilitate a sense of unity with all things. Or perhaps Ritalin, when administered in certain contexts, has mystical potential as well. One can discover many fascinating mysteries between the data-driven lines of psychedelic research papers.

validity of this conversion has been challenged. In a 2021 paper, Matthew Johnson, a prominent psychedelic researcher at Johns Hopkins, wrote, "Across a wide range of body weights (49 to 113 kg) the present results showed no evidence that body weight affected subjective effects of psilocybin."[8] The fact that weight may be an insignificant variable in predicting the intensity of psilocybin's effects points to a uniquely bizarre quality of the mysterious fungal alkaloid, as weight heavily influences the effects of most drugs.

Following Griffiths' 2006 paper, Johns Hopkins focused on psilocybin-assisted therapy to treat depression, smoking cessation, and end-of-life anxiety in people facing terminal cancer diagnoses. In 2016, the university published results concurrently with research from New York University on end-of-life anxiety, concluding that a single dose of psilocybin "decreased clinician- and patient-rated depressed mood, anxiety, and death anxiety, and increased quality of life, life meaning, and optimism." Six months after dosing, about 80% of participants continued to demonstrate alleviation in depression and anxiety. Again, nearly 70% considered their psilocybin session among the five most meaningful experiences of their lives.[9]

In 2020, Johns Hopkins published the results of another study in *JAMA Psychiatry* that followed participants diagnosed with major depressive disorder (MDD) through a therapeutic protocol structured around two psilocybin sessions. Four weeks post-treatment, 71% of participants continued to show a clinically significant reduction in symptoms, and 54% were considered to be in remission.[10]

Johns Hopkins' third major application of psilocybin-assisted therapy focused on addiction to nicotine. The ten participants in the preliminary trial smoked an average of nineteen cigarettes a day for thirty-one years. Half had had minimal psychedelic experiences in their past, while the other half were "psychedelic-naïve," never having tripped before the trial. Each subject underwent a fifteen-week protocol involving cognitive-behavioral therapy, mindfulness training, guided imagery, and two psilocybin sessions with the option of a third.[11] In 2014, Johnson, who conducted the study, published remarkable results: 80% of the participants had abstained from cigarettes for six months following the treatment. This figure more than doubled the efficacy of leading interventions like nicotine replacements and behavioral therapies.[12]

The powerful results of Johns Hopkins' psilocybin research and the university's key role in inspiring similar studies around the world led to the establishment of The Johns Hopkins Center for Psychedelics and Consciousness Research in 2019, the largest university-based psychedelic research site in the history of the United States. At the time of writing, the center's tremendous financial backing of about $17 million dollars funds psilocybin research in the three aforementioned areas as well as in treatment of anorexia nervosa, post-treatment Lyme disease, co-occurring depression and alcohol use disorder, and Alzheimer's disease.

I'm not much of a numbers-and-figures guy, but the Johns Hopkins results are mind-blowing. What blows my mind even more is that Griffiths found a way to usher mysticism into a respectable position amid the scientific research institution. Given scientists' historical disdain for such "unscientific" concepts, this marks a radical transformation, indeed.

The Mystical Experience

Though instrumental in bringing scientific legitimacy to mysticism, Griffiths was not the first scientist to focus on mystical experiences. These visionary states have interested academic researchers for more than a century, and it's from the seeds they planted that Johns Hopkins' research sprouted.

Some of the earliest academic work on mysticism came from American psychologist and philosopher William James. Often considered "The Father of American Psychology," James was the first major psychologist of the West to take profound religious experiences seriously rather than pass them off as a form of mental disturbance. James believed mind-altering substances could induce such states, and he wrote about his perspective-shifting experiments with nitrous oxide—the "laughing gas" dentists administer to lucky patients—as early as 1874. James' thinking crystallized in his opus, *The Varieties of Religious Experience*, which contains a passage that is all but required for inclusion in books about psychedelics: "Our normal waking consciousness, rational consciousness as we call it, is but one special type of consciousness, whilst all about it, parted from it by the filmiest of screens, there lie potential forms of consciousness entirely different . . . No account of the universe in its totality can be final which leaves these other forms of consciousness quite disregarded."[13] In short: non-ordinary states of consciousness are both real and important in one's consideration of the universe.

James' work in the phenomenology of mysticism, along with that of British philosopher Walter Terence Stace in 1960, laid the groundwork for a man named Walter Pahnke to craft a psychedelic bridge. In 1962, during his graduate studies at Harvard Divinity School, Pahnke, under the supervision of Timothy Leary and Richard Alpert, designed a double-blind experiment on twenty graduate divinity students. (Both Leary and Alpert (who later became the great Western guru Ram Dass) would make headlines the next year when the university fired them for administering psychedelics with a "lack of scientific rigor.")

On Good Friday, Pahnke gathered the divinity students in Boston University's Marsh Chapel, where half received an active placebo of niacin and the other half received psilocybin. The goal of the study, known colloquially as the "Marsh Chapel Experiment," was to ascertain if psilocybin could induce a mystical experience in religiously predisposed individuals. To report on such an intangible notion, Pahnke crafted a 147-item assessment called the Mystical Experience Questionnaire.

According to Griffiths' 2006 paper, Pahnke's questionnaire covered seven domains of the mystical experience:

1. Internal unity (pure awareness; a merging with ultimate reality)

2. External unity (unity of all things; all things are alive; all is one)

3. Transcendence of time and space

4. Ineffability and paradoxicality (claim of difficulty in describing the experience in words)

5. Sense of sacredness (awe)

6. Noetic quality (claim of intuitive knowledge of ultimate reality)

7. Deeply felt positive mood (joy, peace, and love)[14]

Due to their high scores in the majority of the categories, Pahnke determined eight out of the ten individuals who'd received psilocybin had mystical experiences. Their average scores in every category exceeded those of the placeble group.[15] One member of the psilocybin group, Huston Smith, who would go on to become one of the leading religious scholars in the United States, recalled his Marsh Chapel session as "the most powerful cosmic homecoming I have ever experienced."[16]

Pahnke concluded, "Those subjects who received psilocybin experienced phenomena which were apparently indistinguishable from, if not identical with, the categories defined by our typology of mysticism."[17] Translation: psilocybin can catalyze a genuine mystical experience—the same conclusion Griffiths arrived at in 2006.

Pahnke's questionnaire has undergone numerous revisions. A thirty-item version created in 2013 by researcher Katherine MacLean remains one of the most widely used assessments for measuring mystical states in scientific research. This version is central to Johns Hopkins' psilocybin research, which MacLean helped establish and guide.

Mystical Healing and Battling the Ineffable

The mystical conclusions of Pahnke and Griffiths give rise to an important question: Why does it matter?

Do psychedelics turn people into mystics? Would that be good? Might it be impractical?

I'll offer some answers: No. Perhaps. Probably.

As for why it matters? For starters, it's interesting. When it comes to mystical experiences, we're talking about some of the most profound stories of transformation in human history, the *I-see-the-light!* stuff found in mythological and sacred texts of diverse cultures throughout the world. But the real reason it's a hot topic in the psychedelic field is because Johns Hopkins, along with other institutions surfing the revival-era wake, present evidence that the mystical experience is the reason many people undergo profound transformation after as little as a single psilocybin session. After Griffiths' inaugural psilocybin study, the mystical-healing explanation has been applied to research on other psychedelics and plant medicines, including ketamine, 5-MeO-DMT, and ayahuasca.[18]

Interesting as it is, all this data tells us squat about how mystical experiences *feel*. An added challenge is that one of the defining qualities of mystical states is "ineffability," meaning people find them impossible to describe.

Researchers toss around "ineffable" so often in today's psychedelic world that I've become sick of hearing it, and when I do, I think, "You're not trying hard enough." Although we cannot describe psychedelic perceptions exhaustively, we can do better than listing seven qualities and applying a percentage.

Think about how humans describe love. If we break it down to neurotransmitters and glands, do we get closer to understanding what it feels like? To comprehending its transformative power? The answer is, of course, a rhetorical "no," and we are left to describe the subjective feelings associated with the intangible concept. Doing this directly, however, could end up sounding like a teenage dude writing a Valentine's Day poem to his crush, vulnerably expressing he's "feeling emotional" and quoting Tom Cruise in *Jerry Maguire*.*

Evocative descriptions of transcendental concepts like love and mystical consciousness come through figurative language. Rather than trying and failing to label something, we can use metaphor, simile, hyperbole, allegory, and symbolism to evoke the ineffable. One might also ditch words altogether and communicate through painting, dancing, or shredding on a vintage Les Paul. Scientists can point to the value of mystical states, but authors, painters, dancers, and musicians are better equipped to communicate their value in ways the heart can apprehend.

Huxley met this linguistic challenge head-on in *The Doors of Perception*, his classic 1954 book chronicling his first psychedelic experience. In wide-reaching descriptions of a world seen through mescaline-filtered eyeballs, he alluded to timeless philosophical and spiritual concepts of Greek philosophy, Buddhism, the Hebrew Bible, and dozens more sources, detailing expansive layers of abstraction while consistently returning to his perceptions of the world's nonphysical dimensions.

In a memorable section, Huxley paused to observe a garden chair. "That chair—shall I ever forget it? Where the shadows fell on the canvas upholstery, stripes of a deep but glowing indigo alternated with stripes of an incandescence so intensely bright that it was hard to believe that they could be made of anything but blue fire. For what seemed an immensely long time I gazed

---

* Honestly, if any teenager at this stage in history has even seen *Jerry Maguire*, that's a huge win for the endurance of pop culture, and a huge loss for the teenager who spent time watching that lame flick.

without knowing, even without wishing to know, what it was that confused me. At any other time I would have seen a chair barred with alternate light and shade. Today the percept had swallowed up the concept. I was so completely absorbed in looking, so thunderstruck by what I actually saw, that I could not be aware of anything else . . . It was inexpressibly wonderful, wonderful to the point, almost, of being terrifying."[19]

These words evoke a more vivid sentiment than the word "ineffable."

Regardless of how one describes psychedelic states of mystical awareness, the perceptions and visions accompanying them can be powerful enough to transform a person to the point of forever seeing the world anew. It's something we probably didn't need science to "prove." Can't we read the religious texts of the world and recognize the profundity of spiritual visions? Regarding psychedelics, couldn't we get the message by listening to holders of Indigenous lineages who have used plant medicines to heal their communities for generations?

It's like seeing a scientific paper entitled, "Meditation Correlated with Reduction in Stress." As much as this researcher may laud themselves on this scientific discovery, they could have saved their institution time and money by reading a book on Buddhism instead.

The Western perspective places more trust in percentages than the words of brilliant thinkers and visionaries throughout history. Given that rating scales like the Mystical Experience Questionnaire are a form of people describing their subjective experiences—albeit with numbers and symbols—science's insistence on its epistemological supremacy seems ridiculous. But alas, science structures the Western world, and clever researchers have found ways to bridge such nonscientific concepts as mysticism into the literature, garnering academic interest in the healing power of psychedelic states. Ineffable as these experiences may be, I hope people will continue to describe and express them creatively.

Default Mode Network and the Entropic Brain

In 2009, a team at Imperial College London led by neuroscientist Robin Carhart-Harris studied the brains of research subjects on psilocybin. In 2014, based on their complex scans, the team presented a hypothesis that psilocybin decreases activity in key regions of the brain's default mode network (DMN), a dominant system where concepts of identity and the "narrative self"—a.k.a. the ego—are stored. "As the highest level of a functional hierarchy," the authors wrote, "it [DMN] serves as a central *orchestrator* or *conductor* of global brain function."[20]

Reduced DMN blood flow results in a "phase transition" into a decentralized "entropic brain state" of chaotic formlessness, a pre-egoic "primary consciousness" of "unconstrained cognition" from which "secondary consciousness" of DMN dominance emerges.[21] "In primary states, cognition is less meticulous in its sampling of the external world and is instead easily biased by emotion, e.g., wishes and anxieties," the authors wrote.[22] Likewise, "processes are more flexible in primary consciousness."[23] Unsurprisingly, depression is correlated with "hyper activity and connectivity within the DMN."[24]

With the support of a therapist, the entropic brain state allows new neural pathways to form, decreasing the DMN's dominance in determining one's view of oneself and the world. Carhart-Harris hypothesized the entropic brain state forms the basis of mystical experiences, for the DMN's decreased dominance yields connection to one's primordial birthright at a neurological level.

Psilocybin Therapy Outside the University

At the time of writing, Johns Hopkins no longer holds the distinction of leading all major psilocybin therapy research. Dozens of private and public corporations have joined the field, influencing how the history of the second wave is being written.

The first major for-profit company to enter psychedelic research was Compass Pathways. Founded in 2016, Compass turned its sights toward psilocybin-assisted therapy. In 2018, the company's double-blind, placebo-controlled Phase 2 study of psilocybin-assisted therapy for Treatment-Resistant Depression (TRD) received Breakthrough Therapy designation from the FDA. This Federal process is "designed to expedite the development and review of drugs that are intended to treat a serious condition and preliminary clinical evidence indicates that the drug may demonstrate substantial improvement over available therapy on a clinically significant endpoint(s)."[25]

In November 2022, Compass published the results of their Phase 2b trial, which gathered data from 233 participants. After three weeks, just under 30% of the 79 participants who received a single psilocybin dose of 25 mg were in remission—impressive results, given the severity of TRD, but not the astonishing figure many had expected. Of the 233 participants, 77% experienced adverse events, including nausea, headache, dizziness, and suicidality.[26] The company's investors were not impressed, evidenced by a large dip in the value of Compass stock. Still, the results were strong enough for the FDA to grant Compass approval to take their research into Phase 3, the final phase required for FDA approval of a new prescription medication.

On the other side of Compass's for-profit model is the nonprofit Usona Institute, founded in 2014 with a mission of "alleviating depression and anxiety in people for whom current medical treatments fall short in offering relief and a better quality of life."[27] In 2019, the FDA also granted Breakthrough Therapy status to Usona's trial investigating psilocybin therapy to treat Major Depressive Disorder, a condition suffered by over 17 million people in the US alone. Bill Linton, who cofounded Usona with Malynn Utzinger, was inspired to start the company after a close friend suffering from terminal cancer participated in Johns Hopkins' end-of-life anxiety trial and experienced profound relief.

Similar to the Compass study, Usona participants are given one dose of 25 mg of psilocybin in the context of extensive therapy. Unlike Compass, Usona developed seventeen acres in Madison, Wisconsin, into a beautiful, retreat-like center where they intend their future psychedelic research to take place. According to their website, "With therapy at the core of our approach, Usona Institute will bridge medical research with integrative practices in healing," and the center "will support the development of best practices that consider the needs of diverse communities around the world."[28]

If trials like those of Compass and Usona continue to demonstrate the significant results researchers anticipate, psilocybin could become rescheduled as an adjunct medication for therapeutic treatments of at least two forms of depression. Current research forms a precipice upon which the psychedelic future is balanced.

Non-Therapeutic Applications of Psilocybin

Various institutions are also researching psilocybin's applications outside a therapeutic context. In 2017, Yale University launched neurological research into its potential to treat obsessive-compulsive disorder without a lengthy therapeutic protocol, and in 2022 they published a promising case study on one participant.[29] Results of another small-scale Yale study, published in 2020, showed potential for psilocybin's efficacy in treating migraine disorders.[30] Yale researchers are also looking into psilocybin as a treatment for cluster and post-traumatic headaches.[31]

At University of California San Diego, psilocybin is being investigated for the treatment of phantom limb pain, the confounding phenomenon where people who lose a limb continue to feel pain as if the limb is still there. Albert Yu-Min Lin, who is leading the research, lost his right leg in an off-road vehicle accident. He experienced pain that "was all consuming, but coming from a part of the body that literally no longer existed."[32] Desperate for relief, Lin self-experimented with taking psilocybin in the desert. He combined the effects with the "mirror therapy" technique, which treats phantom limb pain by tricking the brain with reflective illusions of the affected limb. Lin was amazed by what happened. "The pain was gone," he told reporters. "It was a profoundly spiritual moment. My mind had a map of my body and it was experiencing severe feedback issues . . . the psilocybin allowed the mind to reject the old map and create a new one. Now, I occasionally have a jolt of pain, but it's mostly gone."[33]

Lin believed his experience was more than a fluke. He launched a study to help other phantom limb sufferers heal, and thanks to the funding he received, thirty amputees are participating.[34] Like Yale's research, Lin's study is less interested in therapy than in learning about psilocybin's effects on the brain, specifically how it processes (and sometimes creates) pain.

Confronting Death

Unless you're a pro at avoidance, you can't spend much time thinking about psychedelics without thinking about death. After all, the train of the current revival of research was turbo-charged by studies from Johns Hopkins and NYU demonstrating a single dose of psilocybin could significantly alleviate the existential anxiety individuals faced after receiving terminal cancer diagnoses. Kerry Pappas, one of the fifty-one participants of the Johns Hopkins study, had been diagnosed with Stage 3 lung cancer, and psilocybin eliminated the tremendous anxiety she had felt. "It's amazing," Pappas recalled during a *60 Minutes* special. "I feel like death doesn't frighten me."[35]

Dinah Bazer, who participated in the NYU study after being diagnosed with ovarian cancer, told *The Verge*: "I was totally consumed with anxiety for two years . . . It was running my life and ruining my life." When she envisioned her fear as a physical mass in her body while on psilocybin, she "became volcanically angry and screamed 'get the fuck out,'" and the mass was gone.[36] Neither Pappas nor Bazer found the Fountain of Youth, but both made peace with their mortality. The implications of these transformations are more remarkable in lived experience than anything a peer-reviewed article can communicate.

The existential philosophers recognized fear of death as one of humanity's primary emotions. German philosopher Martin Heidegger wrote of our death denial in *Being and Time*. He argued we are afraid to face death, so we distract ourselves from thinking about it, sacrificing authenticity along the way. Most religions tell us where we're going after we die, but we still feel terrified, for there is nothing more unknown than what, if anything, awaits us across the final threshold. Isn't it intriguing how consistently so many of us avoid thinking and speaking about such a fundamental inevitability?

Some participants of psilocybin studies have experienced an insight that countless psychedelic users have had before them: the *certainty* that consciousness continues after death, and we need not fear what will transpire. It's one thing to read a sacred text describing the after-death state; it's a different thing to experience it directly.

Outside of academia, at least one influential person turned to psychedelics to assist the actual process of dying. That person was Aldous Huxley, who in 1963 asked his wife, Laura, to inject him with 200 micrograms of LSD—two standard "hits" or "tabs"—on his deathbed. In a letter to Huxley's brother a few days later, Laura wrote that the people in the room all said "that this was the most serene, the most beautiful death. Both doctors and the nurse said they had never seen a person in similar physical condition going off so completely without pain and without struggle."[37]

She added, "We will never know if all this is only our wishful thinking, or if it is real, but certainly all outward signs and the inner feeling gave indication that it was beautiful and peaceful and easy."[38]*

While Huxley's testimony has inspired many, it was not until 2022 that it hit home for Roland Griffiths. During a routine colonoscopy, Griffiths' doctor discovered a tumor. Within days, it was clear the tumor was metastatic, and Griffiths was diagnosed with terminal Stage 4 cancer at the age of 76.

Speaking to *Wisconsin Public Radio* in 2023, Griffiths shared that a friend had recently sent him Laura Huxley's book. After having remained silent about his personal psychedelic experiences throughout his Johns Hopkins leadership, he decided to open up about how psychedelics helped him accept his diagnosis with the equanimity he helped many other cancer patients experience.[39]

"I did have a significant experience after my diagnosis," Griffiths said. "It was with LSD, and I went into it as an opportunity to dialog with the cancer."[40]

For twelve hours, he asked the cancer two primary questions. "One is, what's going on here? Do I have to die? And the answer was, 'Yeah, this is the way it's supposed to be.' And then I asked, how am I supposed to be with this? Am I doing what I should be doing? And the answer came back, 'Yes, you're doing exactly what you should be doing. There's something you have to say about this.' And that felt good to me."[41]

Speaking to the *New York Times*, Griffiths shared that in spite of his prognosis, "Life has been more beautiful, more wonderful than ever." With the aid of his psychedelic experiences and his thirty years of meditation practice, he recognized "the best way to be with this diagnosis was to practice gratitude for the preciousness of our lives."[42]

He was unsure if there is an afterlife, but he didn't discount the possibility. "What I do feel very strongly is that we're living within a mystery that

---

* I have to mention the remarkable synchronicity that as Huxley was crossing death's gateway on LSD, the wide eyes of the world were transfixed on their televisions, for John F. Kennedy had just been shot. I don't know if this coincidence means anything, but it's too fascinating not to acknowledge.

far outstrips our science and our ability to understand what's going on." He added, "And I find that to be enthralling."[43]

Above all, Griffiths regarded his diagnosis as an opportunity to wake up. "I want everyone to appreciate the joy and wonder of every single moment of their lives . . . There is a reason every day to celebrate that we're alive, that we have another day to explore whatever this gift is of being conscious, of being aware, of being aware that we are aware. That's the deep mystery that I keep talking about. That's to be celebrated!"[44]

On October 16, 2023, Roland Griffiths passed away. He was 77 years old. If one day some philanthropist constructs a Psychedelic Research Hall of Fame, a prodigious exhibit would be necessary to honor Griffiths' influence. His compassion and brilliance earned him widespread respect, and his attitude toward his death revealed he had embodied his research conclusions into a way of life. More people will miss him than he could know, but as the psychedelic history books continue to be written, his legacy will live on.

Farewell, María Sabina

There's a saying, sometimes attributed to the great Sufi poet Rumi, that instructs people to "die before you die." An astonishing potential of psychedelics like psilocybin is that of opening the gateway to the liminal space between life and death, allowing us to prepare for our meeting with the scythe-wielding skeleton when the moment arrives. Though the West prefers to resist death's inexorable approach, contemplations on our common destination need not be macabre. Respecting the impermanence of our mortality can spark the realization that every moment is indeed precious; although we all pass away, life continues to flourish.

The questions psilocybin raises are limitless, as evidenced by the seemingly infinite directions research into this fungal compound is taking. While little has been concluded objectively, no compound has been researched as extensively as psilocybin in the first two decades of the revival. Time will tell whether it proves efficacious for treating the many conditions of interest. Regardless, psilocybin continues to factor centrally in the mainstream adoption of psychedelics.

María Sabina passed away long before second-wave psilocybin research began. We can only speculate how she would feel about its therapeutic applications, which are a far cry from the traditional *veladas* she facilitated in Mexico. Given her dismissal of Westerners' attempts to find God through the magic mushroom, I can't help but wonder if she would interpret Johns Hopkins' focus on the mystical experience as an extension of the same trend.

The spirit of the holy *children* may have been lost to the ages, replaced with percentages and brain maps. If that spirit cannot be resuscitated, I hope we will continue to remember that no Johns Hopkins researcher or mycologist banker has played a more crucial role in the Western world's inquiry into psilocybin-assisted healing than the legendary Mazatec *curandera*, María Sabina.

4

LSD: Transformation in Death and Rebirth

"When the light turns green, you go.
When the light turns red, you stop.
But what do you do
When the light turns blue
With orange and lavender spots?"

—Shel Silverstein, "Signals"

Of all the psychedelics, *lysergic acid diethylamide*, better known as LSD or "acid," is the most famous in the West—or infamous, depending on whom you ask. It may be surprising to learn that as often as it is mentioned in the context of the revival, LSD has been slow to reenter research laboratories. The specific stigma LSD carries continues to obstruct its mainstream acceptance.

It wasn't always that way. LSD's history began in the 1930s when a small team of Swiss chemists at Sandoz pharmaceuticals aimed "to isolate the active principles of known medicinal plants to produce pure specimens of these substances."[1] One of those chemists was young Albert Hofmann, who'd joined the company soon after graduating with distinction from the University of Zurich's medical school. Hofmann was lauded for his research into the chemical structure of chitin, nature's second-most-abundant polysaccharide. After a few years studying Mediterranean squill, Hofmann turned to ergot, a fungus that grows on rye. Ergot's isolated alkaloid *ergotamine* had already produced a pharmaceutical to treat migraines. Recognizing American and English chemists had begun isolating alkaloids from the already-isolated ergotamine, Hofmann persevered in spite of his boss's warnings of ergot's instability.

Ergot had a polarizing history. On one hand, it was responsible for dozens of endemic outbreaks of poisoning throughout Europe dating to the Middle Ages. On the other, its medicinal properties were recognized as early as 1582, when midwives used it to induce uterine contractions. It was not until the 1800s that scientists aimed to extract its medicinal properties, leading chemists of the Rockefeller Institute of New York to isolate the common nucleus of ergot alkaloids, which they named "lysergic acid."

Knowing lysergic acid was profoundly unstable, Hofmann applied innovative technologies and successfully combined lysergic acid with propanolamine, an amino alcohol, to synthetically produce ergobasine, the alkaloid behind ergot's induction of uterine contractions. This was a significant discovery, but Hofmann wasn't finished. Recognizing the alkaloid's "interesting pharmacological properties," the young chemist focused on new lysergic acid compounds.[2] When he produced the twenty-fifth compound in 1938, he could never have anticipated how profoundly it would shake up the structures of the Western world.

Hofmann's intention with LSD-25 was to produce a circulatory and respiratory stimulant, but the animals on which Sandoz tested it appeared restless under its influence. It was determined to have no basis for further research, and Sandoz abandoned LSD-25.

Hofmann continued his ergot research, yielding a discovery that produced hydergine, a medication for improving circulation and cerebral function in the elderly. Although it became Sandoz's "most important pharmaceutical product," Hofmann continued thinking about LSD-25. More than four years after Sandoz abandoned it, Hofmann was led by a "peculiar presentiment" to reproduce LSD-25 for further testing, and on April 16, 1943, his synthesis was interrupted "by unusual sensations." He described "a remarkable restlessness, combined with a slight dizziness," and he returned home and "sank into a not unpleasant intoxicated-like condition, characterized by an extremely stimulated imagination." He described how, "In a dreamlike state, with eyes closed, I perceived an uninterrupted stream of fantastic pictures, extraordinary shapes with intense, kaleido-scopic play of colors."[3]

Theorizing he'd accidentally absorbed a minuscule amount of LSD-25 through his fingertips, Hofmann realized "it must be a substance of extraor-dinary potency."[4] He decided to conduct a bold self-experiment. On April 19, Hofmann consumed 250 micrograms of LSD-25, embarking upon his-tory's first intentional LSD trip.

Hofmann's brief notes from the experiment documented how forty min-utes after ingestion, he felt "dizziness, feelings of anxiety, visual distortions, symptoms of paralysis, desire to laugh." Shortly after, he found himself in the throes of a "most severe crisis."[5] Unable to write and struggling to speak, he rode his bicycle home, escorted by his assistant Susi Ramstein.*

Back in his home, Hofmann feared he had poisoned himself. "Everything in the room spun around, and the familiar objects and pieces of furniture assumed grotesque, threatening forms. They were in continuous motion, animated, as if driven by an inner restlessness."[6] He recalled, "A demon had invaded me, had taken possession of my body, mind, and soul. I jumped up and screamed, trying to free myself from him, but then sank down again and lay helpless on the sofa. The substance, with which I had wanted to exper-iment, had vanquished me."[7] He felt all but certain he was losing his mind, and he feared he would not come through the episode alive.

When the family doctor arrived, however, he found no abnormal symp-toms in Hofmann's physiology apart from dilated pupils. The chemist's fears relaxed, and the diminishing effects "gave way to a feeling of good fortune and gratitude."[8] Relieved, Hofmann found pleasure in the sensations.

"Kaleidoscopic, fantastic images surged in on me, alternating, variegated, opening and then closing themselves in circles and spirals, exploding in col-ored fountains, rearranging and hybridizing themselves in constant flux. It was particularly remarkable how every acoustic perception, such as the sound of a door handle or a passing automobile, became transformed into optical perceptions. Every sound generated a vividly changing image, with its own

---

* Hofmann's bipedal transportation on LSD immortalized April 19 as a psychedelic holiday, celebrated today as "Bicycle Day."

consistent form and color."[9] The following morning, Hofmann noted, "a sensation of well-being and renewed life flowed through me," and the world "glistened and sparkled in a fresh light."[10]

Hofmann knew he had discovered something extraordinary, especially given the profundity of a microscopic dose. "I was aware that LSD, a new active compound with such properties, would have to be of use in pharmacology, in neurology, and especially in psychiatry, and that it would attract the interest of concerned specialists. But at that time I had no inkling that the new substance would also come to be used beyond medical science, as an inebriant in the drug scene."[11]

The Roots of LSD Stigma

Most of us know what happened next: in the 1960s, the hippie countercultural movement adopted LSD as a sacrament. The acid trip became a rite of passage for the youth, facilitating immersion into a new way of being. The counterculture's resistance to the Vietnam War mirrored their rebellion against the cultural norms of the United States, and through LSD-influenced radical expression and rock 'n' roll, the hippies dreamed of a utopia of peace, harmony, and freedom they believed they were creating.one acoustic ballad at a time.

Unsurprisingly, the US government didn't like the hippies. The Johnson and Nixon administrations sought to destroy the movement, spending significant resources to spread mistrust of flower power adherents. At the end of the decade, the hippie dream met its destruction through two primary events: the notorious Manson murders involving LSD-zonked youths brutally and remorselessly killing nine people in California, and the violent conclusion of the Altamont Free Concert in 1969, where members of the Hells Angels Motorcycle Club, hired to handle security, stabbed an eighteen-year-old to death during the Rolling Stones' set. Nixon's focus on solving the "drug problem" prevailed with the passing of the Controlled Substances Act in 1970, sealing LSD's criminalized status and bidding adieu to the utopian dream.

So began the War on Drugs, and LSD's associations shifted from wonder to depravity. Propaganda convinced the masses that a single hit of LSD could scramble your chromosomes, prompt permanent madness, and cause the sanest person to commit heinous acts of violence. These messages were so potent that they endure to this day, and two important chapters of acid's early history were removed by the government's focus on criminalization: LSD's value in therapy and medicine, and its sketchy use by the Central Intelligence Agency (CIA).

Project MK-Ultra

One of the great ironies of the 1960s was summed up nicely by John Lennon: "We must always remember to thank the CIA and the Army for LSD. They brought out LSD to control people, and what they did was give us freedom."[12]

The hippie movement might never have started without the notorious CIA program known as Project MK-Ultra. Launched in 1953 under the leadership of Sidney Gottlieb, MK-Ultra was the CIA's top priority for over a decade. Much of its history remains ambiguous, for in 1973, when word of the secret program was getting out, CIA director Richard Helms ordered the destruction of all associated records. As fate would have it, however, his minions missed an enormous cache of documents, and when a whistleblower found and released them, a portrait of the freaky operations reached the public.[13]

MK-Ultra was launched at the height of Cold War paranoia. The CIA believed the USSR had developed interrogation and mind-control tactics through various techniques like hypnosis and sensory deprivation in tandem with psychoactive chemicals like LSD. To thwart other nations and develop their own techniques, the CIA ordered a boatload of LSD from Sandoz laboratories and conducted secret experiments on human subjects, many of whom were unwitting.

Some of the more inhumane MK-Ultra subprojects involved covertly administering LSD and other drugs to vulnerable citizens and incarcerated populations. The CIA gave the drug to prisoners, promising them more recreation time and reduced sentences. They gave it to mentally impaired individuals at psychiatric hospitals. They hired prostitutes to trick johns into following them to a "safe house," where the prostitute would dose them as CIA agents watched through a two-way mirror. Some subjects endured the effects in horrible settings, and others were forced to take LSD every day for months. It was all justified in the name of America beating "them commies" once and for all.[14]

What the CIA didn't expect was that certain individuals would discover LSD's positive potential. One of those individuals was writer Ken Kesey, who took part in an MK-Ultra-funded experiment at the Menlo Park Veterans Administration Hospital in Palo Alto, California. Kesey found LSD so profound that he got a job as a night attendant in the hospital's psychiatric ward. He'd take LSD and talk to the patients, and his conversations inspired his most famous novel, *One Flew Over the Cuckoo's Nest*.

Kesey started smuggling LSD out of the facility and giving it to friends. Together, they'd explore their consciousness and find creative expression for their wild trips. When his second novel, *Sometimes a Great Notion*, was about to be published, he and his crew, who called themselves the "Merry Pranksters," purchased an old Harvester School Bus, named it "Furthur,"* painted it with trippy, colorful designs, and embarked upon a legendary journey across America. Under the influence of copious quantities of acid, they blasted music and bellowed through megaphones from Furthur's roof, boisterously announcing their presence to the nation.[15] This 1964 journey is often regarded as the origin of the hippie movement, bridging the post-World-War-II countercultural Beat generation inspired by Jack Kerouac's *On the Road* with the LSD-fueled revelry soon to assemble in the heart of San Francisco. It was all made possible by the CIA's obliviousness to the powers they wielded.

Though the US government preferred to villainize the hippies over acknowledging their sketchy program's role in creating the counterculture, MK-Ultra is hardly a secret at this point. The second part of LSD's pre-1960s history was more effectively erased, and it likely would have stayed that way had it not been for the revival.

The Psychedelic Underground

One might assume that in the decades of prohibition preceding psychedelics' surge in mainstream popularity, psychedelic therapy did not exist in the West. After all, isn't this stuff so exciting because it's new?

---

*   They intended to name the bus "Further," but when one of the Pranksters misspelled it as "Furthur" on the front of the bus, they decided to roll with it—probably because they were tripping.

There's an important difference, however, between the consensus stories of the past and reality. Our memories are limited, our egos thrive on filtering information, and our emotional biases lead us to believe certain things while ignoring others. When you combine these limitations with such things as parental and institutional impacts on our individual belief systems and the mass media's influence on our perception of history—well, it would be almost impossible not to fall victim to humanity's ignorance of the big picture.

The big picture I'm referring to is that psychedelic therapy didn't spontaneously emerge out of the void. While Western society's current degree of interest in the healing potential of psychedelics is undoubtedly novel, lesser-known histories underlie the revival, and understanding those histories provides important context for nuances and complexities in these treatment modalities. The pre-Columbian roots of psychedelic healing stretch deeper than those of the oldest Sierra Redwood, and amid the repressive prohibition of the War on Drugs, psychedelic therapists continued facilitating sessions in secret, exploring how to heal with these medicines in the "psychedelic underground."

This underground evades precise definition. It is a catchall phrase for a breadth of approaches from a swath of facilitators with a wide array of skill sets. By nature of their enterprise, underground practitioners are discreet. Unless one infiltrates their innermost sanctum, few specifics can be known.

What is known is that many of the core pieces of psychedelic therapy were developed, nurtured, and sustained in the underground. These practitioners knew how important these methods of healing were, even if Uncle Sam and mainstream society considered LSD use worthy of a prison sentence. When research organizations and universities started pushing through Federal blockades and launching psychedelic therapy trials, they found a preexisting network of anonymous healers from whom to learn best and worst practices.

Still, the psychedelic underground was not the beginning, but rather a continuation of first-wave Western psychedelic research the US government nearly succeeded in burying.

First-Wave Psychedelic Therapy

From the 1950s to the 1970s, several countries researched LSD's mental health applications. The most well-known experiments were conducted in the early 1960s by Timothy Leary and Richard Alpert at Harvard. Their fascination with the spiritual potential of psychedelics inspired suspect experiments in which they administered psilocybin to students in unsupervised settings. When holistic doctor Andrew Weil, a Harvard undergraduate at the time, was rejected from taking part, he exposed the psychologists' tactics through a series of articles published in the *Harvard Crimson* newspaper. Leary and Alpert were fired, and they went on to conduct more far-out experiments beyond the university's aegis, attracting no shortage of negative press along the way.[16]

Infamous as they became, Leary and Alpert weren't the only academics studying LSD. In Maryland, a team of researchers at the Spring Grove State Hospital developed protocols for LSD-assisted therapy. Among the team's influential members was Stan Grof, who facilitated more than four thousand LSD therapy sessions in the 1960s and early 1970s.

At Spring Grove and beyond, LSD was used to treat depression, anxiety, psychosomatic diseases, and addiction. Dozens of research papers were published, many of which showed considerable efficacy. Several studies administered LSD to groups going through Alcoholics Anonymous (AA) programs. One study from 1962 found that of the fifty-eight AA members who received one session of LSD therapy, thirty-four remained sober six to eighteen months later. In comparison, only four of the thirty-five participants who hadn't received LSD achieved the same result.[17]

Grof published several books on his work at Spring Grove. His seminal text *LSD Psychotherapy* detailed many psychedelic therapy guidelines still applied today, including the use of eyeshades, the importance of music, and the non-directive approach focused on evoking the participant's innate capacity to heal.

Eyeshades and Music

A recurring facet of psychedelic therapy established in the early days of LSD research is the client's use of eyeshades during their trips. Eyeshades encourage an internal experience, opening possibilities of insight into the workings of subtle and typically inaccessible layers of the psyche. Psychedelics alter perception of the external world—if you talk to folks at a music festival, you're bound to hear someone's account of seeing a tree as if for the first time or receiving divine messages from patterns in the clouds. In psychedelic therapy, external fascination is often regarded as distraction. Losing yourself in the beauty of a painting could be valuable, but it may prevent you from facing things you habitually avoid.

With eyeshades on, clients have little choice but to experience their inner world and attend to whatever arises. There's no predicting what this will be, but therapists usually suggest whatever comes up is emerging for a reason. The psychedelic session isn't about making sense of the experience—that's what integration is for. Psychedelic sessions are about surrendering control to the process unfolding, and eyeshades encourage clients to let the long, strange trip flow.

The use of eyeshades in psychedelic therapy is the physical expression of the modality's alignment with an age-old spiritual adage: *true change comes from within*. Eliminating the visual world establishes conditions for transformational insight into how our day-to-day minds tick. Our familiarity with routine patterns can block realization that the patterns don't define *who we are*. They are habits of the mind, embedded as neural pathways through complex influences related to one's development.

Eyeshades comprise only half of an important relationship between two procedural pillars that first-wave psychedelic researchers established. The second pillar is the use of music as a guide. Music plays such an influential role that some practitioners refer to it as an "invisible" or "hidden" therapist. When paired with psychedelics, music can be so influential that the client can no longer differentiate between the songs and the inner journey itself. In a sense, music can *become* the trip.

Facilitators tend to choose playlists or sequences of songs for specific individuals. They take clients' preferences into account, structuring the grooves to guide the client through rhythms and crescendos that suit their struggles and goals. For someone facing heavy fears, gentle ambient or classical music might be ideal, whereas electronic music thick with chunky bass might be best for someone aiming to evoke intense emotions.

"Music in psychedelic therapy provides a meaningful structure for the experience and creates a continuous carrier wave that helps patients to overcome difficult parts of the sessions and to move through impasses," Grof wrote in *LSD Psychotherapy*.[18] Johns Hopkins neuroscientist Frederick Streeter Barrett asserted combining music and psychedelics may lead to "a change in neural circuitry that may be stuck in patterns of negative emotional bias . . . And that may be just enough to give someone access to new perspectives on their selves and their lives and begin on the road to healing."[19]

Even with music's recognized centrality in psychedelic therapy, a relatively paltry amount of research has been done on it. Mendel Kaelen decided to fill that void. Hailing from Holland, Kaelen earned a master's degree in neuroscience from the University of Groningen before getting a PhD at Imperial College London, where he studied under Robin Carhart-Harris. At Imperial, he realized his passions for music and psychedelic research need not remain separate.

"I realized music is almost the only stimulus that patients have during the peak effects of the drug," Kaelen said in our interview. "I realized we need to look into this and start talking about it."

Kaelen continued, "The main function of music is to support the therapy process in a nonverbal, experiential way. Music can do that by providing a profound sense of acknowledgement, reassurance, and love along with a feeling of deepening into difficult experiences. In that deepening, various layers of memories and thoughts are revealed that you may not have been able to access before. The ways music can support therapy are broad, but in essence, music is so effective because it's nonverbal. Providing this nonverbal framework allows parts of yourself to be brought to the forefront without interpreting them or adding words that box things down into particular categories and move you away from the felt sense of the experience."

It's not as simple as popping on some tunes and letting it ride. Specific music pairs well with specific psychedelics for specific people, calling for creativity and intuition in the curation of playlists. My friend Pierre Bouchard, a highly experienced psychedelic therapist and music aficionado, told me, "A general practice that I have is to start with gentle music. You might reductively call it spa music—something soothing and open that doesn't have too many of its own opinions. As people start to have an experience, I play something that deepens them into that experience. I think of it as sonic attunement, where you're mirroring them musically."

Kaelen shared a similar approach. "Music can guide the experience in different directions. It has the capacity to convey a sense of awe, a sense of transcendence, or a sense of religiosity. You may have a mystical-type experience, but sometimes it's not a mystical experience the person needs. They may need emotional catharsis or getting to the root of a certain trauma. What may be needed is an emotional breakthrough experience, or a sense of deep forgiveness, or a feeling of profound safety and security. The question is how can we use music as a therapeutic tool to guide the experience of each client in a person-centered way, where a therapeutic experience occurs?"

On top of these challenges, the pause between songs can interrupt the journey's fluidity. Grof recognized this in the 1970s, noting, "It is quite common that clients have difficulties with the periods when the music stops and the records or tapes are being changed; they complain that they feel suspended in midair, and sense a painful gap in the experience."[20] Streaming services work better than the cassette tapes of Grof's era, as they typically have a "fade" feature for smoother transitions, but even these can be jarring and disrupt a sequenced flow. Further, if the therapist senses the current song isn't appropriate for the emotional state of the client, they have two choices: let the song run its lengthy course, or disrupt continuity with a sudden change. Neither is a good option.

Recognizing this issue, Kaelen pivoted from academic research to entrepreneurship. In 2019, he and a team established the company Wavepaths, and two years later, the company released an innovative "person-centered music product"[21] designed to facilitate a continuous carrier wave without obstruction. Wavepaths is essentially a web-based digital instrument that facilitators control, allowing them to select a specific medicine, dose, and emotional focus, all of which guide the music selection. The system doesn't play prearranged playlists. It is *generative*, which means the algorithm draws from thousands of "artist composed stems"—basically, blips of music and tones provided by numerous musicians—to produce an uninterrupted stream that has never been heard before.

Kaelen argues therapists have two primary choices with music: use it to mirror the state of the client and deepen their experience, or use it to guide the client toward a different emotion. Wavepaths empowers therapists to do both. Instead of having to ride out a song or disrupt the process by abruptly changing it, users can slide a dial toward an intended emotional effect, and the algorithm draws from the library of stems to shift the wave in that direction.*

Another important function music serves is keeping the journey alive after the effects wear off. Listening to the playlist in the days, weeks, or years following a journey can bridge the distant emotions and insights into present, embodied experience. Because it can be difficult to remember a trip and even more difficult to reconnect to the emotions it evoked this function of music is immensely important.

And it makes sense. Can you think of a song that transports you back in time, summoning nostalgia-tinted memories of specific people and places? Music has a mysterious way of magnetizing emotions and memories into a close relationship over which time's decomposing trends exert little influence. Understanding the innate power of music can equip psychedelic therapists and voyagers to derive enduring value out of sessions.

"Working with music therapeutically is an art," Kaelen said. "It's something that takes time to master. Wavepaths is founded on the conviction that music has the potential to facilitate life-changing experiences."

To Kaelen, music itself is a psychedelic agent, carrying all of these potentials with or without the use of a drug. Like LSD and psilocybin, music kindles an inner experience that can catalyze emotional breakthroughs and realizations.

Ego Death

Though psychedelic experiences appear to share mysterious commonalities with death, it's extraordinarily unlikely you will die under their influence. In fact, one of their more amazing properties is that most psychedelics *can't* kill you on a physiological level the way too much heroin, alcohol, or Tylenol

---

* I'm not getting paid by Wavepaths to write about them, by the way. I'm writing about them because I've used the product, and I am deeply impressed with what it can do and how helpful it could become for psychedelic therapy.

can.* What they can kill is your entire understanding of your identity and the reality you live in, and if that happens, may the Force be with your personal experience of psychedelic "ego death."

Ego death is a slippery term, largely because "ego" is one of those words people toss around as though its meaning is as clear as the word "socks." In this context, ego refers to the conscious mind as a constellation of desires, fears, neuroses, and beliefs. It is the seat of personality and identity, our individual yarn ball of conceptual strands about who we are and where we came from. Given that we are limited humans, many of these concepts are delusional, constraining our sense of identity to narratives with no basis in reality outside our skulls. While the ego helps us navigate the world as autonomous beings, it also blocks out aspects of the world that threaten our beliefs and values.

When people say psychedelics cause ego death, they're saying psychedelics can unravel structures of identity and belief. While this can be liberating, people can mistakenly think ego death is the goal of psychedelic use. This idea assumes a negative conception of the ego. The ego is necessary, helping us traverse an overwhelming planet by filtering out the large majority of reality and conceiving of ourselves as continuous *somethings*. Without that ability, we'd be hosed.

When our fears, beliefs, and self-narratives become calcified, our egos become isolated fortresses. That's when ego death becomes therapeutic. As rigid concepts loosen, we open to new possibilities. We remember to take ourselves and our private universes less seriously. In the words of Carhart-Harris and his research team, "Moreover, it is the ability of psychedelics to disrupt stereotyped patterns of thought and behavior by disintegrating the patterns of activity upon which they rest that accounts for their therapeutic potential."[22]

---

*   This is particularly true of classic psychedelics like psilocybin and LSD, neither of which have been linked to a fatal overdose in and of themselves. This is particularly *not* true of MDMA and ketamine, both of which have been linked to fatal overdoses outside therapeutic settings. And though no one has fatally overdosed on LSD or psilocybin in isolation, both have contributed to deaths when combined with contraindicated substances, and both have contributed to accidental deaths due to loss of touch with reality, such as drowning or falling from a great height.

On the other hand, overidentifying with the ego can be a recipe for a rough journey. When ego death comes beckoning, a rigid ego becomes a gazelle fleeing a lion. Unlike the gazelle, however, the cornered ego can resist its annihilation, no matter how agonizing the struggle. It will be shaken up, perhaps traumatized, but the ego can endure as long as its driver is unwilling to let go of the wheel.

Another issue arises when people think a psychedelic-induced ego death is permanent. "My ego died on LSD, so I'm egoless now, channeling pure energy through this body," says a finance bro rebranding himself as a guru. That's an issue because it's total bullshit. His former ego may have died, but as he returns to baseline consciousness, a new ego forms, and part of its new foundation is the *belief* it's an egoless guru. Such self-delusion can put others in harm's way, for this egoless guru's ego blocks out threatening feedback. For example, this finance bros might recommend taking time to integrate his LSD insights before giving it to others and claiming he can heal them, to which the egoless ego would reply, "You're projecting, bro. That's your stuff, not mine."

We all have egos, and while psychedelics can shatter them, we eventually return to consensus reality.* In that return, new ego structures form, even if our new ego disguises itself as a transcendent being with godlike powers drawn from peering through the codes of the matrix.† The ego is not a villain, and being "egoless" is not healthy. It would be better to cultivate a balance of appreciating the ego without overidentifying with it—recognizing that, like physical objects, its apparent fixedness is an illusion.

---

* There are some rare exceptions, however, where people have died on psychedelics. Typically, this has to do with physiological factors, such as contraindicated chemicals in the bloodstream, dehydration, overhydration, unreported hypertension, or other factors related to lack of care and harm reduction in the setting. It is also more common with plant medicines, especially iboga, which brings risks most others do not.

† Many psychonauts refer to consensus reality as "the matrix." It's a reference to the aforementioned Keanu Reeves film, and it's often paired with these folks claiming they "took the red pill" that Laurence Fishburne gave Reeves to escape the imprisoning simulation. While some red-pill takers may indeed have seen the truth (whatever that is), many others have simply constructed a new matrix of self-delusion. These phony prophets annoy me a lot, for, they clearly think they're enlightened when really they're spreading their delusions like an Agent Smith virus.

For those who maintain this healthy balance, psychedelic ego death presents an opportunity to become "reborn" into a more actualized version of themselves, freed from the limiting confines of their distorted thoughts. For this to occur, integration is essential. A therapist or guide can help the individual build a new, healthier ego structure than the one that buckled under the weight of the psychedelic. This process may take months, if not years. It may be difficult and painful, but it is an unparalleled opportunity for transformation.

If one isn't willing to release their attachment to what they believe most fervently about themselves and the universe, ego death can feel like actual death that one is powerless to stop. Such a terrifying nightmare, however, could become a revelation with the support of a skilled facilitator. The facilitator anchors the frightened journeyer to a safer reality than the hell of their fears' construction, reminding them that even in such desolation, they are not alone. The facilitator doesn't aim to change the person's experience, but instead helps it transpire in a supportive context so the person can relax their resistance. After all, experienced practitioners know that if the journeyer gets stuck thinking "This is bad! This shouldn't be happening!" all the way through, their egoic resistance will emerge stronger, leaving their bodies locked in an unending struggle against a pervasive threat of danger.

If facilitators fail to understand and appreciate the phenomenology of ego death, they put the client at risk. They may, for instance, interpret the journeyer's terror to mean something has gone wrong, and when the client intuits the therapist's fear, their panicked sense of "Something awful is happening!" will amplify, increasing the potential for a traumatic outcome.

We struggle to release our deepest wounds because we have spent our entire lives identifying with them. No matter how clearly you realize the invalidity of self-narratives built from these wounds, the ego clings to the stories it knows best. Its grip rarely releases easily, and when a psychedelic all but forces it to happen, it can feel like the Grim Reaper has arrived. Understanding this pattern empowers people to enter psychedelic journeys equipped to allow ego death to unfold naturally, opening the possibility of ego liberation. To help ground these abstractions, psychedelic researchers and writers have turned to religion and mythology.

Death, Transformation, Rebirth

Perhaps the clearest expression of the bridge between LSD, music, and early researchers' evocation of world religions is the Beatles' song "Tomorrow Never Knows." John Lennon sang the iconic opening words* in the explosive conclusion to *Revolver* in 1966, drawing directly from the work of Leary, Alpert, and fellow Harvard psychologist Ralph Metzner in their influential book, *The Psychedelic Experience: A Manual Based on the Tibetan Book of the Dead.* Throughout the text, the three authors relate the psychedelic experience to the Tibetan Buddhist concept of the bardo. The bardo is the liminal space consciousness enters after death, the navigation of which determines the quality of one's reincarnation or, for the most adept, liberation. The Harvard writers used the urtext on the subject—the *Bardo Thödol*, better known as *The Tibetan Book of the Dead*—as a foundation for their guidebook to help people navigate the frightening bardo-like realms into which LSD can transport users.

For devotees of Tibetan Buddhism, the purpose of meditation is to prepare for the bardo. For the Harvard researchers, LSD opened training opportunities by transporting people to bardo states before the death of their physical body. In such liminal spaces, psychonauts could gain insight into their mind's hallucinatory projections of desires, attachments, fears, and regrets. According to the authors, "All individuals who have received the practical teachings of this manual will, if the text be remembered, be set face to face with the ecstatic radiance and will win illumination instantaneously, without entering upon hallucinatory struggles and without further suffering on the age-long pathway of normal evolutions."[23] Skillful navigation, they argued, could catalyze liberation from egoic attachment and suffering, prompting a "rebirth" into a more expansive state of consciousness.

If the *Bardo Thödol* is too "out there" for the Western mind, mythology can offer some signposts for these otherworldly journeys. The theme of death and rebirth is found throughout countless cultures, religions, and works of art. In the second half of countless films, the protagonist undergoes death and rebirth in some form. It could be loss of hope, like George Bailey in *It's a Wonderful Life*,

---

*   It saddens me to report that due to copyright issues, I am barred from reprinting Lennon's words. If you do not know the words I'm referencing, I strongly recommend listening to "Tomorrow Never Knows" right now.

who walks drunkenly to a bridge with suicidal intent before his guardian angel intervenes. It could be hopeless defeat by a powerful nemesis, like when King T'Challa gets tossed over a waterfall by Michael B. Jordan in *Black Panther*, only to be revived by his mother, sister, hard-to-get crush, and token White companion, who give him the medicinal "heart-shaped herb."* It could even be legitimately dying, like Harry Potter getting struck by Voldemort's killing curse in *Harry Potter and the Deathly Hallows* or Neo getting shot by Agent "Mr. Anderson" Smith in *The Matrix* before literally resurrecting to defeat the bad guy.

No matter how the motif is expressed, the hero conquers death through a *rebirth* into a more powerful form, at last capable of accomplishing the goal the former self was unable to achieve. It was not the individual who died but the limitations of their former self, the cessation of which made space for the reborn self to, as the kids say, *level up*.

Movies can be viewed as modern myths. If one applies the framework of Swiss psychiatrist Carl Jung, their mythological roots point to death and rebirth as a motif common to the acultural human psyche. The motif is successful in films not because it's a clever idea, but because it speaks to a foundational truth that resonates within us all. We are all capable of dying and being reborn in another form, and those who doubt this would likely doubt it less after ingesting a large enough psychedelic dose.

Beyond modern movies, myths of death and rebirth have been essential to humanity's self-understanding since antiquity. Every culture has their unique variation of the common tale. Consider the Greek myth of Persephone, daughter of Olympians Zeus and Demeter, who was abducted into the underworld by Zeus's brother Hades, who was in love with her. The grief of Demeter, goddess of harvest and fertility, was so great that the seasons ceased to change, and all flora perished. Zeus bargained with his brother to allow Persephone to return to Olympus with her mother, and although Hades

---

* Black Panther's heart-shaped herb must be reference to psychedelic plant medicine. When someone takes it, their consciousness is transported to the ancestral plane, where they are granted insights and powers. It's on this plane where T'Challa draws the strength necessary to defeat B. Jordan in a good old-fashioned superhero brawl.

agreed, he tricked Persephone into eating pomegranate seeds, which bound her to the underworld each autumn and winter.

Persephone's cyclical descent into the underworld and ascension to Olympus represented the seasonal cycles of wintry death and springtime rejuvenation. The myth was so foundational to their culture that the Eleusinian Mysteries, the Greeks' most important religious rite of initiation, centered on Persephone's cyclical journey. And wouldn't you know it, there's speculation, and even evidence, suggesting the mysterious brew the Greeks consumed during these secretive ceremonies contained the fungus from which LSD was derived.

Ergot Dance Party at Eleusis

In 2020, Brian Muraresku, a Catholic lawyer with a BA in classics, went on Joe Rogan's podcast to talk about his new book, *The Immortality Key: The Secret History of the Religion with No Name*. Millions of listens later, the book became a bestseller, introducing a mainstream audience to the bizarre, suspect, and fascinating field of what might be called "entheogenic anthropology."

Muraresku embarked on a *Da-Vinci-Code*-esque quest to uncover evidence that the kykeon, the concoction around which the Eleusinian ceremonies centered, was a psychedelic brew. The Eleusinian Mysteries, which took place for nearly two thousand years, transpired at the sacred site of Eleusis—near Athens—via two annual celebrations. The "Lesser Mysteries" took place at the threshold of spring, and those who'd completed the Lesser Mysteries were deemed worthy of the "Greater Mysteries," which occurred over ten days in September. The Greater Mysteries climaxed when the initiates drank the kykeon and entered a sanctuary called the Telesterion, commonly theorized to symbolize entry into the underworld. Initiates would "die" inside the Telesterion and emerge "reborn."

No one knows for certain what transpired in the Telesterion, for initiates were sworn to secrecy under the punishment of death. Evidently, initiates kept the secret, for their testimonies spoke to unanimous adulation of the ritual's power and importance. Nearly every prominent Greek, from Aristotle to Sophocles to Homer, participated, the latter of whom asserted the ritual was designed "to lead us back to the principles from which we descended . . . a perfect enjoyment of intellectual [spiritual] good."[24] The mysteries were so highly regarded that several Roman leaders took part, including the great Emperor Marcus Aurelius, whose legacy remains strong through the film *Gladiator* and the popular trend of quoting his Stoic philosophy on social media. Roman statesman Cicero wrote, "Among the many excellent and indeed divine institutions which your Athens has brought forth and contributed to human life, none, in my opinion, is better than those mysteries."[25]

All was well until Christianity spread through the Roman Empire. The end was nigh in 391 CE when Roman emperor Theodosius I, seeing the mysteries as a pagan threat to the Church, ordered the closing of sacred sites. Four years later, Alaric I, military leader of the Germanic Visigoths who had served Theodosius until the emperor's death in 395 CE, rode into Eleusis with his Christian compatriots and dealt the finishing blow, razing much of the sacred site to the ground.

How did Eleusis produce such consistent and profound transformations? What did initiates do in the Telesterion? Did they dance? Have deep conversations? Revel in a wild Athenian orgy? We will never know for sure, but Muraresku's bestselling claims reappropriated a theory several psychedelic leaders espoused decades before him: the kykeon contained ergot from the barley that grew in the region, lending it properties similar to LSD.

These pre-Muraresku theorists were Hofmann, Wasson, and Boston University professor Carl Ruck. Their 1978 book *The Road to Eleusis* laid out their argument of an LSD-like kykeon to explain the transformative power of the mysteries. Believe it or not, academics of the late 1970s didn't like this theory. They may have gotten pissed off, if they'd taken the book seriously. Instead, they scoffed the way tenured professors often scoff at new theories that challenge assumptions upon which their livelihood relies. If a psychedelic brew factored centrally into ancient Greek and Greco-Roman culture and religion, then the history of Western civilization and religion, cemented over nearly two thousand years of scholarship, would need to be revised down to its very foundation.

Ruck got the worst of the backlash. Boston University tarnished his reputation and blocked graduate students from entertaining curiosity about his research, all the while forcing him to stay put due to contractual obligations. While obscure writers had kept entheogenic anthropology alive, Muraresku's appearance on Rogan's podcast brought the line of inquiry into the mainstream. The Robert Langdon-esque lawyer even took the theory further and argued the psychedelic kykeon inspired the original Christian Eucharist, which would mean that the most important ritual of Western history's most dominant religion can be traced back to a psychedelic sacrament.

If the theory is valid, it marks an important revelation: despite what the War on Drugs propaganda got people thinking about LSD and psilocybin, psychedelics played a key role in the formation of Western civilization. This would further the evidence that human beings have a natural impulse toward inducing altered states to connect with sacred realities, regardless of their culture. This revelation would position the anti-psychedelic values of the West more at odds with human history than in line with a "superior" moral perspective.

Even if it's not true, the Eleusinian Mysteries provide a model for ritualistic context and symbolic meaning as important factors for transformation. With or without ergot, the mysteries ground the death and rebirth motif as a ceremonial practice structured to mobilize transition into higher levels of self-actualization. The validity of arguments about psychedelic dance parties in the Telesterion are unnecessary to recognize the metamorphic implications of dying before you die.

LSD in the Second Wave

When LSD became a Schedule I drug in 1970,[*] the US Government ignored reality to determine it had no medicinal value. This effectively obliterated all medical research into the compound. Uncle Sam gripped LSD in a stronger chokehold than any other psychedelic, and he's hardly loosened his grip today.

However, not all countries hold LSD in such a punishing stranglehold. Fittingly, Switzerland, the country where Hofmann discovered the molecule, has led the revival of research into LSD's therapeutic potential. In 2008, a team of Swiss researchers received approval for a pilot study on LSD and end-of-life anxiety, the first clinical LSD trial in more than thirty-five years. That study, which

---

[*]   LSD was actually first banned by the US government in 1968, and the state of California banned it two years earlier than that. The Controlled Substances Act of 1970, however, established the conditions for its Schedule I classification.

ended in 2012, found participants' anxiety decreased significantly during the treatment, and the decrease remained consistent at the one-year follow-up.

As LSD research continues in Switzerland, clinicians have found legal loopholes to offer LSD-assisted therapy to specific patient populations. Peter Gasser, a kind, soft-spoken psychiatrist and psychotherapist, told me there are currently more than fifty therapists doing LSD therapy in Switzerland. In the years since Gasser gave LSD to his first patient in 2014, he and his colleagues have provided the treatment to about one thousand patients.

Speaking on LSD's long-term benefits, Gasser said, "It's not only symptom reduction like antidepressant drugs, which, when you stop taking them, you see symptoms getting high again after a while. With LSD, it's more likely that symptoms stay down, in the sense that LSD has the power to *transform*."

Switzerland's research has diminished the LSD throttlehold in other nations as well. Researchers in the UK are looking into LSD's potential as a remedy for neurodegenerative diseases. Their hypothesis draws from a growing body of research showing serotonergic psychedelics like LSD promote *neurogenesis*, inducing growth in atrophied brain cells like those found in the brains of people suffering from Alzheimer's.[26]

Researchers in the Netherlands are researching LSD's potential to treat chronic pain. In a paper published in the *Journal of Pharmacology* in 2020, the authors reported a low dose of 20 micrograms increased volunteers' overall pain tolerance 20% more than a placebo group. This percentage was comparable to common opioids and significantly longer lasting. Although some physiological side effects were noted, none aroused concern, and low doses of LSD were determined to be reliably safe.[27]

Despite the abundant psychedelic research conducted since the Johns Hopkins 2006 paper, LSD wouldn't be given to a human research subject in the United States until 2022. With the help of leaders like Gasser, a biotech company called MindMed launched a Phase 2b double-blind, placebo-controlled trial studying LSD for the treatment of Generalized Anxiety Disorder.* It's not a therapy study, instead requiring two "dosing session

---

*   Perhaps to evade attracting LSD-attached stigma, MindMed gave their molecule the name "MM-120."

monitors" to sit with participants who receive either a placebo or one of four LSD doses ranging from 25 to 200 micrograms. Because LSD's effects last longer than most psychedelics, sessions take twelve hours to complete. Fortunately, researchers learned not to repeat the methods of MK-Ultra, and participants hang out in a comfortable office as groovy music plays instead of a white-walled room, jail cell, or wiretapped safehouse alongside double-agent prostitutes and peeping Toms working for the CIA.

Hofmann's Eleusinian Vision

In his 1992 lecture entitled "The Message of the Eleusinian Mysteries for the Modern World," Hofmann appealed to Friedrich Nietzsche's *The Birth of Tragedy* to explain how the Greek mysteries exemplified humanity's "Dionysian" impulse toward formlessness. The rituals dissolved subject/object, humanity/nature dualisms of logical thought into ecstatic unity, celebrating the interconnectedness of all things. The intoxication-induced mystical experience was central to these rites and equally essential to civilization as the "Apollonian" worldview of rational materialism and fixed form.

There's no need to read Karl Marx to recognize the Apollonian worldview dominates Western capitalist culture. Amid such rationalism, the West lacks any noteworthy Dionysian rites structured to catalyze inner transformation. The impulse toward ecstatic intoxication, however, remains apparent in packed clubs on Saturday night, Coachella, and all along Bourbon Street and the Las Vegas Strip. Unfortunately, no transformative framework in the vein of the Eleusinian Mysteries. Hofmann argued that for psychedelics to help create a better world, intentional contexts are essential, for betterment comes not through taking a drug but through inducing a meaningful experience whose value transcends the constraints of capitalist dogmas.

"The fundamental significance of a mystical totality-experience for the healing of humankind, afflicted by a one-sided, rational, materialistic worldview, has lately been emphasized by leading representatives of psychology and psychiatry," Hofmann noted in his lecture. "Yet even more significant is that overcoming our dualistic worldview is considered to be a prerequisite and fundamental step for the healing and renewal of occidental civilization and culture, not just in medicine, but in ever-wider circles of our society, even the ecclesiastical."[28]

Hofmann believed that the Judeo-Christian worldview is, like society, enraptured in a dualistic worldview of the "Creator and the created," the "Heavenly and the human." Unlike this paradigm wherein "a godly power enthroned in Heaven is worshipped," the Eleusinian Mysteries exemplified accessible transformation "effected within individual people, a visionary glimpse of the ground of being, which converted her or him into a mystes or an epopetes, into an initiate."

Albert Hofmann passed away in 2008 at the age of 102. In his later years, he felt at peace walking through his beautiful garden, and he enjoyed a quiet and contemplative life. Shortly before Hofmann died, Gasser had the opportunity to inform him that his research team had received approval for the first study on LSD since first-wave research was shut down. "He said he was waiting for a long time for LSD to reenter medicine," Gasser recalled, "and he hoped that it would continue."

Despite the history of his "problem child," Hofmann remained hopeful LSD would reach its positive cultural potential. Grof shared the chemist's view, writing in his foreword to Hofmann's memoir, "I personally believe that in the future LSD will be seen as one of the most influential discoveries of the twentieth century and that Hofmann's 'problem child' will again be seen—as it should have been seen all along—as a 'wonder child' that had to grow up in a dysfunctional society."

Hofmann hoped Western culture would one day incorporate psychedelics like LSD in Eleusinian-inspired rites that honored the molecule's transformative potential. In such contexts, psychedelic-induced death-rebirth experiences could invite modern humans to actualize their slumbering potential. Separation of psychedelic use and intentional rituals is endemic of capitalism's itemization of reality, reinforcing borders blocking people from peering into the nature of reality. Hofmann believed reverence for the sacredness of psychedelic compounds allowed their potential to manifest fully. Otherwise, psychedelics become another drug defined by practical value in a medical paradigm, if not another means of escaping a culture desperately in need of radical transformation.

Will the revival prove more successful in honoring and catalyzing LSD's transformative power than first-wave research? Or will Hofmann's "wonder child" again become the "problem child" sending psychedelic research awry? Time will tell. Regardless, the remarkable molecule *lysergic acid diethylamide* occupies an indelible position in the ongoing psychedelic history of the West.

5

MDMA and Nonlinearity

"It is now some years since I detected how many were the false beliefs that I had from my earliest youth admitted as true, and how doubtful was everything I had since constructed on this basis."

—René Descartes, *Meditations on First Philosophy*

A noteworthy feature of classic psychedelics like psilocybin and LSD is their hallucinations. While *3,4-Methylenedioxymethamphetamine*—better known as MDMA—can cause visual distortions, it is not not known for its hallucinogenic effects. The classic psychedelics mimic the neurotransmitter serotonin, acting as agonists to the brain's 5-HT2A serotonin receptors. Rather than acting as a serotonergic agonist, MDMA is believed to prompt the brain to release serotonin in excess, causing a tremendous elevation in mood that concludes with a feeling of depletion as serotonin reserves are exhausted.

MDMA also induces a significant release of the neurotransmitter nor-epinephrine, responsible for increased arousal and alertness, and blocks the reuptake of dopamine, responsible for motivation and reward-seeking behavior, making dopamine more bioavailable during the drug's window of effects. The ensuing effects of profound well-being, pleasure, empathy, and love common to MDMA earned it the nickname "Ecstasy."*

---

*   It is important to acknowledge that MDMA and what is commonly called "ecstasy" are not necessarily the same. Pure, unadulterated MDMA can induce sensations of ecstasy, but a drug called "ecstasy" is not necessarily pure MDMA. If you're at a festival, for instance, and some drifter sells you ecstasy, it's very possibly something that contains MDMA—though that isn't guaranteed—as well as a host of other chemicals. In short: MDMA is ecstasy, but not all ecstasy is MDMA. The same logic applies to MDMA's other nickname, "Molly."

MDMA is chemically closer to a stimulant than a classic psychedelic. Under its influence, heart rate increases. Tension accumulates in the jaw, leading to involuntary grinding of the teeth. Euphoria can ensue, prompting a feeling of being "on top of the world." Unlike psilocybin and LSD, you can overdose if you take too much MDMA, and its effects on cardiovascular function and thermoregulation contraindicate it with many prescriptions (e.g., Adderall) and diagnoses (e.g., hypertension).

Although MDMA was invented in the early 1900s, it didn't arouse Federal concern until it became a popular "club drug" in the 1980s rave scene. This recreational use resulted from growing interest in MDMA's therapeutic properties in the 1970s. A key figure of this chapter of MDMA's history was the esteemed chemist Sasha Shulgin. Drawing from German company Merck's invention of the compound in 1912, Shulgin synthesized MDMA in the mid-1960s, but he didn't take much interest until a stream of students came to him reporting positive experiences with the substance. Their interest propelled Shulgin to resynthesize MDMA and try it himself in 1976. In a report on its effects published in 1978, Shulgin and coauthor David Nichols described "an easily controlled altered state of consciousness with emotional and sensual overtones."[1]

Influenced by Shulgin's prominent role in the underground, dozens of therapists adopted MDMA into their practice. They recognized its potential as a therapeutic adjunct due to its potency of positive effects and relative subtlety compared to classic psychedelics. They witnessed MDMA consistently relaxing clients' defense mechanisms, opening access to difficult unconscious content like traumatic memories. They also witnessed something different from classic psychedelic effects: MDMA's enhancement of well-being expanded the client's ability to stay with challenging emotions without becoming dysregulated, supporting their capacity to process traumatic memories and release the fear and shame they'd carried ever since.

The individual credited as leading MDMA's incorporation into therapy was a psychotherapist named Leo Zeff. Zeff gave MDMA the nickname "Adam," for he believed it reconnected users with a primordial innocence akin to the Garden of Eden. Zeff and other MDMA therapists believed so wholeheartedly in its healing potential that when they witnessed the rise of the drug's recreational use in raves, they attempted to limit its distribution to avoid its scheduling. But alas, as Nancy Reagan's "Just Say No" campaign extended Nixon's War on Drugs and demonstrated an equal degree of naïveté regarding the complexities of addiction, the Drug Enforcement Agency called for MDMA to be classified as a Schedule I substance in 1985.

Numerous therapists, psychiatrists, and researchers fought back. Many testified on behalf of MDMA's undeniable medicinal value, prompting the judge presiding over the administrative hearings to recommend a Schedule III classification, which would allow it to be prescribed. The DEA ignored them and slapped on a Schedule I label, prompting Harvard psychiatrist Lester Grinspoon to sue the DEA on claims that they had willingly ignored MDMA's therapeutic potential. The argument was strong enough to sway the judge, who lifted the Schedule I designation on the grounds of the DEA's "unpersuasive" case, but DEA operatives flashed a bureaucratic middle finger at the justice system and reclassified MDMA as Schedule I.

Just as the War on Drugs didn't stop people from using drugs, the Schedule I designation didn't stop therapists from using MDMA. They moved the work underground, maintaining secrecy to avoid criminal prosecution. In 2004, Myron Stolaroff published *The Secret Chief Revealed*, divulging how Zeff continued to lead the MDMA charge in the underground after the DEA paved the road to victory with bricks of deception. Zeff reportedly trained thousands of therapists to administer MDMA, and his approach heavily influenced the nonprofit organization that shepherded MDMA therapy from the fringes to the mainstream. The results of this nonprofit's research have provided strong evidence supporting the claims of the early MDMA therapists, further establishing that former DEA administrator John C. "Jack" Lawn was indeed as big of an asshole as MDMA's history suggests him to be. If you have prior knowledge of the revival, you already know the nonprofit I'm referencing is the Multidisciplinary Association for Psychedelic Studies, better known as MAPS.

MDMA-Assisted Therapy for Post-Traumatic Stress Disorder

Ever since Rick Doblin founded MAPS in 1986, the nonprofit has centered on a mission to foster medical, legal, and cultural contexts for the use of psychedelics and marijuana through nonprofit research and education. Its primary focus has been to change the DEA's ruling on MDMA and create legal pathways for its therapeutic applications. As the revival's waves grew larger, MAPS's FDA-approved clinical trial studying MDMA-assisted therapy for the treatment of post-traumatic stress disorder (PTSD) has gained significant momentum. At the time of writing, the study's groundbreaking results has received positive coverage from mainstream media outlets ranging from *Fox News* to the *New York Times*, the latter of which ran a front-page article on MDMA therapy in 2021 with the gripping headline, "The Psychedelic Revolution Is Coming. Psychiatry May Never Be the Same."

Traditionally, PTSD has been treated through cognitive methods. The focus has been on *memory*, and various approaches have been developed to heal memories associated with traumatic events. Long-prevailing models include cognitive-behavioral therapy (CBT), eye movement desensitization reprocessing (EMDR), exposure therapy, and pharmaceutical drugs like SSRIs. MAPS reported that 40–60% of individuals with PTSD do not respond adequately to traditional approaches, and many of the pharmacological treatments bring unwanted side effects and must be taken daily over lengthy periods, if not indefinitely.[2]

This gets at one of the reasons the revival of psychedelic therapy has struck a cultural nerve: the mental health field has been reconciling its failings for some time, and there's a consensus that significant change needs to occur. So, when reports came of patients with treatment-resistant PTSD taking ecstasy in a therapist's office and radically boosting those percentages, interest and desperation outmatched stigmas and taboos.

The rigorous standards of MAPS's MDMA-assisted therapy protocol earned the respect of the scientific community. Their clinical trials met the imperatives of the establishment, including the gold standard of "double-blind, placebo-controlled," meaning neither therapist nor participant knows whether the substance administered is MDMA or a placebo until the study concludes. If the results of the medicine being tested demonstrate significant statistical difference from the placebo, then the drug, over any other possible factor, can be determined as the key to those results.

MAPS's results have repeatedly demonstrated statistical significance. Their Phase 2 reports told an astounding story: two months after treatment, 56% of participants in the MDMA group no longer met diagnostic criteria for PTSD. Twelve months after treatment, the percentage had increased to 68%, indicating participants got *better* over time. These results led the FDA to give MAPS's trial Breakthrough Therapy designation in 2017.

An important feature of their results is the finitude of the treatment. Unlike taking a medicine such as an SSRI every day for years, the MAPS protocol concludes after fifteen sessions over five months. Participants receive MDMA in only three of those sessions, with the remaining twelve focusing on preparation and integration.

MAPS proved their Phase 2 results were no fluke. Due to the increased number of participants in the trial, Phase 3 was broken up into two subphases called MAPP1 and MAPP2. Each subphase took about one hundred participants through the protocol. In 2021, *Nature Medicine*, one of the world's top scientific journals, published the highly anticipated results of MAPP1: 88% of participants in the MDMA group experienced a clinically significant reduction in PTSD symptoms. Of that 88%, 67% no longer met criteria for a PTSD diagnosis.

The Strategic Focus of MAPS

In *A Manual for MDMA-Assisted Therapy in the Treatment of PTSD*, author Michael Mithoefer, a leading MAPS therapist and architect of their protocol, wrote that "important insights and healing often arise through a nonlinear process that may shift and resolve in unexpected ways."[3] A similar statement may be made about MDMA's journey through the U.S. bureaucracy since its 1985 scheduling. Perhaps it's due to MAPS's leaders' understanding of nonlinearity that they achieved what surely struck many as impossible in the Reagan era. To usher MDMA through decades of dense cultural stigma, MAPS shifted their strategy as the culture changed and focused on a bipartisan issue powerful enough to change the minds of the masses.

Rick Doblin is often lauded as the strategic mastermind behind MAPS's success. An enthusiast for all psychedelics, Doblin decided to focus on MDMA not only for its efficacy in trauma therapy, but because its effects are gentler than classic psychedelics, reducing the possibility of adverse events. Knowing statistics wouldn't sway popular opinion to the same extent as stories, Doblin led an effective strategy to concentrate MAPS's early efforts on a high-needs population that garners significant empathy from the masses: military veterans.

After returning home, countless veterans suffer far more than any legitimate standard would deem acceptable. Despite getting applauded at ball games, they frequently face crippling psychological torment after returning from deployment. Although the Department of Veterans Affairs (VA) connects them with resources, veterans' pain is often rooted deeper than those resources can reach, leaving them to live in a constant state of hypervigilance and anxiety that renders them incapable of adjusting to the patterns of contemporary culture.

I don't want to reduce MAPS's strategy to a political ploy, because their leaders care about healing. Still, Doblin and his team were wise in bringing psychedelic therapy to veterans to bridge a political divide and evoke bipartisan support. The need for better treatments for traumatized veterans is so great that the population proved themselves willing to set aside the propaganda they were fed about MDMA as a "dangerous club drug" known to "burn holes in your brain" and instead view it as a breakthrough psychiatric medication.

MAPS's strategy was so successful that they gradually expanded their participant criteria to include survivors of other forms of trauma, such as sexual assault and domestic abuse. If the FDA reschedules MDMA, as MAPS predicts it will, MDMA-assisted therapy will become available to every qualifying individual who suffers from PTSD, regardless of the condition's origin.* As important as the Johns Hopkins psilocybin studies were in reviving psychedelic research, no organization has shifted public perception on psychedelics' healing potential as significantly as the Multidisciplinary Association for Psychedelic Studies.

Psychedelics and Relationships

Although the psychedelic research and therapy I've discussed so far focuses on the individual, people have taken psychedelics outside clinical settings to connect with friends, families, and lovers since the mid1900s. Indigenous peoples have imbibed plant medicines in community for far longer. The element of

---

*   By "qualifying individual," I'm referring to the strict criteria MAPS has had to enforce to maintain safety in their study. I imagine some of these criteria will relax over time, but as it currently stands, there are several contraindicated conditions and differential diagnoses whose risk factors would prevent people from receiving MDMA treatment, even if they have treatment-resistant PTSD.

a *shared experience* is missing from individual psychedelic therapy, sacrificing many benefits in its absence.

In the 1980s, many therapists discovered that MDMA can help people deepen their intimate relationships. In her book *Good Chemistry*, psychiatrist Julie Holland recalled, "I've known since the mid1980s that MDMA is particularly suited to couples work. I have spoken to therapists who were using it before it became illegal, and the two things nearly all of them told me were that it was good for processing trauma, and it was great for couples therapy."[4]

These early MDMA therapists found the molecule's heart-opening, oxytocin-releasing effects helped couples soften rigidity, creating a fruitful container to process pressing issues without getting ensnared in *he-said-she-said* reactivity. Similarly to how it helps trauma survivors process painful memories without becoming overwhelmed, MDMA helps couples explore their personal and shared wounds while remaining connected to empathy and love.

In 2020, MAPS published the results of a pilot study on MDMA-assisted therapy for six couples in which one partner had PTSD. According to Candice Monson, the study's lead researcher, "MDMA may allow people to talk about painful experiences without experiencing the pain again. The therapist can guide couples to talk about very difficult things that they've either experienced themselves or experienced together—against the other or with the other—with a greater sense of understanding, openness, connection, and empathy."[5]

Co-therapist teams guided couples through a seven-week protocol involving fifteen sessions of cognitive-behavioral conjoint therapy (CBCT), two of which featured MDMA. In the dosing sessions, each partner took 75 mg or 100 mg of MDMA with the option of a supplemental dose after ninety minutes. According to MAPS's press release, improvements were observed in "PTSD symptoms; participant depression, sleep, emotion regulation, and trauma-related beliefs" along with "adjustment and happiness."[6] As with the PTSD study, MAPS reported no significant adverse effects.

Reflecting on Monson's study, Holland observed, "The novelty, the bonding that occurred around taking a medication that alters your consciousness, the readiness of the couple to go through an adventurous experience together—it all added to the effectiveness of the treatment."[7]

Sometimes, all that's needed is for each person's inflexibility to relax enough to witness the other's point of view, release their self-righteousness, and say, "I hear you, and it makes sense you feel that way." We humans are a stubborn bunch, and a medicine that temporarily alleviate this tendency strikes me as invaluable in terms of how we relate to each other.

Psychologists have long theorized that our relationship patterns are less guided by free will than we may think. Attachment theory, developed by British psychologist John Bowlby in the 1950s and expanded and reinterpreted by others such as Mary Ainsworth and Erik Erikson, explains relationship patterns through a developmental lens. In short, our relationship to our primary caregiver as infants and children influences, if not determines, our style of relating to intimate partners. That's why people often repeat a dynamic with a string of romantic partners: they are playing out unconscious patterns wired into their brains since childhood.

According to Bowlby, there are four primary attachment styles: anxious, avoidant, disorganized, and secure. Becoming aware of one's attachment style helps shift cyclical, conflict-drenched relational dynamics and expands the capacity to give and receive love. MDMA can provide release from an attachment pattern's ruthless grip, helping one observe their default impulses before reacting. In the resulting space, we can tend to the difficult emotions beneath the impulses instead of letting our wounds run the show.

Painful childhood memories can be extraordinarily difficult to acknowledge, for they are often shrouded in shame. MDMA can help alleviate the burden of shame by facilitating understanding and compassion. Traditional attachment theory holds that relational wounds must be healed in relationship, meaning individual therapy and journeying will fall short of doing the work with a partner or partners. Given the continued acceptance of this premise, psychedelic-assisted couples therapy could become an important modality in the future of the revival.

Trusting the Process

If psychedelic healing had a guiding mantra, it might be: *trust the process.* Rudimentary as the words seem, they serve as an effective metaphysical anchor for people voyaging through non-ordinary states. The mantra is simple enough to remember even in a far-out land of discombobulation, and it points toward equanimity with whatever's happening. A modified version of "trust the medicine" can remind someone who is fifth-dimensionally confused that as unpleasant as things feel, the psychedelic is taking them where they need to go, and they are safe to relax and surrender the impulse to maintain control.

People of Western cultures often desire straightforwardness and concrete explanations. We take medicines for specific results, swallowing antibiotics to treat infections and gulping down analgesics to ease pain. Psychedelic effects are never so straightforward, and the unpredictable directions they yank, twist, and deliver consciousness commonly inspire psychological resistance. If trusting the process is like becoming Superman, psychological resistance is kryptonite. The more fervent the resistance, the more it assumes the form of Lex Luthor thwarting Superman's noble intentions. As Superman prevails over his adversary, however, we can nullify our inner defiance by releasing attachment to linearity as a necessary healing condition.

The Inner Healer

What exactly is this "process" I keep talking about? Is it something that just happens? Or does someone or something *make* it happen?

It appears to be some of both. To help explain such a cop-out answer, the psychedelic therapy field established the concept of an *inner guide*. Psychedelics do not create this guide; it lives within us, and psychedelics invite it to the forefront. This guide has been given many names—inner healing intelligence, innate capacity to heal, and innate healing wisdom—but it's best known as the inner healer.

Because this notion can sound like New Age nonsense, therapists ground it with analogies of physical healing. When I was twenty-three, for example, I slipped off a rope swing and broke my left patella in half. It hurt a lot. The orthopedic surgeon put two rods through the half-patellae and fastened a tension band to press them together. From there, all I had to do was keep my leg straight and elevated, and after I'd watched every episode of *Lost* and eaten many Hawaiian pizzas, the halves had fused together into one bone. Now, I have a perfectly working kneecap. How amazing is that? The body's innate capacity to heal itself is an incredible phenomenon we all too often take for granted.

With the inner healer, the idea is that a similar innate mechanism heals the mental and emotional levels of our being. Since mental and emotional wounds are more abstract than broken patellae, that mechanism manifests abstractly as well. But the basic rule is the same: when we create optimal conditions to support a healing process, healing naturally unfolds.

The thing is, we tend not to create optimal conditions for our inner wounds to heal. Often, we ignore or reject these wounds via distraction, addiction, obsession, denial, or whatever else convinces us they aren't there. These defense mechanisms work better at the mental level than the physical: if you ignore a broken knee and go for a jog, your body is going to let you know that's a bad idea; if you ignore a painful memory and crack open a cold one or twelve, your mind may be fully on board.

The idea is that psychedelics invite the inner healer to the forefront. When optimal conditions such as a safe setting, a compassionate therapist, and excellent music are set to allow one's inner wisdom to guide the session, the process becomes one of *trusting what comes up* rather than forcing something to happen. Such trust allows the inner healer to work its magic on the abstract planes of suffering. In MAPS's treatment manual, Mithoefer explained that MDMA therapy "is enhanced by the participant's trust that the inner healing intelligence in conjunction with the medicine will bring forth whatever experiences are needed for healing and growth, so anything that arises is viewed as part of the healing process."[8]

In the work of Carl Jung, the libido parallels the inner healer concept. Jung's understanding of *libido* differed from that of his mentor Freud, whose sexualized conception has maintained a lasting cultural impact as evidenced by such classic films as *Austin Powers*. Jung's conceptualization of libido encompassed broader psychological energy and drive, teleologically directed toward a state of wholeness. Jung recognized an innate, unconscious intelligence aimed toward self-regulation and balance, allowing libido to flow in positive directions. Through a Jungian lens, the inner healer can be seen as libidinous energy freed from unconscious restraints, guiding the psyche toward integration of fragmented parts.

Another helpful analogy comes from biology. In 1972, Chilean biologists and neuroscientists Humberto Maturana and Francisco Varela observed a property in many living systems to maintain and renew themselves, even amid environmental strife. They called this trend *autopoiesis*, the system's natural movement toward its fullest expression. This process may be blocked, as in the case of a rooftop constructed over a budding tree,* yet the principle of autopoiesis entails that the reinstatement of proper conditions will allow an organic process of growth to resume. The same can be said for the inner healer.

Although helpful, the correlation to physical healing eventually breaks down. The physical mechanisms of my patellae fusing together, supported by the conditions of surgery, rest, and Terry O'Quinn's nuanced portrayal of John Locke, followed predictable, observable patterns. It's more difficult, if not impossible, to observe mental phenomena, and the inner healer may follow no quantifiable trajectory. Maybe your inner guide brings up a repressed traumatic memory from childhood. Maybe it connects you to your ancestors, who offer insight into your purpose. Maybe you have a vision of a jaguar approaching through the thicket as an anaconda slithers out of its mouth. Or maybe your mind remains black as night, and you feel pain in your stomach and chest that seems interminable. There's no predicting how the inner healer will express itself, and knowing this helps one trust the process.

Nonlinear Healing

Bruce Poulter is one of MAPS's core trainers for new MDMA therapists. With his co-therapist and wife Marcela Ot'alora G., he has led several phases of MAPS's research at their clinic in Boulder, Colorado. When I spoke with Poulter about MAPS's training program, he touched on how important it is for therapists to understand each client's healing process can assume limitless forms.

---

* I'm not sure who would do this or why, but I have to imagine that at some point in history, someone built a roof over a budding tree and subsequently abandoned the developmental plans meant to follow.

"You're starting at point A, you're going to get to point B, and I have no idea what the path will look like," Poulter said. "Even for people with similar trauma histories, the solutions participants come up with are absolutely unique."

A key theme to draw from his explanation is that psychedelic healing is non-linear. This makes things tricky, as Western culture more or less worships linearity.

Practice → Get better!

Wake up → Breakfast → Coffee → Crush Day!

Get job → Buy house → Start family → Midlife crisis → Red Corvette!

Westerners tend to see themselves as traveling forward through chronological time, from current place A toward destination B, and the more they plan their route, the better equipped they are for the journey. Westerners value order and structure, believing the quicker they arrive at point B, the sooner they'll get whatever they believe they currently lack. But as the great Agent Cooper says in David Lynch's *Twin Peaks*, "In the heat of the investigative pursuit, the shortest distance between two points is not necessarily a straight line."[*]

In allopathic medicine, linearity is equally prized. When we of Western orientation have ailments (point A), we see doctors to get cured (point B). We want relief, and we want it now! The same goes for mental health. We see psychiatrists and therapists seeking diagnoses and cures. We want to chart our progress along a straight line of getting better every day, or we want our dang money back!

I'm not suggesting there's anything wrong with linear thinking. It serves us in countless ways. But nonlinearity has value too, and when we stay hyper-focused on linearity, we accustom ourselves to filtering out the expansiveness of inner and outer reality. By extension, we reduce our capacity for wonder, joy, and engagement with life's possibilities.

Linear Narratives and Patterns of Nature

Psychedelic voyagers often return with memories they cannot place in a linear sequence. They lose sense of what happened in what order in a past → present → future paradigm. Such is the nonlinear nature of psychedelic journeying.

---

[*] Cooper should know, as he had a habit of getting sucked into an alternate dimension known as the "Black Lodge," each visit of which provided important clues in his obsessive attempt to find Laura Palmer's killer. If you haven't seen that show, please put down this book and watch it right away.

According to mainstream understanding of Western story structure you may recall from your high school English class, there's something suspect about nonlinearity. Valuable stories, we learn, follow a linear progression of causes and effects in a sequence of beginning → middle → end. In the shape of an arc, this sequence takes the form of rising action → climax → resolution. In screenplay structure, it's Act I → Act II → Act III.

This is usually how stories are told—especially in Hollywood, where anything experimental gets curb stomped before the money-grubbin' producer has time to light his fresh stogie. But this is not the only shape of stories. In her book *Meander, Spiral, Explode: Design and Pattern in Narrative*, Jane Alison deconstructed the "self-evident" supremacy of linear, arc-driven storytelling. She traced the arc to Aristotle, who discovered this causal sequence in numerous Greek tragedies and conceptualized it in *Poetics*. Alison suggests that while the dramatic arc fits tragedies in effectively conveying an emotional swell, it should not be applied to all narratives. Doing so limits our creativity and stifles our frameworks for engaging with and representing the world. Insofar as stories reflect our inner lives, reducing them to a linear arc restricts our inner experiences to such parameters as well.

Alison argues that stories reflect patterns found throughout microcosmic and macrocosmic nature. The dramatic arc reflects a wave in its rising and falling, and other story patterns mirror different natural phenomena:

1. Spiral: "whirlpool, hurricane, horns twisting from a ram's head"

2. Meander: "a river curving and kinking, a snake in motion, a snail's silver trail"

3. Radial/Explosion: "a splash of dripping water, petals growing from a daisy's heart, light radiating from the sun"

4. Branching: "self-replication at lesser scale, made by trees, coastlines, clouds"

5. Cellular: "repeating shapes you see in a honeycomb, foam of bubbles, cracked lake bed, or light rippling in a pool"[9]

While a psychedelic journey can follow a dramatic arc or wave, it may follow any of these patterns at different times, if not simultaneously.

When we unconsciously anticipate an arc in a psychedelic experience, we set ourselves up for disappointment. What if there's no peak? What if there's no resolution? Does that mean the journey was a failure?

If you insist on applying this structure, then perhaps so. After all, you're the one creating the meaning. But if you open your mind to other possible structures—or even the complete abandonment of structure—you equip yourself to flow with the trip and discover significance in its patterns, no matter the shape.

When we project expectations of causality onto the psychedelic journey, we are neither trusting the process nor participating in it. We are applying preconceived notions to a space whose healing power is interwoven with novelty. Within this application is a struggle for control, a fear of surrendering to something foreign to our constructs of reality. You may enter an MDMA session thinking you need to heal a specific trauma by reliving the memory (point A) and feeling the associated emotions to release its charge (point B). That could end up being valid, or your process could take you in infinite other directions, each of which could be vital to your transformation.

Maybe your trip progresses like a stone tossed into a lake as a memory ripples into awareness, leading you to feel its emanations expanding radially through your body. Maybe your experience takes the shape of a DNA strand, as a double helix of desire and fear spirals in interconnected simultaneity. Maybe one thought branches out into another, and another, until your inner healer guides you along the limbs to the trunk of the great tree of your life, and you peer into the roots of who you are. Whatever the case, openness to myriad shapes and patterns allows the inner healer to lead the way.

Nonlinear Origins of Linear Thinking

In a society whose academic institutions are run by hyperrational adherents to the scientific method, it's no surprise that a linear worldview gets indoctrinated into its people. The scientific method, impressed into the Western mind as history's ultimate approach for discovering truths about the world, is, in its rawest form, as linear as processes get: Hypothesis → Procedure → Conclusion. The end.

It's interesting to note that the origins of the scientific viewpoint, widely regarded as stemming from the Age of Enlightenment, are often traced to a man whose thinking was anything but linear: René Descartes, the French philosopher whose books, bangs, and Zappa 'stache earned him the honorific of "Father of Modern Philosophy."

In *Meditations on First Philosophy*, Descartes inquired into the nature of reality through radical skepticism. By doubting everything he could possibly doubt, Descartes aimed to unearth unquestionable truth. In his sixth meditation, he posited a fundamental certainty: *cogito, ergo sum—I think, therefore I am*. Many scholars maintain this declaration marked the beginning of the Enlightenment in its focus on objective truth and reductionism. If that's the case, then the Enlightenment began with Descartes delineating a thinking "I" from the external world, perpetuating a subject-object, internal-external, mind-body dualism that consequentially separated humans from the natural world. Descartes's separation was so fundamental, in fact, that he ascribed no moral value to animals, which he likened to machines without souls.

It's intriguing that the linear scientific method inherited from the Enlightenment would stem from Descartes's nonlinear meditations. Never mind his errors, given the meandering nature of his meditations.

If Descartes didn't convince you, here's a better example. Although many scholars trace the Enlightenment to Descartes's *Meditations on First Philosophy* in 1641, others posit the origin to be Sir Isaac Newton's 1687 science book, *Philosophiæ Naturalis Principia Mathematica*. If Newton set the stage, it would appear Enlightenment thinking did originate with linear thinking, for history remembers him as the rational scientist who came up with the fundamental laws of motion and universal gravitation still taught today.

The thing is, Newton was more complex than textbooks teach. Beneath his white wig was a mind fascinated not only with science but also what is commonly called "the occult." Read up on ole Isaac, and you'll discover he spent upwards of three decades obsessed with such subjects as alchemy and the Hermetic Qabalah, a mysterious and complicated system of esoteric inquiry.[10] The Qabalah's origins are attributed to a mythic figure named Hermes Trismegistus, whom some believe to be the alchemist sage who taught Abraham the ways of God, thereby begetting the lineages of the Abrahamic religions. Newton was obsessed with alchemy and wrote about it at length, exerting great effort to discover alchemy's ultimate goal: the philosopher's stone, an elusive elixir believed to possess powers of converting base metals into gold and imbue its wielder with immortality. Newton's English translation of the Emerald Tablet, a cryptic work of Hermes Trismegistus said to hold the key to the stone's discovery, remains one of the relic's prevailing translations to this day.

This lesser-known avenue of Newton's work proceeded through complex, nonlinear inquiry into the interrelatedness of the seen and unseen, undoubtedly prompting many spiraling journeys into the mysterious nature of reality. It's impossible to know how significantly this esoteric fascination influenced Newton's discovery of the universal laws regarded as valid half a millennium later; Newton shied away from publishing his alchemical works for fear of backlash from the academic community, which, like today's scientific establishment, refused to recognize value in such pursuits.* What we do know is that he wrote more than a million words on the subject,[11] leading economist John Maynard Keynes, who collected Newton's alchemical papers after they were auctioned in 1936, to claim Newton "looked on the whole universe and all that is in it as a riddle."[12]

"Newton was not the first of the age of reason," Keynes said. "He was the last of the magicians."[13]

Back to Psychedelics

Western minds unwittingly inherit a bias that champions linear thinking to such an all-encompassing degree they rarely recognize there are other valuable ways of perceiving the world. How ironic that the agreed-upon origins of these dogmatic models of thought came from individuals who recognized the value of nonlinearity! With such an embedded bias, it's no wonder the West defaults toward applying linear thinking to all forms of healing: if I do *this*, I will fix *this*, because A causes B, and that's a fact, Jack!

---

* Newton faced the added pressure of the Christian monarchy, which regarded such pursuits as heretical. Unlike today's secular skepticism of metaphysics, early-Enlightenment accusations of heresy had a way of riling up people's ids and sending them on murderous rampages to lynch the blasphemer and get home in time for supper.

No wonder we are so easily seduced into buying products or programs to get somewhere better than here. The product is sold as the catalyst to move us from painful present A to better future B, but that's not always how emotional and psychological healing works. Healing can be maddeningly cyclical, and psychedelics amplify this cyclicality. If you don't bear this in mind, you may get caught thinking you're back at the start because you feel depressed again when really, you're coming around to tend to new depths of pain spiraling out from the core issue. You might get caught thinking your healing is hopeless, and you may give in and slip into whatever default grooves of thought and behavior embed your suffering as inescapable reality.

Tibetan Buddhist teacher Pema Chödrön offers elegant phrasing to this notion in her book *When Things Fall Apart*. "Things don't really get solved. They come together and they fall apart. Then they come together and fall apart again . . . The healing comes from letting there be room for all this to happen: room for grief, for relief, for misery, for joy."[14]

In his final book, *Memories, Dreams, Reflections*, Jung wrote, "There is no linear evolution; there is only a circumambulation of the self. Uniform development exists, at most, at the beginning; later, everything points toward the centre." Through his recognition of the psyche's nonlinear circumambulation, Jung made sense of the strange and terrifying dreams, visions, and experiences that afflicted him following his personal, professional, and ideological split from Freud in 1913. In lieu of this insight, Jung recalled, "my inner peace returned." If you remember that healing need not be linear, you can be with yourself, wherever you are, trusting the autopoietic process.

Rick Doblin's Vision

For Doblin, the rescheduling of MDMA for therapeutic use is just the beginning of a long-term vision. "Once MDMA is a medicine, we're going to try to train 25,000 therapists in five years," he told me. "Let's say that we accomplish that, psilocybin gets approved in 2025 or 2026, and other psychedelics follow. I think we're going to have a network of psychedelic therapy clinics where therapists will be cross-trained to work with different psychedelics, and there will be five or six thousand set up in the U.S. in a decade. People's attitudes about psychedelics will change due to all the stories they'll hear about people healing from supervised therapeutic sessions."

Such lofty ambitions might mark the limits of another person's vision. Doblin is not like most people. To call him an optimist would be to understate the lengths to which his optimism reaches.

"When those clinics are set up, we will end prohibition by 2035," he continued. "People will be comfortable enough with marijuana legalization, and we'll legalize all drugs, so long as you get a license to do them. The psychedelic clinics will then become sites of initiation: if you want to get a license, you do a supervised therapeutic session, so you know what you're getting into. Then, you can buy it and do it on your own. If you misbehave while under the influence of a drug, you can lose your license to purchase that drug and have to go through another educational program."

Then came the icing on Doblin's cake: "The hope is that once we develop this legalization and culture of therapy, by 2070, we will have a spiritualized humanity—or at least a significant enough minority—and humanity can create a better world."

Tempting as it may be to pass off such claims as the musings of a quixotic dreamer, it's important to recall that Doblin is the person who started MAPS in the Just-Say-No culture of 1986 with the goal of legalizing MDMA for therapeutic treatment. Surely people passed him off then as unrealistic, but now, nearly forty years later, his impossible-sounding mission is positioned to succeed. Doblin's story proves that enough drive, practical intelligence, and perseverance can bridge an improbable dream into reality. As a fellow dreamer, I'm grateful that an individual who has accomplished such feats focused his unique prophetic telescope on such a future, especially when the present world makes it so difficult to hope that things can get better.

6

Ketamine and Connection

"And when things start to happen, don't worry. Don't
stew. Just go right along. *You'll* start happening too."

—**Dr. Seuss**, *Oh, the Places You'll Go!*

Of the compounds discussed thus far, ketamine stands out as the weird-
est. It's the only psychedelic in this book that belongs to neither the
tryptamine nor phenethylamine class of compounds, and it's the only one
that doesn't interact with serotonin.* If the classic psychedelics are the Sun
in the hallucinogenic solar system, ketamine is Pluto. And as astronomers
debate whether or not Pluto is a planet, psychedelic enthusiasts debate
whether or not ketamine belongs in the category.

A category in which ketamine definitely belongs is *dissociative anesthetics*,
a class of drugs whose effects tend to separate a user's consciousness from the
physical world. At high enough doses, ketamine can safely and consistently
knock out any living being in seconds, making it invaluable for surgery and
immediate alleviation of extreme pain. We know this because unlike other
psychedelics, ketamine is, at the time of writing, a Schedule III substance,
meaning doctors can legally administer and prescribe it. Ketamine's use in

---

* There's a unique benefit to this: ketamine is the only psychedelic unaffected by SSRIs, allowing safe consumption of both in tandem. For everything else, they have to ween off SSRIs,
which can be extraordinarily difficult and take months. Taking SSRIs alongside MDMA, on
the other hand, can lead to "serotonin syndrome," a potentially life-threatening reaction to
an overabundance of the neurotransmitter in the system. One need not worry about such a
reaction with ketamine, the molecules of which offer a friendly wave toward serotonin as they
carry on to their neurological designation.

nontherapeutic capacities is so important that it belongs to the World Health Organization's list of "Essential Medicines."

People commonly ask, "Isn't ketamine a horse tranquilizer?" I'm not sure how it earned that reputation. Sure, ketamine is powerful enough to tranquilize the mightiest stallion—heck, it's powerful enough to tranquilize John Wayne riding that stallion toward the dusty town over yonder. Veterinarians use ketamine to anesthetize a wide variety of animals because it's safe, cheap to produce, and consistent. But it was never solely a veterinary drug. Since its creation in 1962 and after its FDA approval in 1970, ketamine has also been used to anesthetize humans in various settings, one of which was the Vietnam War. With ketamine, American medics could relieve the immense pain and fear of the wounded on the battlefield, allowing quick medical treatment that spared soldiers from excruciating agony.

When ketamine is administered intravenously or via intramuscular injection, its effects take hold within minutes. At high enough doses, you can wave goodbye to consciousness. Within a lower range of "sub-anesthetic" doses, however, ketamine induces otherworldly psychedelic experiences, where the individual remains semiconscious as their observing "I" travels through an immaterial, dreamlike landscape. One's sense of the physical world dissolves, and the abstract reality they traverse often feels more fundamentally *real* than the everyday life left behind. About an hour or so later, the individual returns to their body feeling disoriented, suspended between worlds, struggling to walk, talk, and be a human until their mental and physical functionality returns over the next few hours.

It was discovered that these far-out journeys have profound antidepressive effects. Research on ketamine's therapeutic health applications continues to grow, but ketamine's future doesn't depend on FDA-approved research. Psychiatrists can prescribe it "off-label" for mental health conditions other than those for which it's been approved, such as treatment-resistant depression. Hundreds of ketamine clinics have sprung up in several nations around the world, establishing ketamine-assisted therapy as the revival's first legally accessible psychedelic treatment outside clinical trials and a sought-after mental health treatment.

Effects of Various Doses

Ketamine is administered in a variety of ways. In medical and therapeutic settings, it's typically given via intravenous, intramuscular, or subcutaneous injection. It's also administered sublingually through lozenges, troches, or oral solution, all of which require people to swish the pretty-dang-gross chemical solution in their mouths for at least fifteen minutes. In recreational settings, it's usually *insufflated*—better known as *snorted*—in powder form.

One of the go-to books on ketamine's therapeutic capacities is *The Ketamine Papers*, a collection of essays from forefront therapists and clinicians. In a gargantuan essay on ketamine therapy, seven doctors and academics led by psychiatrist Eli Kolp separated its therapeutic effects into four dose-dependent categories:

1. Empathogenic Experience

2. Out-of-Body Experience (OBE)

3. Near-Death Experience (NDE)

4. Ego-Dissolving Transcendental Experience

Empathogenic experiences are typical of low doses. People remain aware of their bodies and their sense of self as they relax into a state of euphoria. Defense mechanisms ease, allowing for the possibility of talk therapy wherein the client can access thoughts, memories, and fears typically blocked from awareness.

Out-of-Body experiences are common to medium-level doses, where people find themselves entering what appear to be different realms. Consciousness is perceived as distinct from their body, animated with otherworldly visions.

Near-Death experiences are associated with high doses. They catalyze ego dissolution and departure from one's body. People may relive their past and become aware of how their words and actions have affected others. These journeys can be blissful, terrifying, or both, depending on one's relationship to their mortality.

Lastly, Ego-Dissolving Transcendental experiences are associated with similar high-dose ranges as those of NDEs but differ in that one doesn't endure a sense of death but rather transcends concepts of space and time.

One may feel connected to something greater—i.e., the Cosmos—and sense an inherent sacredness in all things.

In the latter three categories, people usually lose their capacity to speak, making talk therapy impossible. Still, many researchers maintain that such ketamine journeys have inherent value, such as expediting one's psychospiritual growth and granting renewed meaning in life and a higher degree of responsibility for one's choices. These experiential categories can relieve individuals from the burden of limiting self-concepts, allowing them to identify with what might be deemed their "true" or "higher" self.

Applications of Ketamine-Assisted Therapy

Ketamine-assisted therapy is used for a variety of purposes. In the aforementioned essay from *The Ketamine Papers*, Kolp et al. wrote that when administered in high doses in therapeutic settings, it can treat:

- alcoholism

- opioid dependencies

- stimulant dependence

- post-traumatic stress disorder

- neurotic depression

- anxiety disorders

- phobic neurosis

- obsessive-compulsive disorder

- histrionic personality disorder[1]

Another important application of ketamine therapy is treating acute suicidality. Even with therapy, it can be nearly impossible to help someone out of a suicidal mindset. Ketamine can catalyze direct contact with novel existential possibilities, bridging the theoretical realm into the immediacy of one's emotional state and giving the therapist something new to work with—the client's experientially grounded hope of feeling happier. Even temporary immersion in a better world can remind someone straddling the edge that possibilities exist beyond the limits of their convictions, reminding them that the darkness in which they have been immersed need not author their entire story.

Ketamine disrupts the individual's default state of consciousness, which, in the throes of depression, is characterized by affliction and rumination. Such disruption allows the individual to reconsider their everyday mindset with added pliability. To quote leading ketamine educator Phil Wolfson, there is an "awakening of future prospects with the newness, flexibility, and openness of an improved experiential state."[2]

Unlike psilocybin, which has been shown to induce a sustained anti-depressive effect after a single therapeutic dose, ketamine usually requires multiple administrations. "Repeated administration, whatever the route, tends to extend the effect and gives rise to what can be termed a cumulative effect," Wolfson wrote, "and is complemented and most likely further extended by being a component part of an extended psychotherapeutic modality."[3] Ketamine can kickstart healing for people who have given up hope. For lasting transformation, however, one may have to delve deeper into the roots of their suffering than what a ketamine session or two can offer.

Regardless of the level of depression, we can all use an occasional retreat from our heavy baggage. Without taking active steps to facilitate such retreats, many of us tend to get walled up in our personally crafted fortresses of solitude. Consciously observing those walls evaporate and give way to an expansive perspective can have tremendous transformative value if we allow ourselves to relax into wherever we find our consciousness traveling.

Control and Surrender

When you take ketamine, you rapidly lose control. Many people fear taking psychedelics because they fear losing control. Control yields predictability, and predictability yields stability, while having no control yields a sense of powerlessness. Who wants to feel that?

But fear of losing control can cause problems when it becomes obsession with maintaining control. What factors underlie that obsession? What will you do when life throws some uppercuts you never saw coming?

Although often framed as an enemy, uncertainty—like nonlinearity—can enrich one's life. There's such *aliveness* in wandering outside on a sunny afternoon with no idea what or whom you'll encounter around the bend. If you've ever traveled for an extended period, you probably know the best moments happen when there's no plan. Applying predictive models can limit the future to what is comfortable and known; discomfort and unfamiliarity give rise to growth.

That's not to say compulsively maintaining control is *bad*. For some people, it's an adaptive response to trauma. Think about Sam, the retired Navy SEAL. In response to the awful experience he had as a child, he developed defensive strategies to block the memory and the emotional weight it carried. The thing is, the experience endured as a *somatic memory* stored in his nervous system. Although the traumatic episode happened in the past, the sense of having the experience—or the threat of having it again—remained present and alive. So, at a young age, he developed hypervigilant strategies requiring enormous energy to maintain rigid discipline to fight off everything that could possibly reignite the sense of powerlessness attached to the memory.

Trauma survivors often develop mental algorithms to eliminate possibilities outside their domain of influence to ensure the traumatic event never reoccurs. Staying in control allows their nervous system to remain regulated; losing it entails getting flooded with panic and helplessness in the face of something too overwhelming to withstand. For individuals stuck in this pattern, the belief that they require control to feel safe was likely true at some point in the past; however, it's often less true in the present. Even when one's circumstances have become safer, the trauma looms. Fear of uncertainty creates monsters out of the unknown, rendering tranquility all but impossible.

My friend Jason Sienknecht, a seasoned psychedelic therapist, spoke of ketamine's protective quality for people with trauma. "I had one client with complex PTSD, and in the middle of an IM ketamine-assisted psychotherapy session, she was able to reframe the trauma caused by her ex-husband, who had sexually abused their daughter many years ago. She saw this trauma as a tornado, and she was able to hold it in her hand and not get swept into it. She could then look at it from different angles, and she felt protected and centered the entire time. After this session, whenever memories of this trauma resurfaced, she no longer felt overwhelmed by feelings of anger and helplessness."

Maintaining control can be a protective mechanism, closely guarding homeostasis and rejecting anything threatening. Psychedelics disrupt homeostasis, presenting an important risk to people who resist unpredictability. If they take ketamine and realize they are losing their grip on their reality, their inner fire alarms may blare. They may want to run. They may freeze in terror. If the setting lacks support, things will get worse, and the experience may reach no resolution.

When a trauma-informed facilitator cares for clients, such terrifying experiences can become transformative. Skilled facilitators can provide the support the person needs to navigate the gauntlet of overwhelming emotions, helping them recognize that, as terrifying as things may feel, they are safe. With safety reestablished, the nervous system can relax, allowing consciousness to expand beyond the stricture of a fight/flight/freeze response. The client can recognize the terror as an amplified manifestation of a pattern that governs their control-driven life. Even if no specific insight comes, a therapist can help the journeyer restore inner calmness amid distress. If the client makes such restoration of calmness an ongoing practice, they will gradually widen the range of what they can tolerate without getting hooked by a reactive state.

Then again, you can't tell someone who directs every hypervigilant moment toward eliminating uncertainty to simply take a psychedelic and trust in the unpredictability. It's too superficial to say if they stop gripping and let go, they will release the anxiety that's defined their lives. Telling them to trust the process is instructing them to abandon their most essential defense mechanism, which has been embedded into their neurons for a very long time.

As a therapist, being client-centered entails honoring the utility of hypervigilance, understanding its origins, and patiently aiding the restoration of relaxation. Psychedelic therapists need to earn the client's trust and prepare to stick with them as fully and skillfully as possible if the client's worst fear takes hold, for if it does, the psychedelic could make it feel more monstrous than ever.

It takes extraordinary courage for trauma survivors to take a psychedelic; doing so is no less than turning toward their deepest fears in hope of finding reprieve. Facilitators must have compassion for such courage, rather than acting like "letting go" is some simple thing we all can (or even should) do. But when safety and trust are established through preparation, the client's reward for this courage could be lasting transformation.

Group Psychedelic Therapy

Because psychiatrists can prescribe ketamine for mental health treatment, it has yielded unique opportunities for innovation. One example is the emerging modality of group psychedelic therapy. In the Telesterion of ancient Greece, consciousness-altering ceremonies not only took place in groups, but the group context was essential for transformation to manifest. This has been true throughout cultural history, as the exploration of plant medicines in part IV will make clear.

Many first-wave psychedelic researchers administered psychedelics in groups. In the Marsh Chapel Experiment, preparation took place in groups of four, and on the psilocybin dosing day, the seminarians sat in the chapel together.[4] In LSD research on alcoholism, the group context of Alcoholics Anonymous was a key feature in the patients' recovery.

Two elements of Alcoholics Anonymous are widely known: the importance of recovery in groups and connecting to a "higher power." LSD was incorporated to assist in the latter. After all, Bill Wilson, the founder of the program, once sought to incorporate LSD into the program. When he took acid in 1956, Wilson found it induced the spiritual experience he believed essential for recovery.

"I am certain that the LSD experience has helped me very much," Wilson wrote. "I find myself with a heightened color perception and an appreciation of beauty almost destroyed by my years of depression . . . The sensation that the partition between 'here' and 'there' has become very thin is constantly with me."[5]

Wilson's vision of LSD-assisted Alcoholics Anonymous didn't catch on. A.A. was already established, and other leaders rejected what they deemed hypocrisy between aspiring to become substance-free and taking a substance to get there. Nevertheless, first-wave LSD research points toward LSD's safety and efficacy for treating alcohol addiction in groups.

Perhaps future leaders will take up that torch, but for now, researchers like psychiatrist Scott Shannon are exploring group ketamine therapy. Shannon was an early-1980s MDMA therapist and the clinic he cofounded in Fort Collins, Colorado, now hosts ketamine therapy groups for various patient populations.

"I believe group therapy is the future of psychedelic medicine," Shannon told me. He explained that groups lower the individual cost, which promotes increased access to treatments, and the communal context provides a sense of connection that can be difficult to find in our individualistic world.

Natalie Lyla Ginsberg, MAPS's global impact officer, has co-conducted research on group psychedelic healing processes. She's found that in populations facing cultural and intergenerational trauma,* psychedelics "can be helpful in helping you see a bigger picture perspective. It's not often that we create the appropriate containers for people to have these shared, intimate, and vulnerable experiences. Psychedelic ceremonies can create spaces where people are able to be with other people in their trauma, and that group process can trigger powerful visions, insights, and healing."

Considering how plant medicine ceremonies of numerous cultures throughout history have taken place in communities, group psychedelic therapy bears more similarity to traditional practices than individual psychedelic therapy. Can the West learn from traditional practices while simultaneously honoring the unique context of therapy? Since plant medicine ceremonies were central to many cultures, what functions could group psychedelic therapy bring the Western world? What potential healing are we eliminating by focusing on individuals?

Roots to Thrive

One clinic bridging the gap between traditional healing ceremonies and group psychedelic therapy—primarily ketamine at the time of writing—is the nonprofit Roots to Thrive. The Vancouver Island clinic's medical lead, Pam Kryskow, exuded vibrant enthusiasm for their work during our conversation. Roots to Thrive's approach isn't as simple as gathering people in a room, giving them ketamine, and letting it ride. "We started in boardrooms in the basement of the hospital on the weekend which we beautifully transformed - like yoga retreat centers," Kryskow explained. "Since then, we've been invited onto Snuneymuxw land and have the honor of running the program out of four beautiful ceremony rooms."

---

* As its name suggests, intergenerational trauma is trauma passed down through generations. For example, a traumatized veteran may develop hypervigilant coping strategies, which, left untreated, will be implicitly taught to their children. A more extreme example would be a population who survives genocide. That population faces terrible mental health challenges as a result—and surely a distaste for the oppressors—and their trauma-based coping mechanisms and perspectives are passed down the generational line.

While most Western clinics are run by doctors, nurses, and therapists, Roots to Thrive's interdisciplinary team includes spiritual care counselors, energy workers, and Indigenous Elders like Geraldine Manson of the Snuney-muxw First Nation, who share the wisdom of their lineages to broaden community members' perspectives and facilitate connections between differing worldviews.

"There's no hierarchy on our team," Kryskow said. "If I'm the one that's available and we need extra pillows, I go get the pillows. I don't defer that because I'm a medical doctor. Everybody pitches in."

The team brings a ceremonial approach to the psychedelic sessions. "Our Indigenous Elder starts it out with a clearing for the cohort," Kryskow explained. "There are intentions, prayers, photos, et cetera. After sharing, the medicine is ceremonially given."

Kryskow knows they aren't inventing a new process. She understands the ritualistic use of plant medicines in communities began way before the revival, and the one-on-one therapeutic model is a significantly more recent development reflecting the individualistic ethos of the West. Roots to Thrive's approach doesn't eschew the contemporary context, but the team recognizes that medical doctors are just one piece of a primordial healing paradigm.

"The healing happens faster because it's happening in community," Kryskow said. "I think that's fundamentally what most of us are craving: connection, love, and acceptance. That's what this group process provides." Community bonding is not restricted to the three psychedelic sessions of the twelve-week ketamine program. The team recognizes the importance of practicality in integration, and so each week, a different team member teaches a specific skill participants can apply to their lives, and participants tend to hold one another responsible for doing the work in a mutually supportive way.

Perhaps community-based models of psychedelic therapy can help the West heal the wounds of excessive isolation. Maybe they can remind us that we need not endure our struggles alone, and we can heal in connection to others facing similar obstacles.

As more psychedelics become accessible, researchers and therapists will continue incorporating them into group therapy. Groups could help people realize that their pervasive isolation is less a birthright than a culturally indoctrinated condition that betrays fundamental needs. There's value in self-sufficiency, but once the rugged individualism of the pioneers overrode the importance of community, Westward expansion manifested a destiny of inward regression. Their tracks on the Oregon Trail have faded, and the alienating echoes of their mentality ought to fade in kind.

The Illness of Isolation

In the US, the emphasis on carving your own path and making a name for yourself has left people feeling lost and alienated. If they do not ascribe to American values, they may feel they have no lifeline, for no broader system of meaning supports them. If you think about it, rugged individualism could not have been the ethos of our archaic ancestors. To try and survive in the wild on your own would have been foolish. Early *Homo sapiens* recognized the evolutionary advantage of community, where responsibilities were shared, and members worked together to ward off threats and gather necessary materials and sustenance.

Communities keep us accountable. If someone veers from the value system, the community can work together to help that individual reorient. Such supportive rehabilitation stands in stark contrast to the US penal system. Instead of promoting buy-in to a greater community, the penal system threatens the mental torture of imprisonment to keep people in line. It's a behaviorist, consequentialist model, eschewing consideration of causes apart from a generalizable "free will." This neither works—unless the unspoken goal is to fill up prisons, of course—nor does it align with contemporary models of the psyche that recognize the influence of trauma, environment, and relationships on behaviors like violence and addiction.

A helpful demonstration came through the famous Rat Park studies on drug addiction at Simon Fraser University in the 1970s. These arose in response to previous addiction research that gave morphine drips to caged rats, resulting in every rat consuming morphine until their bodies withered and their hearts stopped. The seemingly clear conclusion was that opiates were inherently addicting.

A new group of late-1970s researchers wondered, "Was the opiate inherently addicting, or was the addiction fueled by the rats' solitary confinement, which was so shitty that morphine was the only possible source of relief? Did the morphine meet a primordial need that the terrible environmental conditions obstructed?" These researchers focused on two apparatuses: one had rats in isolation, and the other arranged them in communities of fifteen to twenty. The results supported the researchers' hypothesis: while the communal rats still consumed morphine, they did so to a significantly lesser extent than the rats living in isolation. The researchers concluded addiction was less of a disease than a byproduct of "the cage you live in."[6]

The studies' influence remains strong today, when intellectual movements like critical race theory emphasize how social, political, and environmental factors influence behavior and worldview. Still, the US justice system doesn't take such factors into account. It reduces all human behavior to "personal choice," eliminating environment, trauma history, and interpersonal connection from consideration.

When we spoke, Deb Dana explained that "a traumatized nervous system gets pulled out of regulation into a survival state, gets stuck there, and can't find the way back to regulation." If disconnection is a key variable in conditions like trauma and addiction (which is often a trauma-based coping mechanism), it's intriguing to note that connection is a fundamental element of the mystical experience that the researchers at Johns Hopkins have argued to be the prime mover in psychedelic healing. The long-term smokers participating in Matt Johnson's study may not have connected directly with a community under psilocybin's influence, but they often reported connection to something beyond themselves. Ketamine seems uniquely helpful in restoring one's connection to something beyond one's ego, given its capacity to separate consciousness from the body.

I'm not surprised by conclusions demonstrating community and connection as important elements of well-being. What is surprising is that these conclusions weren't obvious from the start. Suffering in the Western world runs so deep that symptom-reducing pills like SSRIs and benzodiazepines rarely feel like enough. To heal our wounds, something must shift, and whether this manifests in one's daily habits, relationships, career path, or anything that keeps hammering down depressive brain structures, the shift must endure. Otherwise, the pseudo-transformation will prove nothing more than another quick fix.

I'm optimistic that the grip of rugged individualism is loosening. As it does, the healing value of authentic connection will move to the center of Western healing models. The kinds of connections psychedelics like ketamine can facilitate could be instrumental in speeding up this cultural shift, especially if attention is paid to the group experience.

Rites of Passage

Perhaps group psychedelic therapy could motivate this cultural shift by reawakening a broader healing process whose archetypal nature is suggested through its recurrence across cultures and time: the *rite of passage*.

Depth psychologist Bill Plotkin understands rite of passage to indicate movement from one state of being into another. A rite of passage is an initiation, often into a more integrated role in society. Without rites of passage, numerous social structures throughout history would have ceased to function. Given the importance of the Eleusinian Mysteries, for instance, I imagine Greece would not have maintained its broad influence and power for so long without their central initiatory rites.

If your history is similar to mine, your rite of passage into adulthood consisted of getting told you were an adult on your eighteenth birthday, and your initiation into the workforce involved receiving a college diploma and getting told to find a job. Predominant Western religions have rites of passage—the Jewish bar and bat mitzvah, the Catholic confirmation—but how often do you hear folks describe these experiences as deeply transformational? The descriptions I've heard usually go something like, "I did it because everyone at my school did, and I got some pretty lame presents."

These are different than, say, a teenage male consuming sacred plant medicine while community leaders conduct a traditional ritual to signify passage from one life stage to the next. Take, for instance, the *huskanaw* ritual of the Powhatan people—known also as the Virginia Algonquians of Tsenacomoco, who occupied the land surrounding what the British called Jamestown. After two days of ceremonial dancing, the *weroance*—the community leader—guided young boys, who were painted white, into remote parts of the woods to lie as if dead beside a tree. As their mothers grieved, the *kwiokos*—whom the West would regard as "the shaman"—carried the boys through a gauntlet of whips and clubs, protecting them from the blows, and laid them beside another tree. After the community feasted around the motionless boys, they were then carried into the depths of the woods to be confined, nearly naked, in a wooden cage. The boys would remain in the cages for nine months, enduring changing weather and imbibing little food or drink apart from *wysoccan*, a "mad potion" that induced vivid dysphoria, violent spasms, and horrifying hallucinations. The key ingredient of *wysoccan* was *Datura stramonium*, better known as jimsonweed, whose reputation as one of the most terrifying plant medicines in existence earned it a nickname of "devil's snare."

The *wysoccan* wiped out the boys' memories of childhood. If they returned to the village and so much as recognized a childhood friend, they were sent back to undergo the *huskanaw* again. Boys sometimes died on the second *huskanaw*, but those who emerged were "reborn" as social and military leaders in the community. Some of them became *kwiocosuk*, for *wysoccan* led them to meet the wrathful god Okee, who called them to service on the outskirts of the village.

The *huskanaw* wouldn't meet ethical standards of Western medicine. But for the Powhatan, the ritual served the higher good of the community and the land. If the goal of a rite of passage is to catalyze a shift in the initiate, many prevailing Western rites fall short, whereas the initiates in plant medicine cultures undergo a transformation of consciousness to become an adult prepared to serve the community.[7]

To enter a higher plane of development, the former self must die. This process can take countless forms, the most extreme of which brings the actual possibility of physical death, forcing the initiate to make peace with their inescapable mortality. But the primary transformational power comes through the facilitation of ego death, opening space for a new, more powerful self to be born.

Psychedelic writer and ceremonial magician Julian Vayne wrote about a wild ketamine-assisted rite in his book, *Getting Higher: The Manual of*

Psychedelic Ceremony, called the "Temple K Initiation Rite." I'm uncertain if this rite has historical precedent or if Vayne and his friends invented it, but it involves a participant voluntarily mummifying their body in black cling film, snorting ketamine, and wrapping their face in the film, leaving only a hole for breathing. The mummified individual enters the depths of a "K-hole," a dissociated emptiness void of sight and sound. When bodily control returns, they find their body constricted until the guide cuts the cling wrap, and the individual emerges as if reborn. Such death-rebirth rites are psychological corollaries of the mythical Greek phoenix, the bird that erupts into flames before resurrecting from its own ashes.

Rites of passage are ancient technologies of human development which ceremonially facilitate personal evolution. Admitting this is speculative, I'm of the belief that the preponderance of the "immature masculine" in Western society has to do with an absence of rites of passage to initiate boys into manhood.* When does that happen? At the first legal shot ordered at the dive bar? At first wallop of the wooden paddle just before the beer bong tube is jammed through the quivering lips of the teenager desperate to avoid further ridicule?† At the first successful stifling of tears?

I wonder if psychedelics could structure novel Western rites of passage geared toward the facilitation of meaning, belonging, and maturity. Perhaps a structured, therapeutic psychedelic group process could encourage sufficient intention for people to undergo psychological and spiritual rebirth, encouraging release of immature patterns through initiation into higher stages of development and service.

Michael Pollan has pointed out that in the 1960s, LSD created a unique rite of passage for the youth. "Rites of passage are typically organized by

---

*   Few examples of the immature masculine were as disturbing as that of film producer and convicted rapist Harvey Weinstein, whose bloated face seemed to encapsulate the pattern's grossest manifestations when it accompanied widespread media attention beginning in 2017.

†   A noteworthy exception to the fraternity hazing stereotype was Kenyon College, a liberal arts school whose coed fraternity "PEEPS" had been known to offer noncompulsory LSD during its initiation rituals—until 2020, when the college suspended PEEPS for three years after catching wind of such use. (Source: Ronan Elliott, "PEEPS suspended for three years following LSD distribution," Kenyon Collegian, April 3, 2020, kenyoncollegian.com/news/2020/04/peeps-suspended-for-three-years-following-lsd-distribution/.)

community elders for the adolescents to make the transition from the world of children to the world of adulthood," Pollan told me. "They go through a series of ordeals—it might be a vision quest, a hunting ritual, or a drug experience—and then they're welcomed into adult society, having passed through the gauntlet. With psychedelics in the sixties, the adults didn't organize the rite of passage. The kids did themselves, and where they ended up was not the adult world, but a place of alienation from the adult world with a desire to create a new culture, characterized by different ways of dress, different ways of speaking, different manners. I think that the rite of passage they'd been through—the acid trip—had a lot to do with it."

Huxley contemplated similar questions. *Brave New World* may be his most famous novel, but his final novel, *Island*, focuses more on rites of passage. Huxley's first psychedelic trip took place between the two books, and its influence on his hopes for civilization shows in *Island*. In contrast to the pleasure-driven dystopia of *Brave New World*, *Island* presents an imagined utopia through the fictional island of Pala. A central element of Pala's culture is a coming-of-age ritual with the "*moksha*-medicine," a psychedelic fungus that grants its users temporary clarity on "what it's like to be what in fact you are, what in fact you always have been."[8]* In case any ambiguity surrounds Huxley's point of reference, Hofmann received a letter from the author in 1962 addressing the chemist as "the original discoverer of the moksha-medicine."[9]

In Pollan's eyes, there's an indelible relationship between psychedelics and rites of passage. "I see the high-dose psychedelic trip as a rite of passage in that it's transformative," he said. "You start in one place and you end up in another. You're passing through a liminal state, where consciousness is changed, and that facilitates the growth experience that you're supposed to have." How to create conditions sufficient to facilitate group-based transformative rites in the West remains to be discovered. One controversial individual who explored the terrain, however, was Mexican psychiatrist Salvador Roquet.

---

*   In Hinduism, Jainism, Sikhism, and Buddhism, the term moksha refers to liberation from saṃsāra, the suffering-laden cycle of death and rebirth.

Salvador Roquet

According to *The Ketamine Papers*, Roquet was the first person to introduce ketamine to Western psychiatry. He brought a large supply to Baltimore's Spring Grove State Hospital in 1972, and Stan Grof recalled feeling trans-fixed as he listened to Roquet's descriptions of his patients' "fantastic voyages through a wide range of other realities—extraterrestrial civilizations and parallel universes, the astrophysical world and the micro-world, the animal, botanical, and mineral kingdoms, other countries and historical periods, and archetypal domains of various cultures."[10]

In Roquet's gonzo, *Clockwork-Orange*-esque approach, he'd gather participants in a room and administer numerous psychedelics—often a sequential com-bination of LSD, peyote, psilocybin, ketamine, and even *datura*, a powerful plant medicine known to induce destabilizing and horrifying hallucina-tions along with numerous unpleasant physical effects, of which even the most seasoned psychonauts usually steer clear. Once the effects kicked in, Roquet, played intense, evocative music while projecting images and videos of graphic violent and sexual content. Colored floodlights flashed chaotically, contributing to a sensory overload that lasted for eight hours. In the end, Roquet claimed patients emerged in a space of peace and tranquility, where they could rest in psychedelic savasana and their integration began.[11]

"The personality of each participant is reintegrated around the insights gained during the first stage of the session," Roquet reported. "The tone of the session is confrontation with ongoing problems in the individual's life situation."[12]

Grof expanded, "His intention was to induce in his clients profound experiences of ego death followed by psychological rebirth."[13] Whether Roquet's methods were justifiable or too extreme remains a controversial topic—though a scathing critique of Roquet on the podcast *Cover Story* in 2021 tilted the pendulum toward the latter. But Roquet claimed no patient was ever harmed and that 85% of the 2,000 people he treated reported positive results.

A rogue figure of Western psychedelic history, Roquet attracted respect from some and ire from others. Regarding the latter, he once hosted many Mexican doctors and therapists for dinner and spiked their food with psilo-cybin mushrooms. Unsurprisingly, they were pissed, and Roquet's esteem in the community diminished. He was arrested in Mexico in 1974, imprisoned for five months, then arrested and imprisoned again in the US in 1976. His model wouldn't fly these days, but in it we can note an exposition of rite-of-passage criteria in a Western therapeutic context, where ego death/rebirth was the goal and, according to the practitioner, the consistent result.

A Trip Outside the Walls of Therapy

Ketamine's therapeutic application has transformed its former reputation as a dangerous drug of abuse. Nevertheless, ketamine use is not limited to the therapy office, and the same applies to other psychedelics. The variety of psychedelic experiences that transpire in homes, parks, and concert venues remain a controversial subject in the revival, with some arguing use should be limited to medicinal contexts and others maintaining humans should have the freedom to change their consciousness at will. Regardless of one's position, the broad category of *"recreational psychedelic use"* requires consideration for a realistic understanding of humanity's relationship to these molecules.

II

PSYCHEDELICS IN EVERYDAY LIFE

7

Recreational Use

"Western tradition has a built-in bias against self-experimentation
with hallucinogens. One of the consequences of this is that
not enough has been written about the phenomenology of
personal experiences with the visionary hallucinogens."

—Terence McKenna, *The Archaic Revival*

There is ample evidence to suggest that humans have an instinctual desire
to change their consciousness. Throughout human history, numerous
cultures have consumed plants to alter their mental state, from Andean peoples chewing coca leaves to elevate mood to the Chinese of the Tang dynasty
imbibing opium for vitality. Even anti-psychedelic cultures of the contemporary West accept that a huge percentage of citizens consume alcohol, nicotine,
and cannabis not to mention ocean-filling quantities of coffee.

With recent research demonstrating the widespread medicinal benefits of
psychedelics, people who would never have previously considered tripping
are seeking psychedelic therapy. As helpful as this is in dismantling the negative reputation these drugs have carried since the 1960s, therapeutic use is a
drop in the river of motivations. Beneath the data and glowing media reports,
the human desire to see the world through an augmented lens remains an
innate motivation in research rooms and everywhere beyond.

Nontherapeutic psychedelic use is generally labeled "recreational." Given
the inaccessibility of psychedelic therapy due to its cost and tortoise-paced
journey to legality, I'd bet my most beloved fountain pen that in the last five

years, far more people have taken psychedelics recreationally than in the office of a therapist.

Nevertheless, when recreational use is mentioned in scientific papers, it's generally used as a point of contrast to elevate the research methods' legitimacy. In the Johns Hopkins paper on psilocybin and mystical experiences, for instance, Griffiths contrasts the "epidemic of hallucinogen abuse" of the 1960s with the study's "rigorous double-blind clinical pharmacology methods." The article's penultimate paragraph states that hallucinogen abuse is exacerbated when the drugs are "readily available illicitly."[1]

It is true that psychedelics can be abused. It's also true that alcohol, caffeine, sugar, exercise, sex, television, and online shopping can be abused. Linking availability and abuse as a self-evident principle commits a false cause fallacy. Abuse of *anything* is exacerbated when it's widely available because more people have access.

It's extremely rare for a psychedelic research paper to acknowledge even a single example of safe and responsible recreational use. Because of such exclusion, psychedelics in general are not being destigmatized nearly to the extent that medicinal use is being destigmatized. A binary exists between therapeutic and recreational results, and the psychedelic users of the latter category continue to bear the burden of indoctrinated judgments while those fortunate enough to be accepted as research participants are championed by Netflix and *Newsweek*.

Is the medical approach inherently "better" than recreational use? Or can psychedelic journeys outside the therapist's office yield transformation of proportionate power to those chronicled in the research literature? Before jumping to conclusions, let's make sure we agree on what "recreational" means.

Recreational versus Therapeutic

The term "recreational" is like the word "epic"—people misuse it all the time.* These days, "recreational" might as well be replaced with "not in a therapy office or research lab," yet it accounts for a significantly wider

---

* No, college freshman, that beer bong you just did was not epic. If you want to learn what epic means, get down from that keg, sober up, and read the *Epic of Gilgamesh*.

range of uses than psychedelic therapy. Common contexts of recreational use include concerts, music festivals, museums, watching a movie, hiking, camping, connecting with a partner or loved one, celebrating with friends, dancing the night away at a rave, grieving alone at home, meditating, jamming with the band, and exploring Joshua Tree National Park until you find the perfect tree that just *speaks* to you. These lists extend indefinitely.

Psychedelic science's tendency to contrast their models with recreational use has been an effective strategy to legitimize psychedelic medicine. To gain positive regard from the anti-psychedelic masses, therapeutic use must be presented as categorically distinct from the legacy of the hippie counterculture, thus manufacturing a scapegoat representing everything wrong with psychedelic use. Meanwhile, "upstanding" scientists clad in white can become the visual representation of how great these molecules really are.

Fortunately, Pollan didn't reinforce this hierarchical division in *How to Change Your Mind*. His psychedelic exploration began years before he had given these compounds serious consideration, when a tech guy named Bob Jesse sent him Griffiths' mystical experience paper. Pollan ultimately adopted Jesse's skepticism of the distinction between "therapeutic" and "recreational," especially as it pertains to the latter being "bad." Jesse's interest in the subject, after all, burgeoned through his psychedelic use at raves in the 1990s, which is as "recreational" as it gets.

During an interview, after Pollan had "carelessly deployed the term 'recreational use,'" Jesse called for the term's reexamination, saying, "Typically, it is used to trivialize an experience. But why? In its literal meaning, the word 'recreation' implies something decidedly nontrivial." Quick to remind Pollan that recreational doesn't mean "frivolous, careless, or lacking in intention,"[2] Jesse warned against establishing psychedelic medicalization as the primary path of incorporation into society. He was more interested in actualizing their spiritual potential than reducing them to a diagnostic paradigm.

I followed up on this discourse with Pollan. "The lines between recreation, therapy, and spiritual use are not so easily drawn," he explained. "People might go in seeking a fun experience and then have a spiritual experience. As I learned from Bob Jesse, you shouldn't dismiss a recreational experience." He added, "The word 'recreation' is about *re-creating* ourselves, making ourselves better in some way, and not just seeking thrills. I know plenty of people who have had profound experiences that they approached in a recreational way."

One problem with the recreational label is its generality. There are about as many potential uses of psychedelics as there are people in the world, and these uses vary in terms of intention, setting, and outcome. Someone could take LSD at a festival and travel through a cosmic portal opened by Jack White's savage guitar solo,* while another could take it in a congregational setting to find God. Either could prove transformational, and to claim these uses are categorically inferior to wearing eyeshades in an office beside a contemplative therapist strikes me as a pompous, infantilizing ethical leap.

When determining a setting for psychedelic healing, one must ask at least two questions: What external influences help catalyze transformation, and what container will allow the journey's full, uninterrupted expression? When the answers are restricted to "therapy office," an extraordinary number of possibilities are extinguished.

One reason the therapeutic/recreational binary exists is that the breadth of recreational uses bring a breadth of risks. A great thing about psychedelic therapy is the degree of control it provides. It essentially closes out the world, curating a narrow range of stimuli conducive to "going inside." For many, this is essential, because their trip may be so emotionally intense that a crowd of strangers appears more like a horde of demons who definitely know they're high. It's all but impossible to predict if freaky visions will enter the scene, and when they do, it's already too late to turn back.

Psychedelic therapists create and hold space for the journeyer to lean into heavy emotions. They provide support when needed, reassure clients of their safety, and help them surrender to whatever is happening. If emotional emergence is stifled through lack of safety in the setting, the emotion may get "stuck" in some unresolved limbo, leaving the individual to feel as if the reel of a blood-pumping action movie cut off before the climax. Psychedelic therapy aims to reset the reel for a satisfying conclusion.

---

* Speaking from personal experience, this is an incredible way to tap into LSD's boons.

Another reliable thing about the therapeutic model is that psychiatrists and nurses can screen for contraindicated conditions—and there are many. All psychedelics are currently contraindicated with schizophrenia, for they can worsen symptoms like visual and auditory hallucinations. Less well known is that some psychedelics, like MDMA and ketamine, are contraindicated with hypertension because they raise blood pressure. At a clinic, vitals can be assessed and monitored, and requisite medicines are available in case of an emergency.

Helpful as psychedelic therapy is, researchers aren't keen on acknowledging its limitations. What if someone has an emotional breakthrough on MDMA and is overcome with a somatic demand to express it through dance? They may find the therapy office stifling. Perhaps they'd benefit more from grooving beside a flame-shooting mechanical octopus blasting electronic beats at Burning Man, where they can ecstatically release their emotional shackles through a spontaneous flow of energy.*

As the Western world investigates the healing potential of these substances, perhaps therapy shouldn't monopolize the space of possibility. Yet if one elects to take psychedelics outside the therapy office, they should inform themselves about the risks.

Music festivals, for instance, are home to a constant barrage of unpredictable stimuli. If you take a psychedelic, who's to say whether the music will jive with you? Who's to say the dreadlocked drifter beside you won't aggressively ask you for DMT as your ego dies? A bad trip—or "challenging experience," as some call it—is significantly more likely out in the wild than a comfortable office with therapeutic support.

Often, all one needs to navigate a challenging trip is the presence of a friend. It's ill-advised to take psychedelics with people you don't trust, like the sketchy crew who offered you "Molly" and and exclaimed, "It's good stuff! Trust us!" with eyeballs bulging. Even the staunchest defenders of recreational use encourage people to take steps that eliminate common pitfalls.

---

* In case you're wondering, there is indeed a flame-shooting, music-blasting mechanical octopus vehicle known to roam the Nevada desert during Burning Man. It's called El Pulpo Magnifico, and I believe it legitimately deserves the adjective of *epic*.

Harm Reduction

There's an industry built on promoting safe drug experiences called "harm reduction." Harm reduction comprises a "range of health and social services and practices that apply to illicit and licit drugs."[3] Such services, summarized on the Harm Reduction International website, include "drug consumption rooms, needle and syringe programmes, non-abstinence-based housing and employment initiatives, drug checking, overdose prevention and reversal, psychosocial support, and the provision of information on safer drug use."[4]

I'll start with drug checking. You want to be as informed as possible about what you're taking, because plenty of street drugs are riddled with contaminants, the most notorious of which is the opioid Fentanyl. Fentanyl has been found in many drug types sold illicitly, including ketamine and MDMA. It's extremely powerful at microscopic doses, cheap to produce, and highly addictive, making it a popular additive for those who manufacture and distribute drugs with no care whatsoever about human life.* Fentanyl dramatically increases the possibility of a fatal overdose. Unless you're in cahoots with the chemist, you never *really* know exactly what you're getting when you buy illegal drugs, as the substance could have gotten contaminated by any hand it touched en route to your expensive little baggie.

Harm reduction organizations provide resources for drug testing to help prevent accidental overdoses. While the technology is imperfect, there are affordable, reliable, and simple kits that clarify if harmful contaminants like Fentanyl are present and whether the "Molly" you bought is clean MDMA or some sketchy concoction. Anyone can legally purchase these kits online.

There's a big push from nonprofit organizations like DanceSafe, a harm reduction leader, to make drug testing more accessible, especially at festivals and raves where drug use is as common as neon glowsticks. Unfortunately,

---

* This does not apply to all drug dealers and manufacturers. Some LSD manufacturers, for instance, have been known to focus on positive intentions in their synthesis, praying over a batch that it may help people awaken to their full potential. But manufacturers and dealers who sprinkle Fentanyl into their supply to get people hooked and make more money, unconcerned with how many customers fatally overdose, are the kind of morally bankrupt pricks who give drugs a bad name. (Source: Joe Moore, "William Leonard Pickard – LSD, Fentanyl, Prison, and the Greatest Gift of All: The Natural Mind," April 19, 2022, in Psychedelics Today, podcast, MP3 audio, 1:34:57, psychedelicstoday.com/2022/04/19/william-leonard-pickard/.)

the US legal system makes this difficult. Cover your eyes and ears, fans of President Biden, if you don't want to learn about his responsibility for the law that most directly obstructs harm reduction in places where drug use is commonplace: the Illicit Drug Anti-Proliferation Act of 2003, then-Senator Biden's revision of 2002's "RAVE Act." The clever acronym stands for Reducing Americans' Vulnerability to Ecstasy—although the "R" might more accurately stand for "Raising."

After it was passed, the act created a widespread fear that blocked festival and rave organizers from providing medical and harm-reduction-oriented infrastructures at events. DanceSafe's long-standing executive director, Mitchell Gomez, told me, "It was basically designed as an expansion to the Federal 'crack house' laws "which said, 'If you own a building, and the primary purpose of that building is drug use, you can be held liable for that drug use even if you were not directly involved in the drug trade on the property.'" After a few DEA attempts to charge electronic music promoters under the "crack house" laws failed because the promoters didn't own the buildings, the RAVE act came to the Senate floor.

"It was partly pitched as a social justice expansion of the 'crack house' laws," Gomez explained. "The idea that poor African Americans who owned these buildings were being charged while rich white kids throwing raves couldn't be charged struck people as unfair. My solution would have been to get rid these terrible laws that were almost universally very poorly written. But that's how it was."

The act spread fear through the electronic music community. According to Gomez, that fear endures like a "goblin hiding in the shadows." Event organizers are concerned that services like drug-testing booths could be interpreted as breaches of the law and summon Uncle Sam's wrath. Gomez has even had venues block DanceSafe from giving out free water and providing "chill-out areas" for people to rest, claiming such services could be considered evidence of support for MDMA use.

"Weirdly, there have not been any successful prosecutions," Gomez added. "There's been very few charges under the RAVE Act—and all were part of larger investigations around larger drug issues." He believes the act has become a "convenient excuse" for organizers to make more money, such as charging for water instead of paying for harm reduction services. Regardless, Gomez recognizes it as "a law that basically allows people to have a cover for why they aren't allowing harm reduction services." For this inconvenient Federal promotion of danger, the nation can join the chorus crying, "Thanks, Biden!"

The Zendo Project

While DanceSafe focuses on all drugs, other harm reduction organizations focus specifically on psychedelics. The most prominent is the Zendo Project. Zendo was founded at Burning Man in 2012, and it has maintained close associations with MAPS ever since. Its founders were avid festivalgoers who recognized that a lot of people take psychedelics in such settings. Given the overwhelming stimulation of festivals, it's common for tripping attendees to wind up freaked out, especially if they weren't prepared, took more than intended, or took something different than what they believed they were taking.

What does one do in such a situation? What if they've been abandoned by their crew? What if their attempted calls for help are strangled by an unnamable force reaching through the ether and shredding the fabric of reality beneath their sparkling shoes?

Zendo was created to meet these needs. At festivals, volunteers construct safe, serene tents styled to simulate Japanese meditation halls. At individual stations decked out with mattresses, blankets, cushions, stuffed animals, and other comfortable accoutrements, trained "sitters" support "guests" having a rough time. Basic necessities like water and food are available, and anyone can come at any time and stay as long as they need. Zendo's organizers maintain close ties with festivals' medical staff and escort guests to their facilities if necessary. Often, that's unnecessary, for someone convinced they're dying from LSD may benefit more from psychological support than a sedative.

Zendo teaches that challenging trips can become transformative. The theory, mirroring that of psychedelic therapy, holds that challenges express elements of the guests' inner landscape that influence their lives more than they realize. Sitters are trained not to interpret a guest's expressed experience or "fix" them by offering solutions; rather, the sitter, like a therapist, helps the guest feel safe and comfortable enough for their inner healer to guide their process. Volunteers meet guests *where they are*, no matter how far out that may be. If a guest is convinced the entire festival is a vast, nefarious conspiracy against them, the volunteer doesn't respond, "That's dumb. *Of course* that's not happening!" Such a response would likely convince the guest the sitter is *in on it*. Instead, the sitter could respond, "That sounds really scary," encouraging the guest to elaborate and respecting their perspective as valid and non-pathological.

Zendo Project is a great starting place for those seeking an entry point into psychedelic healing. It was my personal gateway: volunteering at Burning Man in 2018 was the first time I encountered people whose job title was "psychedelic therapist." I volunteered again at Burning Man in 2022, and during an 11:30 pm to 5:30 am shift, I sat with a guest who'd been having a harrowing experience every moment of their four days in the desert. They'd recently been discharged from the military after more than a decade of service, and the preponderance of pyrotechnics and large vehicles at the event triggered them into a hypervigilant state. They'd taken MDMA the evening of my shift, and in the Zendo tent, they lay comfortably beneath a blanket and eyeshades as they processed how certain art installations had evoked memories of military training and combat. When tears came, they cried; when joy sprang, they laughed. I did very little apart from validating their experience, encouraging their reflections, and making sure they felt comfortable. It's a beautiful position to get to hold for another person.

The principles Zendo teaches can be applied to all psychedelic experiences. Everyone has the capacity to offer their supportive presence to another. Curating safe and comfortable spaces goes far in enhancing positive outcomes for all sorts of trips. As we fumble through in the nuanced challenges of integrating psychedelic healing into society, the Zendo Project reminds us that the heart of psychedelic healing is genuine care for our fellow humans.

Psychedelic Education and Reframing Propaganda

DanceSafe, Zendo Project, and other harm reduction organizations also focus on educating the public about psychedelics. Their leaders understand that due to the enduring impact of the War on Drugs, the public's perception is often informed more by anti-psychedelic propaganda than fact.

Take, for example, the widespread story that MDMA "burns holes in your brain." I recall several friends during the late 2000s telling me this was an undeniable scientific fact. I can't blame them, because that's exactly how the media presented this myth, but it turns out the hole-in-the-brain thing took hold thanks in large part to Oprah Winfrey. In 2001, on her massively popular show, Winfrey compared images of brain scans of Lynn Smith, who had used ecstasy and many other drugs, with brain scans of a "normal" patient. Smith's brain appeared to have big holes in it. Conclusion? Ecstasy burns brain holes. Winfrey and her scientist guest spoke, and millions of people believed them.

Eventually, the assertion was debunked. The "holes" were parts of Smith's brain showing reduced blood flow. There was no way to tie the reduction specifically to ecstasy, and the shift in cerebral blood flow was not abnormal in the ways Winfrey's "experts" claimed. While MDMA does affect cerebral blood flow during the experience and for a few weeks after, researchers have not found evidence it causes lasting brain damage.[*] One person, however, refused to accept this possibility.

In 2002, *Science* magazine, a top-of-the-hierarchy academic journal, published an article by neurologist George Ricaurte on "severe dopaminergic neurotoxicity" in primates to whom researchers had administered MDMA. Ricaurte concluded that a single recreational dose of MDMA obliterates neurons linked with the neurotransmitter dopamine, and by extension, a single dose could catalyze development of disorders related to dopamine dysfunction, like Parkinson's disease. Here it was, in the fine print of trustworthy *Science* magazine: if you take ecstasy, you will probably get Parkinson's.

It turns out Ricaurte was full of hogwash—so much so, in fact, that his article was *retracted*. As reported in a 2003 *Wired News* article by Kristen Philipkoski, "The Sept. 27, 2002 study warned that even one typical recreational dose of MDMA could cause severe brain damage. Scientists around the country applauded the study and warned young people not to experiment with ecstasy. Now Ricaurte says it was a case of mixed-up bottles."[5]

---

[*]   That's not to say it's necessarily safe to take MDMA frequently for years. Frequent use of any powerful drug for prolonged periods will affect the brain. There's a colossal difference, though, between an infrequent MDMA user—such as someone who takes it three times in a therapeutic protocol—and someone who takes it every week.

That's right. In 2003, when Ricaurte failed to replicate the results, it came to light that he'd "mistakenly" administered *methamphetamine* to the primates due to mislabeled containers. Was this an innocent accident for Ricaurte, a qualified Johns Hopkins Medical School employee? Or did Ricaurte's position as a "longtime opponent of Ecstasy"[6] have something to do with the coincidence that his article was published as MAPS's research proposal was finally nearing FDA approval, effectively stalling Doblin's efforts?

Philipkoski wrote that even after the redaction, Ricaurte doubled down on his claims, arguing his incompetence didn't invalidate his other studies showing MDMA was bad. She quoted Doblin, "This [retraction] shows that Ricaurte is completely overzealous in trying to promote the harmful effects of MDMA, and he has ignored evidence to the contrary."[7] Fortunately, history has proved Ricaurte to be the buffoon, for MAPS's data have been so strong, consistent, and respected by the scientific community that you would have to completely disregard the validity of the scientific method to deny MDMA's medicinal potential altogether.

These are but a few of many examples of false psychedelic narratives presented as "scientific fact." Other examples include the late 1960s myth that LSD permanently scrambles a user's chromosomes, that LSD gets stored in the spinal fluid, that MDMA drains spinal fluid, and that a single dose of a psychedelic will make you permanently insane. Thanks in large part to the educational efforts of harm reduction organizations, the truth behind these propaganda-fueled lies is increasingly known, and we can hop aboard the reality train to conduct some real research.

Recreational Healing in Relationships

The distinction between recreational and therapeutic use doesn't mean the latter cannot apply to the former. One common recreational reason to take psychedelics is to connect with friends and loved ones on a deep level.

My friends Shannon Hughes and Rob Colbert, a powerhouse couple of psychedelic therapists, educators, and researchers, coauthored the qualitative study "Evenings with Molly: Adult Couples' Use of MDMA for Relationship Enhancement." The eight couples they interviewed represented a "hidden demographic of MDMA users who find benefit in self-managed recreational use in the privacy of their own homes." Taking MDMA in intentional sets, settings, and shifts in habitual routines, the couples noted improvements in "communication, intimate bonding, and providing a relationship 'tune up,' among other durable positive changes."[8]

Throughout the article, Hughes and Colbert questioned the primacy of therapeutic models, writing, "Adults in this study suggested their use represented an exchange between two people in a healthy relationship, which stands in contrast to how the psychotherapeutic-medical model assumes a diagnosed patient needing supervised care for treatment of mental and emotional distress." In contrast to stigmas suggesting drug use is inherently "escapist," the authors added, "The commitment of the relationship and maturity of intention that participants reported reflect critical differences of their use compared to that typically represented in the literature for deviant, illicit, or recreational users."[9]

Helpful as they can be, psychedelics won't cure all relationship woes. Colbert told me, "MDMA never fixed any relationship, period. But I have seen it open people's hearts to reveal their true self, which allowed them to share that true self with others and in turn allowed them to receive love from those who love them for who they are."

How many people use psychedelics to enhance their relationships? One can only imagine, and as the revival continues shifting cultural perception of psychedelics, that number will continue to grow. But psychedelics need not only be used to help partners heal their afflictions. They can also help loving relationships deepen, empowering the relationship's enduring foundation.

Mushrooms in the Sacred Grove

My friends Remy and Eliza call the Great Plains home. Though they'd lived within sixty miles of each other for most of their lives, they didn't meet until Eliza was forty and Remy was forty-nine. After three dates, they'd recognized something wonderful between them, and Remy followed his intuition to invite Eliza to his spacious prairie property to take psilocybin mushrooms together.

Remy's first mushroom experience took place during COVID lockdown a few months before connecting with Eliza. Mushrooms had intrigued Eliza for decades, but it wasn't until Remy's invitation that she decided to "take a leap of faith with this man that I was falling in love with."

On a beautiful summer afternoon, they each imbibed two grams of dried mushrooms, took a blanket and some fruit down to a serene grove, and sat.

Eliza noticed effects within ten minutes of imbibing. She felt like she was falling through a bottomless abyss, but "these tiny moments would be absolutely erased, and I would be back in this light."

As they recounted the afternoon, vivid memories offered entry points into the broader story. "The grasses and the trees were waving in the wind to an invisible orchestra conductor, as if they were in concert with the heavens," Eliza shared. "We all seemed to be a part of it. It was one of the most beautiful experiences I've ever been a part of."

Remy's dose took longer to kick in, but as soon as it did, he told Eliza what he'd known to be true. "I told Eliza I loved her. It felt like the important thing. I verbalized it so comically fast after a lifetime of being the guy who forever can't make sense of it."

Eliza received the words, but she wasn't ready to repeat them, especially under the influence of psilocybin. Remy respected her boundary and told her he'd wait for her. "If we're looking at the mushroom experience as a microcosm of one's life," Eliza said, "then I've had to do a lot of work accepting exactly who I am. You have to love yourself before you're able to love someone else."

Eliza shared a significant moment of self-love. "I remember looking down at my thigh and exclaiming, 'My thighs aren't fat!' It sounds comical, and it kind of was, but I'd shared with Remy early on that I had struggled with an eating disorder for fifteen years. In that moment, it felt like I had done five years of intense therapy in one go. I could look at myself for who I was, this beautiful creature that didn't have to hate herself anymore."

As he observed her, Remy saw Eliza's face become very old. "It wasn't a cliched, *this-is-an-old-and-beautiful-person* thing. She was *really* old," he laughed. "But she was this old person that I loved."

In one of those inexplicable synchronicities psychedelics induce, Eliza simultaneously saw Remy as an old man. Initially finding it terrifying, she struggled to look at him, but she realized her fear had nothing to do with

Remy's appearance itself. "I was looking death in the face, or my partner's death, or the potential of staying with someone long enough to witness that," she said. "It was me being able to see him to the end, which is a gorgeous way of seeing someone you're falling in love with."

The meeting of death and compassion accompanied Eliza's inward turn. "I had a moment where I wept for my mother," she shared. "She lost her parents when she was very young in a terrible accident, and she held her mother as she died. The calcification of feelings I had toward her was gone. I saw her as a young woman, as a child, and I felt little separation from her."

Remy's experience didn't traverse as many fears and memories. It centered on the depth of love he felt for Eliza, which he'd never known possible through his many journeys across the globe. "I didn't realize the kind of love you hear about in love songs was real, but I saw that love was possible in a non-clichéd way.

"I'm an open-hearted person," he continued, "but I had tamped it down when I was young. I wanted to be bigger than my neighborhood and grow into someone extraordinary, and love felt like a sacrifice I didn't want to make. I had never fully released that until that afternoon, when I returned to the open-hearted person I always was."

Remy and Eliza named the setting of their fourth date the "Sacred Grove," and in the months following their journey, the grove's significance grew. "I asked her to marry me in that spot, before dawn," Remy recalled. "We got married there a year after our first date."

With a reminiscent smile, Eliza added, "We sit on our deck and look at it all the time. I don't think of it as the mushroom place. I think, 'This is the holy place.'"

Two years later, their love remains strong, although the natural challenges of maintaining an intimate relationship still arise. They noted how helpful it was to revisit their experience. "Talking about it is a way of reviving and celebrating it," Remy reflected. "It's a good exercise to recall it and realize that we're above our temporary challenges. It's good to remember that the windshield can be cleaned, and the gravitas of a bad morning need not define you. You can remember that you saw eternity."

Eliza agreed, though she noted that as much as she can access the feelings, she longs to return to that afternoon. "It felt like where I'd always want to be—open-hearted and receptive to the beauty of the world, ourselves, and the connection that had started between us. There was such clarity of mind. I was able to see without the scrim of the everyday life in front of my eyes."

"It's one thing to go through certain kinds of therapy," Remy said. "It's another thing to have the universe opened up."

Eliza added, "You can *talk talk talk*, get to the core of things, and have emotional breakthroughs, but seeing how beautiful things *really are* roots it in your cells. I hope I get to see that day again, in some way."

A Personal Connection

Listening to Eliza and Remy, I was struck with how vibrant the images and their corresponding emotions remained two years later. Images and emotions are excellent ways to connect to psychedelic journeys, even when the magic feels distant. Remy and Eliza's ability to reconnect to those emotions amid challenges shows that contents of psychedelic journeys are accessible when we take intentional time to tell our stories.

When Eliza and Remy shared their visions of one another as elderly, I was transported to a similar vision I had with my wife after our first year of dating. We had each taken 100 micrograms of LSD in a cabin in the mountains, and in the depths of the snowy night, we walked in robes to a natural hot spring tucked away in the woods. The warm, sulfur-scented water nourished our bodies and hearts as we listened to the silence, gazing at the shadowed outlines of the surrounding peaks. I looked at her, and as she gazed in awe at Orion smiling down from the clear night sky, I noticed the moonlight illuminating the thin wrinkles around her eyes. I saw her as an old woman, and I sensed I was peering into our distant future. I realized I loved her more profoundly than I had ever loved anyone.

In that vision, her beauty appeared ageless. I pictured her sitting on a rocking chair as an old woman, gazing at the splendor outside the frosty window of our future home, and I knew in my heart's core that this love could endure through any hardship, as long as we continued to nurture its flames.

As I recall that moment, a sense of peace and gratitude warms my solar plexus. In the depths of hardship, I can return to that hot spring and reconnect to feelings that mean far more than any doubt or fear. Two years later, it's not easy, but its possibility remains a beautiful gift I received that night from LSD.

Take Care, Take Care, Take Care

If you choose to take psychedelics recreationally, it's helpful to be as informed as possible about the substance you're consuming, the associated risks, and the preparations you can make to promote a smooth excursion into the unknown. Ignoring risks doesn't make them go away. Although the Drug War's myths may be silly, psychedelics', potential to cause harm must not be underestimated.

With proper safeguards, recreational use can give rise to transformations on par with those reported in psychedelic research. But perhaps transformation need not be the ultimate standard for "right use." Maybe psychedelics simply create the conditions for an unforgettable experience of connection with friends, nature, or oneself. You're not necessarily healed afterward, but you'll always look back on the love, laughter, and equanimity with a fond smile. We shouldn't underestimate the value of such experiences. When the Grim Reaper eventually comes a-knocking, perhaps we will realize these were the moments that mattered most.

8

Microdosing

"He who binds to himself a joy
Does the winged life destroy
He who kisses the joy as it flies
Lives in eternity's sunrise."

—William Blake, "Eternity"

The phenomenon of microdosing currently wears the crown of hippest, coolest, and most talked-about recreational psychedelic use. Microdosing is the practice of taking a very small quantity of a psychedelic—usually LSD or psilocybin—on a recurring schedule to improve one's life. By "very small quantity," I mean 5 to 10% of a therapeutic dose.* It's not enough to trip, but according to thousands of people, it's enough to experience significant benefits.

The popularity of microdosing grew in large part due to podcasts. Around 2015, several hosts of popular shows in the biohacking/optimization realm started talking about discovering cognitive, physiological, and emotional benefits from taking very small doses of LSD and mushrooms. This trend started just as the psychedelic therapy wave was gaining momentum, and soon enough, citizens of many nations were hopping aboard the microdosing train, exuberantly proselytizing the benefits of the ride.

---

* For LSD, it's 8-12 micrograms. For dried psilocybin mushrooms, it's about 100-400 milligrams. Since various species of mushrooms vary significantly in potency, however, it's impossible to standardize a measurement across all fungi.

Podcasts, however, were not the prime movers. A particular individual laid the groundwork for microdosing, and his name has become all but synonymous with the practice. The go-to expert on the subject is long-standing psychedelic researcher, writer, and jovial free thinker Jim Fadiman.

The Psychedelic Explorer's Guidance

When people mention Jim Fadiman, they tend to smile. During our ninety-minute conversation, I realized why. Unlike many psychedelic leaders these days, Fadiman never appears to take things too seriously. Of the people I interviewed, no one expressed the carefree spirit of the psychedelic "good old days" as much as Fadiman.

Although he's technically a scientist, Fadiman doesn't lean on scientific terminology. When I asked him to explain how microdosing differs from tripping, he said, "The flowers might be a little brighter, but they don't smile at you and turn into queens of Ancient Egypt. You don't have great breakthroughs, and you don't have giant anacondas that eat you."

Fadiman's introduction to microdosing came through a psychedelic researcher friend, Robert Forte, who'd recommended Fadiman take a tiny dose of LSD to help him break through his writer's block. Fadiman followed the suggestion, and *presto!* Writer's block eliminated!

Fadiman wrote about the potential of these "sub-threshold doses" in his 2011 book, *The Psychedelic Explorer's Guide*, and the phenomenon erupted in 2015 when he appeared on *The Tim Ferriss Show* podcast and discussed microdosing at great length in his soothing, affable manner. The same year, a *Rolling Stone* article described the popularity of microdosing among tech workers in Silicon Valley, suggesting that small doses of LSD could enhance creative problem-solving.[1] Two years later, novelist and essayist Ayelet Waldman published a splash-generating memoir called *A Really Good Day: How Microdosing Made a Mega Difference in My Mood, My Marriage, and My Life*, chronicling her month-long experiment of taking small amounts of LSD to heal her "mood storms," which no therapy or medication had helped. Neither the article nor Waldman's book would have happened without Fadiman.

At the time of writing, microdosers typically follow one of two protocols. The first came from Fadiman, and the second from Paul Stamets, the go-to expert on all things fungi whose tremendous popularity may have earned him the distinction of becoming history's first "celebrity mycologist." Fadiman's was originally a research protocol, and Stamets based his on his own experience.

Fadiman's protocol goes as follows:

Day 1: Microdose

Day 2: Off

Day 3: Off

Day 4: Microdose

Day 5: Off

Day 6: Off

Day 7: Off

Then there's the Stamets approach:

Days 1- 4: Microdose

Days 5 - 7: Off

Stamets' protocol is better know as "The Stamets Stack," because he recommends combining the microdose of psilocybin—which he focuses on over LSD—with lion's mane mushrooms and niacin. Lion's mane has been proved to enhance brain functionality and connectivity, and niacin flushes the body by increasing vasodilation. According to Stamets, these three ingredients produce a synergistic effect that maximizes cognitive benefits.[*]

---

[*] If you take niacin, be warned: you will become itchy, hot, and very red. I learned the hard way that it's a bad idea to take niacin before a public speaking engagement.

LSD or Psilocybin?

LSD and psilocybin are the most commonly microdosed substances, but they are not interchangeable, even at such minuscule doses. Each appears to bring unique benefits and drawbacks.

Fadiman shared what he'd gathered from listening to hundreds of micro-dosers' stories. "Psilocybin is generally considered more emotionally warm. LSD is considered colder and more analytic. If you're microdosing because of social anxiety, psilocybin would be more appropriate. If you're microdosing to improve your grade in organic chemistry, LSD would probably be better. I don't have data for that. I just have a lot of people who talk that way."

Fadiman's distinction resonates with me. I've found psilocybin micro-doses calm my nervous system, allowing me to be more present and heart-centered. I've also found psilocybin deepens meditation, as if the small doses create a portal into a liminal inner space conducive to insight. It seems meditation potentiates the small dose as well, offering the option of entering a deeper psychedelic state.

In contrast, I've found LSD microdoses increase my energy. I'm more enlivened in my body and more physically active. I feel more confident and laugh more frequently. Sometimes my focus increases; other times, I struggle to concentrate. LSD microdoses encourage a mindset of exploration, helping me see the mundane through eyes of creative possibility and joy. To borrow from Waldman's memoir, in my experience, LSD microdoses consistently induce a really good day.

Microdosing Science, The Young Whippersnapper

If anecdotal reports are valid, the massive range of microdosing benefits includes alleviation of anxiety and depression, increased focus, interruption of addictive patterns, reduced stress, improved relationships, hormonal reg-ulation, mood stabilization, enhanced creativity, and discovery of greater purpose in life. People also claim it induces neuroplasticity, allowing brains to rewire with more optimal neural patterns.[*]

---

[*]   As sci-fi as this may sound, there are no chips or devices involved. Neuroplasticity is simply a sciencey term for a brain state that makes it easier to change how you think, behave, and feel.

It all sounds nice, eh? The thing is, scientific studies on microdosing, while continuing to emerge, are in their infancy. For those who regard science as the holy grail of validity, microdosing is no more valid than the latest influencer's "cure" for everything challenging about life.

A primary question microdosing science has thus far attempted to answer concerns the placebo effect. Are the purported benefits of microdosing legitimate, or do they demonstrate people's ability to trick themselves into getting better because they already believe this groovy new practice will help?

One 2021 study out of Imperial College London[2] concluded the benefits of microdosing may indeed stem from a placebo effect. Microdosing enthusiasts ripped on the study, pointing to its flaws—most, if not all, of which the authors acknowledged in the paper. The primary drawback was that steep regulatory and financial hurdles made a rigorous lab-based study untenable, leading the researchers to take a clever "citizen science" approach. They created a "self-blinding" protocol for participants—most of whom had microdosed before—to implement themselves. The procedure involved small plastic bags, pill capsules, and QR codes to allow the researchers to track whether participants imbibed placebos or microdoses. On "dosing days," participants completed a series of mental health questionnaires and brain-games and guessed whether they were on a placebo or a microdose.

Balázs Szigeti, the study's lead researcher, spoke with me about the results. "According to our study, the positive effects reported on microdosing can be reproduced by these 'deceptive placebos' we used. What that argues to me is that the benefits are real, but the mechanism behind those benefits is not related to the pharmacological activity of the microdosing itself. Rather, psychological expectation effects are sufficient to explain it, because we see the same sort of changes in the placebo group as in the microdosing group."

After Szigeti's article, more microdosing studies were published. The most noteworthy were attached to Stamets. Given his belovedness in the psychedelic stratosphere, Stamets leveraged his influence to attract thousands of regular microdosers to fill out daily questionnaires on his team's app, "Quantified Citizen." By 2022, the data had yielded two publications. The first tracked over 4,000 anonymous microdosers and over 4,000 non-microdosing comparators, concluding, "Among individuals reporting mental health concerns, microdosers exhibited lower levels of depression, anxiety, and stress across gender."[3] The second publication narrowed the scope to 953 psilocybin microdosers and over the course of thirty days found "small- to medium-sized improvements in mood and mental health" and "improvements in psychomotor performance that were specific to older adults."[4] Although both were published in the esteemed journal *Nature*, the data didn't eliminate the placebo question, as participants microdosed on their own volition with no placebo control.

Microdosing provides an example of a mental health trend whose enthusiasts don't care about scientific validation. People aren't waiting to microdose until rigorous research proves its efficacy; in fact, much of the science appears to be aiming to prove what people already think. As the mixed reception of Szigeti's results demonstrated, people will continue to believe in the power of microdosing regardless of the conclusions science draws.

Reconsidering the Placebo Effect

Psychedelics have a way of shaking up established structures, including those whose validity seems self-evident. One such structure is science's unquestioned reliance on placebo control.

Placebo control has such a stronghold as the gold standard of drug research that until Szigeti told me it was established in the 1950s, I'd never considered its historicity. "Placebo controls and the recognition of the power of the placebo effect are relatively recent developments," he said. "Initially, placebo was looked at as a threshold of baseline efficacy. Then, people realized it's not a small effect, but a very significant one. And it's an effect you can increase or decrease, depending on the expectations you instill in participants."

That's particularly true with psychedelics, where expectation plays a central role in determining the trip's qualities. Psychedelics induce suggestibility, meaning any input—from an emotionally evocative song to a framed Shiva poster on the wall—could influence the experience, making it damn near impossible to attach anything objective to the drug's physiological effects alone. Many abstract things frustrate psychedelic scientists' attempts to eliminate variables for the sake of inarguable data, and placebo control cannot eliminate that completely.

In psychedelic therapy research, it's pretty obvious whether you got a placebo or a psychedelic. "A placebo control group is there to confuse the participants, but very often they're not confused because they know when they've taken the active medication, particularly in psychedelic studies," Szigeti said. "That opens up a lot of questions around whether or not placebo control really makes sense."

Placebo control makes sense with physiological concerns. If you have a broken finger, you want to know a treatment works at the cellular level. When it comes to psychology, it's trickier. Despite how diligently philosophers like Daniel Dennett have worked to convince people the mind is nothing more than neural circuitry, there's no objective proof of such physicalist reductionism, and I doubt there ever will be. We cannot objectively reduce psychological phenomena like self-reflection and creativity to chemicals and neurons. We can *correlate* them, but ascribing causality like "the brain causes the mind" amounts to an opinion with no more validity than its opposite.*

"Maybe we should stop pretending these placebo-controlled studies work as well as papers often claim," Szigeti said. "The placebo effect is always treated as an enemy in medical studies, but it should be our friend. We should use the placebo effect to boost patient outcomes."

Some folks have suggested psychedelics in general merely amplify a placebo effect. Rick Strassman, a pivotal psychedelic researcher you'll learn more about in chapter 13, told me he believes psychedelics are "super placebos."

"Their effects are extraordinarily dependent upon expectation, suggestibility, selection bias, hope, intention—those factors combined with a drug that amplifies the placebo effect," Strassman said. "And you'll find that they'll do what you want them to do if you steer the experience in the right direction. They'll prove what you believe and what those around you believe."

I can't help but think of my first psilocybin mushroom trip, when my perception confirmed everything the mystics wrote about the essential unity of eternity and presence. Was I peering through the veil of my ego, or were the mushrooms reflecting what I already believed?

----

* It baffles me that after all these years, people still devote their lives to proving whether the chicken or the egg came first, never pausing to notice both laughing at them from the coop.

If psychedelics are indeed super placebos, why not steer placebo effect toward desirable outcomes? If psychedelics will "do what you want them to do," as Strassman suggested, doesn't that make them even more astounding? It would make them more dangerous, undoubtedly, as they could then reinforce the bricks barricading you inside an echo chamber you'd prefer not to acknowledge. But they could also blow up those bricks, opening you to the deeper sense of meaning for which your heart yearns. Perhaps the debate around microdosing and the placebo effect is less an advancement in knowledge than a way of playing into the constraints science has created for itself.

Deconstructing Data

Philosophical speculations aside, Fadiman doesn't buy the placebo explanation. He pointed to the fact that when Szigeti's participants were asked whether they were on a microdose or a placebo, over 70% guessed correctly. "From my point of view, that doesn't look like the double-blind was very successful," Fadiman said with a wily grin.

One of the great things about Fadiman is his free agency. He teaches, lectures, and mentors, but he's not a MAPS guy, a Johns Hopkins guy, or a Compass Pathways guy. He's just Jim Fadiman, and has no problem speaking his mind, smiling like a magician hiding something up his sleeve. One trick he revealed in our chat was his deconstruction of science's obsession with "data" over "anecdotal evidence."

"The word 'anecdote' means someone asked someone a question and got an answer. If you do it in a laboratory, it's called data. How do you measure depression? You measure depression by saying, 'Here's a scale. Here's some behaviors. Rank yourself.' If you do that on a survey, and you have a thousand people respond, that's called anecdotes. If you're doing it in laboratory, and it takes you a year, and you get eight people to respond, that's called data. The data looks exactly like the anecdotes for the things they've tested.

"Psychology, because they're trying to be a serious science, makes their research look a lot like a medical experiment where you measure physical things," he added. "But we're not really good at measuring mental states. If you're doing a pain study, you say, 'How much pain do you have, from one to ten?' and your one to ten is supposed to be equivalent to mine. But we haven't measured anything. What I look at is situations in which there is physical measurement, which makes the whole placebo thing kind of pointless."

Fadiman offered an example. "I gave a talk at Breaking Convention,* and I said, 'If anyone microdoses, let me know. Here's approximately how you could do it that's safe and we think efficacious.' I get a letter about six weeks later from an art historian in London, and she says, 'I know I owe you a report, but I thought you might be interested in this. My periods have always been very difficult. I microdosed, and my period was normal for the first time in my life.'

"I thought, that's astounding! That's measurable. We know what a bad period is, both emotionally and physically. So, I put on my little scientist hat and wrote back and said, 'What did you take? How much? How often?' She wrote back and said, 'I did your protocol—one day on, two days off—for the month, and I haven't microdosed ever since. My periods are normal. You have changed my life. Thank you.' That's the kind of data that I think matters as much as laboratory work."

Fadiman's been collecting these kinds of reports longer than anyone. He shared another he received from a former student. "He'd been on antidepressants for thirty-one years. With the support of his physician, he came off one of his two antidepressants, and then the other with the help of microdosing. Then, he was only microdosing, and he said, 'I have not had a full deck of emotions for thirty-one years, and now I feel like I have all of them back. I'm crying more often for pleasure, happiness, and sadness. It's a little embarrassing to people. But that's the difference.' That, to me, is astounding. We've taken one of the major mental illnesses on the planet for which we have medications which even the manufacturers say aren't useful for thirty percent of the population, and we're looking at someone who's been using them for decades and not feeling terrific about it. Suddenly, he takes this little *nothing* for maybe a month or two, and there's a return of full functioning'. I can't remember seeing the term 'return to full functioning' in the mental health literature."

To sum up his findings, Fadiman said, "The most common statement someone will make after they microdose for depression for a short time is 'I'm *back*. I feel like myself again.' That's the kind of work that I'm interested in."

---

*   A large, annual psychedelic conference in England.

Contraindications of Microdosing

Like psychedelic therapy, the benefits of microdosing can be overblown to a degree that overshadows contraindications. I know several people who have encountered a variety of difficulties through microdosing. Some shared that while their microdose days were pleasant, a crippling crash of energy would follow for days, leaving them incapable of completing their necessary tasks. Others reported that microdosing increased their anxiety to an extent that negated benefits. They sought an explanation for this, but amid the *microdosing-is-amazing!* culture, they couldn't find one.

This microdose-Kool-Aid-drinking ethos rarely acknowledges microdosing can become another way to drown your sorrows. People can become psychologically dependent on their little doses. Due to the culture's growing psychedelic enthusiasm, these folks have ample ammunition to justify their addictive search for relief, telling themselves their protocol of suppression is healing them. A physical expression of healing is lifestyle change. If microdosing yields no changes apart from making you hate your job a little less on dosing days, then maybe it's no different than an evening bong rip before yet another viewing cycle of *Game of Thrones.*

Given the newness of microdosing, we know nothing about long-term effects. Maybe small doses of LSD over an extended period are bad for the brain. Then again, some have claimed that Albert Hofmann took microdoses of LSD throughout his adult life, and he remained sharp as an eagle's talons at the age of 100. Peter Gasser, whom you'll remember as a leader in Switzerland's LSD research, recalled meeting Hofmann shortly before his 101st birthday.

"What touched me most was how bright and open he was. He was not slow or repeating the same things. He was as sharp as you and me. I was deeply impressed by his person." Gasser couldn't say with certainty if Hofmann microdosed LSD in his late life, as the chemist was not a boastful proselytizer. Fadiman, however, believes it's a strong possibility. "There's a snippet from an interview in 2006, where Rick Doblin and a couple of terrific people were

---

*   I still haven't watched *Game of Thrones*. A large reason is that I have friends who have watched all 70 hours three times or more, and I'm afraid it would actuate the same time-obliterating fate for me.

talking to Albert on his hundredth birthday," he said. "At one point, Albert says, 'You ought to try really low doses.' Rick says, 'What for?' Albert replies, 'It would help your thinking.' Rick asks, 'Like, a really low dose?' And Albert says, 'Like, ten micrograms.' Then the subject changes. When I read that, I thought, 'That's one of those moments in world history when something *didn't* happen.' Nobody in that interview group had the slightest interest."

One thing is clear: if Hofmann did continue using LSD, he took it with intention and respect, for he remained a vocal critic of casual LSD use throughout his life. Microdosing may not transform people as dramatically as macrodosing can, but intention can surely enhance its boons.

Mother's Little Helper

With microdosing and with psychedelics in general, what we don't know significantly outweighs what we do. Is microdosing pharmacologically legitimate, or are its benefits attributable to a placebo effect? There appears to be no consensus among the scientific community. In this space of uncertainty, exercising care in your microdosing protocol won't hurt.

Regardless of the validity or invalidity of the practice's benefits, microdosing provides an entry point for people newly interested in psychedelics who don't want to plunge into the deep end just yet. It's a safer and more predictable alternative to taking a full dose, and while it won't induce an ego-dissolving trip, a microdose can offer a taste of the psychedelic state, allowing folks to discern whether they would like to follow the call to adventure or remain in their ordinary world. As long as it's not harming people's brains or prompting them to harm others, who cares if the reported benefits are due to molecule or mind? Maybe what matters more is that microdosing helps people feel better—and perhaps more creative as well.

9

Creativity and Imagination

"Imagination will often carry us to worlds that never
were. But without it we go nowhere."

—Carl Sagan, *Cosmos*

The more one focuses on psychedelic research, the easier it is to forget about
psychedelics' countercultural history. New narratives about neuroscience
and mental health downplay histories of expression and rebellion. As often as
contemporary psychedelic researchers remind anyone listening about LSD's pre-
1970 therapeutic use, most people back then neither knew nor cared about it.
That was especially true in the summer of 1967, when the nation focused on the
LSD-using, VW Bus-driving, acoustic-strumming youth flocking to San Francisco's Haight-Ashbury neighborhood during the Summer of Love.

Far from a mantra of "Psychedelics can cure PTSD," those Californian streets
rang loud with shouts of "Peace!" and "Free love!" set to the tunes of Jefferson
Airplane and the Grateful Dead. At the center of it all, LSD fostered an uprising
of diverse expression against socially indoctrinated codes of behavioral expectations. In response to a post–World War II strangulation of the imagination with
ropes called "civic duty" and "The American Dream," the hippies led a revolution
of creativity, painting the grayscale society with exuberant color.

Amid today's clinical talk, it's rare to hear discussions of Woodstock, Janis
Joplin, the Doors, or anything else emblematic of the '60s. Researchers tend to
bring up these subjects as examples of forlorn miscreants embodying psychedelic
degeneracy. Have scientists and therapists forgotten John Lennon singing "Lucy in
the Sky with Diamonds"? Or are they merely focused on writing a different story?

Creative Problem-Solving

Although psychedelics have a rich history of connection with creative expression, hardly any research has investigated this relationship. One of the few studies took place in 1966, led by our friend Fadiman while he was working at Stanford. He and his crew gathered twenty-six participants of various professions—engineers, mathematicians, architects, and even a furniture designer—and each identified a specific creative issue they'd been facing. After a preparatory protocol, they underwent an experimental session with 200 milligrams of mescaline, which Fadiman compared to 100 micrograms of LSD.[1]

Nearly all participants came up with creative solutions to their problems. Significant improvements were observed in participants' ability to see the problem broadly, capacity for visual imagery, and concentration. Months later, about half of them continued to report positive benefits in their work performance.

The researchers made another interesting discovery: although psychedelics seem to evoke self-exploration and self-transcendence, "the set, setting, dose, expectation, and facilitation can redirect what is assumed to be the natural thrust of these substances." Because the focus was problem-solving over transcendence, intellectual concerns shaped the journeys' trajectories. While cognitive stimulation runs counter to the ego-dissolving principles of psychedelic therapy, such induction suggested possibilities for novel, psychedelic-assisted ways of thinking and creating.

Unfortunately, Uncle Sam cut Fadiman's research short. Those were the days of Lyndon B. Johnson, who doesn't get enough credit for his role in rallying the troops for his successor's War on Drugs. Johnson's Drug Abuse Control Amendments of 1965 established the first Federal control of psychedelics, prompting Sandoz to stop producing LSD. The following year, LSD was criminalized in California, and the increasingly anti-psychedelic government forced young Fadiman to wave goodbye to his supply.

Even amid the revival, the potential of psychedelics to boost creativity remains a niche subject. Creativity, for starters, is more difficult to study than mental health. With depression or PTSD, people fill out scales, and results are tallied. Can you really ask someone, "On a scale of one to ten, how creative are you feeling today?" If you did, would that data mean anything?

Creativity is enigmatic. The more you conceptualize it, the more elusive it becomes, for it flourishes in a state that includes and transcends known concepts. Rather than being ruled by protocols, the creatively inspired individual feels empowered to rearrange conceptual frameworks in a playful space of possibility.

Think of Pablo Picasso. Which painting comes to mind? *Guernica? The Weeping Woman?* Old Crooked Guy Playing Guitar?* We all know Picasso had a unique style, but if you were to search "Early Picasso Paintings" on the web, you'd discover portraits of regular-looking people that you'd never guess came from the Pab-man. That's because he, like countless innovative artists, mastered the techniques of his predecessors before creatively reconfiguring them into Cubism.

What accounts for creative breakthroughs? Can artistic evolution be studied scientifically? Might psychedelics enhance the possibility of an *ah-ha!* moment in a state of heightened innovative potential? A handful of testimonies from famous technological and scientific luminaries suggest they may.

Psychedelic Breakthroughs

A well-known psychedelic origin story tells that Francis Crick, the scientist credited for discovering the double-helix structure of DNA, used LSD to aid his research. Fadiman wrote that Crick and a few Cambridge colleagues took LSD "as a thinking tool to liberate them from preconceptions and let their genius wander freely to new ideas."[2] According to the story, Crick first perceived DNA's double-helix shape while on LSD. Some claim the story is bogus, but Fadiman was confident enough to print it in his book as fact, claiming Crick let his secret be known as death approached.[3]

A more reliable story is that of Steve Jobs, the turtleneck-wearing visionary behind Apple Inc.'s rise to the highest rungs of the Fortune 500 ladder. Jobs once claimed that taking LSD was one of the most important decisions he'd ever made. "LSD shows you that there's another side to the coin, and

---

*   This is not the official title of Picasso's painting.

you can't remember it when it wears off, but you know it," Jobs said.[4] "It reinforced my sense of what was important—creating great things instead of making money,[*] putting things back into the stream of history and of human consciousness as much as I could."

Intriguing as these cases are, it would be nice if there were more examples of psychedelics helping visionary innovators who didn't support "positive eugenics" like Crick or deny paternity of a biological child for years like Jobs. Genius and eccentricity often go hand in hand, eh? While this next creative individual isn't a technological innovator, she has undoubtedly innovated in the psychedelic field, and she fully earns the adjective "eccentric" in its most complimentary expression.

The Queen of Consciousness

Amanda Feilding has maintained keen interest in psychedelics and creativity for nearly half a century. Once dubbed "The Queen of Consciousness" by *New Scientist*,[5] Feilding has been an unsung psychedelic hero, consistently championing their potential through the dark ages of illegality. Through the Beckley Foundation, a UK-based non-governmental organization (NGO) she founded in 1998, Feilding kept psychedelic research and attention alive, refusing to be thwarted by the widespread flak she received.

"Fascinating" is an understated description of Feilding's life. As a teenager, her burgeoning interest in mysticism prompted her to hitchhike toward Ceylon—present-day Sri Lanka—to connect with her Buddhist godfather. She made it to the Syrian border, where she lived with a Bedouin tribe. She is the only person in this book who holds the title of Countess—"Countess of Wemyss and March," to be specific—and through her marriage to James Charteris, 13th Earl of Wemyss and 9th Earl of March—the ceremony of which took place under the Bent Pyramid of Ancient Egypt[†]—Feilding acquired the courtesy title of Lady

---

[*]   I suppose it was a happy accident that Jobs died with more money than several dozen nations.

[†]   I have tried and failed to learn whether "under" means "at the foot of" or "beneath the ground of." While I initially assumed the former, I discovered that the Bent Pyramid's 4,600-year-old chambers opened to the public in 2019. Though Feilding married Charteris in 1995, her history doesn't tell the story of someone who always follows the rules. It remains a mystery, but at the very least, this inquiry led me to discover that the Pharaoh who commanded its building was named "Sneferu," the Seussian phonetics of which afforded me a hearty guffaw.

Neidpath.[6] Feilding is likewise the only person in this book who once had a pet pigeon with whom she shared a telepathic connection. She was also the only person I'd ever heard of who once drilled a hole into their own head, until I learned that Charteris followed suit after their Bent Pyramid wedding. This skull-hole drilling is an ancient human practice called "trepanation," and Feilding trepanned herself at the age of twenty-three to improve cerebral circulation and expand her consciousness. She was such a believer in the procedure that she twice ran for British Parliament on a platform of "Trepanation for the National Health."

In short, Feilding may have secured my vote for Most Interesting Person in the World.

Unlike many big-name psychedelic researchers, Feilding is candid about her psychedelic use, and the benefits about which she speaks are irreducible to a diagnostic paradigm. Speaking to host Joe Moore on the *Psychedelics Today* podcast in 2020, Feilding reflected on a period during the 1960s in which she imbibed about 250 micrograms of LSD a day. During that time, Feilding and her no-doubt fascinating companions experimented with playing *Go*, the ancient Chinese board game, to test LSD's potential to enhance cognition.*

"What I think it [LSD] does," Feilding told Moore, "is, by expanding the network of integrated brain parts . . . you have a richer base from which to see life." She continued, "It's like playing from higher up the mountain. You've got a better view of the board, and intuitively, you can see more patterns."[7]

Feilding didn't present this as an inherent property of LSD. She and her friends had "learned how to use it [LSD] for cognitive functioning at a higher level,"[8] echoing Fadiman's conclusion that specific approaches and parameters unlock these capacities.† Although her desire to organize research on LSD and *Go* has not materialized—not least due to the difficulty

---

* When I imagine Feilding's life, I can't help but imagine it with a Wes Anderson aesthetic. If you've seen such films as *The Royal Tenenbaums* and *The Grand Budapest Hotel*, perhaps you know what I'm talking about. If Wes Anderson happens to be reading this, I'd ask him to consider writing and directing a biopic of Feilding with Tilda Swinton in the lead role, Bill Murray as Charteris, Owen Wilson as a Go-playing friend, and Willem Dafoe as a mysterious occultist Feilding meets on her hitchhiking journey.

† When the topic of microdosing came up, Feilding noted that microdoses of mushrooms did not seem to have the same sharpening effects on cognition as LSD, supporting Fadiman's assertions that LSD microdoses are "more analytic" than psilocybin.

in finding enough skilled *Go* players to participate—she has funded some of the only research on psychedelic-assisted creativity in the revival. A 2022 Beckley-supported study assessed the creativity of participants who'd received either 50 micrograms of LSD or a placebo. The team discovered that LSD changed several creativity measurements compared with the placebo, including a "pattern break" prompting increased novelty and originality.[9] A separate 2021 study found psilocybin brought similar creative benefits and creative flexibility.[10]

As much as I admire this line of scientific inquiry, perhaps it's aiming to prove something that's been known for a long time. After all, psychedelic use in the 1960s inspired some of the greatest music the West has ever heard. And where better to start than . . .

The Beatles

The Beatles' career spanned the full 1960s, and their evolution reflected the seismic shifts of the monumental decade. Like Western society, the Beatles spent the first half of the '60s dressed pleasantly, bopping their mop-tops and having a jolly good time singing innocent tunes—essentially, continuing the 1950s. Everything changed with *Rubber Soul* and *Revolver*.

It was the mid1960s, and things were getting more complex. The band's love songs were joined with the twangs of the Indian sitar, highlighting Eastern culture in Western pop music. The culture was changing, and the Beatles reflected—or perhaps helped facilitate—the movement. As LSD grew in popularity and the Summer of Love approached, they released *Sgt. Pepper's Lonely Hearts Club Band*, singing about the trippy world of "Lucy in the Sky with Diamonds."*

In *Sgt. Pepper's*, the Beatles broke every rule of songwriting, yet each song somehow maintained the signature poppiness that had catapulted the Liverpool blokes to international superstardom. The album wasn't simply a collection of tracks; it was an *experience*, inviting listeners all across the world to see music and life through colorful specs of possibility.

---

* This track is still so closely associated with LSD that one of the substance's nicknames is "Lucy"—even though, despite its initials, the song is actually about a drawing young Julian Lennon described for his dad.

What caused the band's rapid evolution? We're talking less than two years between "Help!" and "Being for the Benefit of Mr. Kite!" Was it their dedication? Producer George Martin's engineering wizardry? Something in the air?

Surely those played a role, and surely LSD did as well.

John Lennon and George Harrison first took LSD in the spring of 1965. It wasn't intentional. They were dosed by John Riley, a dentist hosting the Lennons and Harrisons for dinner. Terrifying at first, the experience became revelatory.

"I had such an overwhelming feeling of well-being, that there was a God, and I could see him in every blade of grass," Harrison later reflected. "It was like gaining hundreds of years of experience in twelve hours."

"God, it was just terrifying, but it was fantastic," Lennon recalled.

Lennon and Harrison decided to trip again, this time inviting their fellow Beatles to join. "John and I had decided that Paul and Ringo had to have acid," Harrison said, "because we couldn't relate to them anymore. Not just on the one level—we couldn't relate to them on any level, because acid had changed us so much. It was such a mammoth experience that it was unexplainable."

Ringo, always on-rhythm with the vibes, was down. "It was a fabulous day," he reflected. The night, however, was less fabulous, as "it felt like it was never going to wear off. Twelve hours later and it was, 'Give us a break now, Lord.'"

McCartney was more reluctant. "It alters your life and you never think the same again," he later opined. "I was rather frightened by that prospect."[11]

Nevertheless, McCartney gave it a go in December of 1965. "It was such a mind-expanding thing," he said. "You noticed and you heard. Everything was supersensitive."[12]

I can't prove it, but I'd bet my Fender Stratocaster that the Beatles wouldn't have produced their revolutionary, paradigm-shifting post-1965 music without LSD. Once acid entered, everything changed. The moptops and suits became long hair and flashy outfits. The love songs became "Tomorrow Never Knows" and "Strawberry Fields Forever." The black-and-white cover of *Revolver* became *Sgt. Pepper's* explosion of color, mirroring the counterculture's rebellion against grayscale society. LSD broke down structures and opened possibilities at every level of the group's creative expression.

All in all, the Beatles were but one of many '60s groups whose members used psychedelics to experiment with new sounds for Western ears. Jefferson Airplane, the Doors, the Byrds, and the Grateful Dead all took psychedelics to reach new creative heights. Once their collective sounds animated the airwaves, Western music would never be the same.

Creative Enhancement Is Different from Creative Genesis

The first time Brian Wilson, genius songwriter, multi-instrumentalist, and vocalist of the Beach Boys, took LSD, he sat at his piano and wrote the iconic opening melody to "California Girls."* Cheesy as the song may be, consider lending a fresh ear to the intro. Rarely has such a beautiful lullaby facilitated entry into a pop song.

A point to draw from Wilson's story is that psychedelics did not generate creative innovation in a vacuum. He was already a gifted, dedicated musician capable of penning international hits without substances. LSD seems to have opened an experimental gateway, allowing him to use his preexisting skills to discover and arrange new patterns. Much like Picasso, Wilson's mastery of established concepts was necessary for their creative rearrangement. This is equally true of the Beatles and the other legendary sixties musicians who experimented with LSD.

If you take LSD and pick up the rusty trumpet you've never played, you won't sound like Louis Armstrong—although you may think you do, which could be worthwhile as long as no one else's eardrums need endure it. The same principle is evident in Fadiman's problem-solving study: those who solved their problem had mastered the preliminary skills required.

I'll add a brief anecdote from my first LSD trip. I spent the summer of 2012 hitchhiking through the Western United States, and a fellow named Densmore who'd generously driven me around in his RV took me from Oakland to Lake Tahoe. At our campsite, we each took two hits a friend had acquired from a sparkly fellow in Berkeley. After an afternoon of swimming

---

* Wilson's masterful 1966 album *Pet Sounds* so heavily influenced Paul McCartney that Beatles' producer George Martin claimed *Sgt. Pepper's* never would have been made without it. (Source: Jerry Crowe, "'Pet Sounds Sessions': Body of Influence Put in a Box," Los Angeles Times, November 1, 1997, latimes.com/archives/la-xpm-1997-nov-01-ca-48891-story.html)

through Tahoe's frigid waters and marveling at the diverse shades of blue, we made a fire and grabbed our acoustic guitars. We'd jammed throughout the week prior, but that night, the creative levee burst. I had no thoughts. My fingers knew precisely where to go, inside and outside of the scales that had previously dictated the borders of my improvisation. Hours flew by, and the inspiration remained until we decided sleep was a good idea.

To ensure we weren't two tripped-out vagabonds convinced our horrible noises were genius, Densmore and I played our recording of the sesh for his friends back in Oakland. They confirmed our jams were indeed gnarly. We were able to shred so thoroughly due to our basic competence and the synchronization we'd already established together.

However, the creative enhancement psychedelics can induce doesn't always mesh with the practical requirements of artistic creation. On Ken Kesey's bus trip, for example, he and the Merry Pranksters filmed their wild antics, intent on creating a consciousness-expanding documentary to express the spirit of Jack Kerouac's novel *On the Road* through the gang's LSD-empowered expression. As it turned out, the footage was chaotic and untethered to the point of nonsensicality, and the reels remained stowed away for decades. It was due to filmmakers Alison Ellwood and Alex Gibney's heroic attempts to salvage some degree of coherence that the world got to witness highlights in the 2011 documentary, *Magic Trip*.

Psychedelics won't transform an uninspired loafer into a creative genius. If this loafer, however, picks up some skills before adding LSD to the mix, they may find themselves traversing imaginative, enlivening creative territory.

The Misunderstood Sibling of Rationality

Many psychedelics produce vivid imagery in the mind's eye. But there's a pitfall in writing about the imagination these days: people don't tend to take it seriously. Imagination is routinely associated with magical thinking, far-flung fantasies, and Disneyland, reflecting Western perspective's implicit hierarchy wherein rationality presides over imagination. Why are rationality and imagination typically regarded in opposition? Why don't more people recognize they coexist as two inherent faculties of the mind, each essential in its own right?

There's no need to rehash the wonders rationality has yielded for humans. Imagination, however, holds the mind's capacity to envision realities yet to exist, toward whose manifestation we may direct our rational efforts. Surely the Egyptian pharaohs had imagined the Pyramids of Giza before they made their overworked laborers lay the first stones.* As its art and mythology both demonstrate, Egyptian culture prized imagination.

Imagination gets a bad rap because people assume its contents are "not real." That may be true if we're defining the "real" as physical matter, but why would we abide such a thin conception? Even if a child's image of a four-headed zombie lurking in the closet doesn't exist in the material world, the image is so real in the child's mind that it initiates a complex physiological response called "fear." To say imagination isn't "real" is to ignore the physical realities it evokes.

Tempting as it is to position rationality as the faculty of science and imagination as the faculty of art, reality is not so simple. Each faculty is essential to both. To quote Albert Einstein, "Imagination is more important than knowledge. For knowledge is limited, whereas imagination encircles the world, stimulating progress, giving birth to evolution."[13] Imagination creates the visions toward whose achievement science focuses its instruments.

On the flip side, novelists filter their stories through rational analyses to establish a structure. The greatness of the *Harry Potter* book series arose not only through a vividly imagined fantasy world but because J. K. Rowling wove intricate plotlines with threads of the wizarding world's lore based on legitimate history, usurping expectations with new surprises that required rigorous planning to come across as effortless.

Jung theorized that the source of consciousness is approached not through rationality but through *imagery*. To Jung, images make up humanity's primordial

---

* In my first draft of this sentence, "made their overworked laborers" read "forced their slaves." I figured I should fact check this assertion, and I'm glad I did, because it turns out the idea of Egyptian rulers building the pyramids with slave labor is an example of "popular imagination" contrasting with historical evidence. I suppose this is the kind of thing that gives imagination a bad name, and it makes sense that historians would be skeptical of imagination ungrounded in rationality. However, Egyptologist Mark Lehner, a primary figure in the slave-pyramid-builders debunking, constructed his evidence based on visits to Egypt, archaeological discoveries, and the vision of their culture his imagination produced thereof.

language, expressing fundamental patterns from which all experience flows. Plato evoked a similar notion in his descriptions of the "Forms," the nonphysical, eternal images of perfection imitated by all material things. While Plato's metaphysics can evoke an inaccessible, heavenlike dreamworld, Jung's therapeutic approach leveraged the imagination to access libidinal energy. This energy, which parallels what is known as chi or qi in traditional Chinese culture, gets blocked by various internal conditions, and Jungian therapy aims to restore its equanimous flow in the mind, body, and spirit. His technique of "active imagination" directed patients to pay attention to what images spontaneously arose through various associations, for he believed the imagery provided insight into the mysterious workings of the unconscious. The more one tries to reason their way to such insights, the more one obstructs the imagination from guiding them deeper.

Imagination plays an important role in recent therapeutic developments. For several decades, Eye Movement Desensitization and Reprocessing (EMDR) has been a leading modality for treating trauma. A central EMDR procedure has patients focus on "spontaneous associations of traumatic images, thoughts, emotions and bodily sensations."[14] As one engages with the imagery, EMDR helps them reprocess the associated trauma, lessening its disruptive charge. EMDR recognizes that imagination is more closely tied with emotion than can be said of rationality. A sudden flash of a memory can induce a wide range of feelings, from peaceful tranquility to harsh rage.

Some memories become so intertwined with emotions that the two can no longer be separated. For people suffering from PTSD, this linkage becomes debilitating. The memory of the trauma plagues the mind, constantly threatening to conjure overwhelming feelings. One would be hard-pressed to reason their way out of such a bind. Rationality helps separate us from our emotions, and in a culture that routinely suppresses emotions, perhaps this partially accounts for its perceived supremacy.

We heal emotional wounds by turning toward repressed pain and allowing the body to release bound-up emotional charges. Imagination, in its close ties with emotion, opens access to our inner landscapes' widest valleys, darkest caves, and every unacknowledged jungle between. Imagination helps us expand what internalized boundaries dictate about how we view our potential.

Connecting and reconnecting with psychedelic-induced images can yield transformation. My friend Bri Bendixsen, a psychedelic therapist and educator, shared a story of a client who'd been suffering from depression for decades. "During a ketamine experience, he saw an image of himself as a being of light underneath a massive mountain of darkness. We did some work around empowering him to see himself as that light even amid this big mountain of sadness or grief, of finding ways to dig out or shine light through when he can."

A turning point in *The Lion King* illustrates (literally) these concepts. Simba, having exiled himself after the death of his father, Mufasa, stands over a reflective pool, which reveals only what his shame allows him to see. The medicine baboon Rafiki disrupts Simba's despair, telling him, "Look *harder*." As the water ripples, Simba sees his reflection transform into Mufasa, and Rafiki says, "You see? He lives in you." The booming voice of James Earl Jones fades in, and Mufasa appears in the clouds, telling his son, "You are *more* than what you have *become*." As the audience's chills peak, Mufasa's voice fades out with the message, "Remember *who you are*."

Through these images, Simba releases his shame and expands his limited narratives of self. Imagination, not rationality, paved the road to healing his trauma, directing him toward actualizing his slumbering potential to become King.*

Imagination as a Spiritual Gateway

During the three years I taught literature and writing at a Jesuit high school in the Midwest, I was often struck by the Jesuit priests' ability to paint a vivid scene through their sermons. I learned that these skills were not innate so much as developed when the youngest Jesuit of the bunch guided me through the *Spiritual Exercises*, a sequence of meditations and contemplations that Ignatius of Loyola, the Jesuit order's sixteenth-century founder, developed during his religious conversion in the Spanish town of Manresa. Without food, money, or shelter, Ignatius begged for basic necessities, and

---

* I can't tell you how many times this scene has come to my mind on psychedelics and plant medicines, often moving me to tears. There's such powerful meaning packed into those beautiful images.

for many months, he spent seven hours a day praying in a cave. In the darkness, he experienced a series of mystical visions that helped establish the foundation for the *Spiritual Exercises* that would become the cornerstone of the Jesuits' unique approach to prayer.

Bolstered by his visions, Ignatius became convinced that God speaks to humanity directly through the imagination. He thus developed a method of "imaginative prayer" aimed toward stirring the heart's emotions and the spirit's visions to deepen one's relationship with God. Designed to be completed over the course of thirty-day retreats, the *Exercises* are structured on a sequence of Gospel stories with which retreatants engage through contemplation. In the Jesuit perspective, contemplation entails visualizing the story's scenes, imagining yourself in it, and paying close attention to specific details. Jesuits teach that through one's imagined details, God communicates to them personally. What matters is one's imaginative engagement with the text, rather than a literal interpretation of the words.

Instead of focusing on interpreting a Bible story's characters as symbols, Ignatius's method focuses on contemplating them with an open heart. I wouldn't read about Jesus healing a leper and think, "I bet the leper represents the darkness afflicting the innocent." I would close my eyes and imagine the leper standing next to me. I'd focus on the bent shape of his body, the protrusions on his cheek, and the suffering in his eyes, and I'd continue until I felt an emotional connection to him. I might engage him in a dialogue and learn about his life. Imaginative prayer invites the heart to join the mind.

I didn't make it through all the *Exercises*. At a certain point, progression required belief in Catholicism's central mystery of the historical, physical event of Jesus Christ's resurrection, which I could only see as a myth. Still, I benefited from Ignatius's approach, and I found it similar (apart from the Biblical focus) to Jung's active imagination and even certain forms of hypnosis. These methods recognize and teach that through visualization, the mind enters a liminal state between waking consciousness and dreams, a state so conducive to insight that it can catalyze transformation.

Psychedelics tend to activate the imagination, and working with the imagination can have spiritual, healing value. Whether or not you believe in a higher power, the imagination can reveal aspects of your inner world asking for reflection over rational analysis. Without imagination, we cannot envision a better future. Without visualizing a new reality, we cannot devise creative solutions to the problems we face. How much joy, connection, and inspiration do we sacrifice by allowing excessive rationality to strangle our imaginations?

The Dark Side of the Boon

There's a dark side to creative genius and imagination which no balanced portrait can exclude. Amid history's bliss-inspired artists, there are countless tortured artists like Vincent van Gogh, who cut off his left ear in a manic-depressive bout, and Sylvia Plath, who ended her own life at the age of thirty by inserting her head into an oven. As lovey-dovey as the 1960s may seem, there was plenty of darkness behind the flowers.

For the Beatles, LSD wasn't a happily ever-after story. For Harrison, the bliss ended when he visited Haight-Ashbury on acid during the Summer of Love and discovered the vibes were less loving than "the manifestation of a scene from an Hieronymus Bosch painting, getting bigger and bigger, fish with heads, faces like vacuum cleaners coming out of shop doorways."[15]

After his visit, there was no going back. "That's when I went right off the whole drug cult and stopped taking the dreaded lysergic acid . . . that's when I really went for the meditation."[16]

Lennon left acid behind after a series of bad trips. "I just couldn't stand it," he said. "We were going through a whole game that everybody went through. And I destroyed meself . . . I destroyed me ego and I didn't believe I could do anything . . . I just was nothing, I was *shit*."[17]

During a 1967 press conference following a seminar led by Maharishi Mahesh Yogi, founder of Transcendental Meditation, Harrison said LSD "enables you to see a lot of possibilities that you may never have noticed before, but it isn't the answer. You don't just take LSD and that's it forever, you're OK."[18]

Brian Wilson's story didn't end with such equanimity. In the late '60s, his mental health began to deteriorate. He became prone to paranoia, and his distress grew debilitating when *Pet Sounds*, his greatest creative achievement, was met with mediocre reviews and middling chart success. By the end of the decade, Wilson was drowning his woes with alcohol, amphetamines, cocaine, and junk food. These habits led to Wilson's long and disturbing relationship with psychiatrist Eugene Landy, who cut Wilson off from the rest of the band, charged him hundreds of thousands of dollars, and prescribed him a smorgasbord of uppers that left him worse off than before.

I don't want to scapegoat LSD for Wilson's woes; it's uncertain how often he tripped. Nevertheless, he lamented having tried it.

"I've told a lot of people don't take psychedelic drugs," he told *Rolling Stone* in 2016. "It's mentally dangerous to take. I regret having taken LSD. It's a bad drug."[19]

Perhaps the most infamous psychedelic-related tragedy of 1960s music is the story of Syd Barrett, the guitarist, songwriter, singer, and cofounder of Pink Floyd. Though Barrett gave the band its name, you won't hear him on *The Dark Side of the Moon* or *The Wall*, for he was removed from the band in 1968 after a stretch of increasingly erratic and concerning behavior. Soon after his episodes began, Barrett appeared to have lost connection with reality.

While there's debate over the accurate version of the story, one certainty is that around the time of his psychotic break, Barrett took a lot of LSD. His flatmates may even have added acid to his morning coffee, locking him in an LSD trip for months. His personality shifted from a friendly, energetic musical visionary to a depressed, unpredictable loner who often sat motionless in a catatonic daze. He'd stare blankly at interviewers, strum a single chord throughout a concert, and sometimes wander around the stage without playing at all. After Pink Floyd gave him the boot, he fell into obscurity, and he lived outside the public eye until his death from pancreatic cancer in 2006.

Some of Barrett's bandmates speculated his heavy LSD use catalyzed undiagnosed schizophrenia. His sister denied these suggestions, claiming he had Asperger's Syndrome and wasn't the recluse commonly believed. Regardless, Barrett's history with Pink Floyd reached a tragic climax in 1975 during their recording sessions for *Wish You Were Here*. The nine-part song "Shine on You Crazy Diamond" was written as a tribute to Barrett, and as the band worked on the track's final mix, an overweight man wandered into the studio. His head and eyebrows were shaved, and he carried a plastic bag. No one knew who he was until keyboardist Richard Wright realized it was Barrett.

The recognition led bassist Roger Waters, Barrett's childhood friend, to break down in tears.

Drummer Nick Mason later wrote that Barrett's conversation was "desultory and not entirely sensible."[20] He was both there and not there. He gave no explanation for why or how he showed up as the band mixed the track dedicated to him. He would have had no knowledge of that fact, as the remaining members hadn't spoken to him in years. He left without saying goodbye, and it was the last time Wright, Mason, and guitarist David Gilmour saw him. Waters saw his old friend once more a few years later in a department store. Before Waters could say anything, Barrett dropped his bags and ran away, leaving Waters to discover the bags were filled with candy.

With set and setting recognized as essential factors in psychedelic experiences, we can't point to LSD as the sole culprit of Barrett's decline. Journalist Jonathan Meades recounted a strange visit to Barrett's flat in the late '60s. He heard awful banging noises, and when he questioned their source, he received a laughter-filled reply from whoever opened the door that it was Barrett having a bad trip in the linen cupboard they'd locked him in.

Don't Underestimate the Risks

While the War on Drugs embellished things to promote fear and distrust, the claim that psychedelics can prompt the mind to unravel is not total fabrication. Psychedelics frequently destabilize people's internal structures of identity and reality. While this can help someone suffocating beneath the weight of their own rigidity, it can be detrimental to someone already tinkering on the threshold of losing their grip, sending them into an oblivion from which they may not return. The way psychedelics inspire the imagination can be liberating, but if it comes at full expense of rationality, one can lose their footing in reality.

III

INTEGRATION AND EXPLORATION

Mescaline and the Garden of Eden

"Within you there is a stillness and a sanctuary to which
you can retreat at any time and be yourself."

—Hermann Hesse, *Siddhartha*

I n *This Is Your Mind on Plants*, Pollan nicknamed mescaline the "orphan psychedelic," because it factored prominently in first-wave psychedelic research before essentially disappearing from the lab and public interest. As you might suspect, mescaline is reappearing in Western research.

In 1897, German chemist Arthur Heffter identified and isolated mescaline as the psychoactive molecule in peyote, a cactus that has been imbibed in sacred, ceremonial contexts among Indigenous peoples of Mexico and the present-day southwestern United States for over five thousand years. In 1919, Austrian chemist Ernst Späth successfully synthesized mescaline in a lab. Although peyote's history was vaster than one can comprehend, in the early 1900s, mescaline's large-scale influence in the Western world had just begun.

The first widely referenced mescaline trip report in the West came from Aldous Huxley. After achieving international fame with *Brave New World*, Huxley became interested in Native American peyote use, leading him to discover British psychiatrist Humphry Osmond's research in mescaline to understand schizophrenia.* In a letter to Osmond, Huxley volunteered to be an experimental subject,

---

* Osmond is one of the many people I mention who deserves more recognition than he gets in this book. To learn more about Osmond's role in starting the first wave, check out *The Acid Room: The Psychedelic Trials and Tribulations of Hollywood Hospital* by Erika Dyck and Jesse Donaldson.

hypothesizing the compound could grant entry into a state of expansive consciousness that the brain habitually filters out. Huxley invited Osmond to his home in California, and on May 3, 1953, he took mescaline under Osmond's supervision.

Huxley's trip catalyzed his interest in psychedelics as a gateway to spiritual enlightenment and knowledge, which would remain a primary focus for the rest of his life. His classic book on his experience, *The Doors of Perception*, is sometimes regarded as having marked the beginning of first-wave Western psychedelic interest. The title came from a verse of mystic poet William Blake's *The Marriage of Heaven and Hell*: "If the doors of perception were cleansed every thing would appear to man as it is: Infinite. For man has closed himself up, till he sees all things thro' narrow chinks of his cavern."*

To Huxley, the Infinite was "Mind at Large," and mescaline was a key to access it. He confirmed his hypothesis in one of his book's most quoted passages: "To make biological survival possible, Mind at Large has to be funneled through the reducing valve of the brain and nervous system. What comes out at the other end is a measly trickle of the kind of consciousness which will help us to stay alive on the surface of this particular planet."[1]

If the brain did not filter consciousness into a "measly trickle" of Mind at Large, we would feel completely overwhelmed. This reducing valve is essential for survival, but it entails a reduction of awareness that separates us from the endless ocean of possible perception. Mescaline loosens hardwired neurological constrictions, yielding a more accurate way of perceiving life's phenomena. To Huxley, this broadened perception had profound spiritual implications, exposing the mystical core of the world's religions in the immanence of the present moment.

Huxley's writing heavily influenced the hippie counterculture. However, LSD replaced mescaline as the go-to psychedelic for facilitating perceptual expansion. Pollan theorized this was because LSD is over a thousand times more potent than mescaline,[2] making it much easier for chemists and distributors to transport in high volumes. Despite mescaline's important role in generating psychedelic interest in the West, it essentially vanished for half a century.

---

* Blake's poem and Huxley's title influenced singer Jim Morrison and keyboardist Ray Manzarek to name their band "the Doors." The Huxley link of the influence chain also inspired Morrison to take a lot of mescaline and LSD.

Mescaline Revival

In 2021, a team of researchers from several institutions administered an online questionnaire to adults who had used mescaline in natural settings. Of the 452 respondents, 68 to 86% reported improvements in depression, anxiety, PTSD, and substance use disorders directly following mescaline use. About one third ranked their mescaline trip as among the top five most meaningful experiences of their lives.[3]

Pharmacologist Matthias Liechti, a lead researcher behind Switzerland's LSD studies, has been investigating mescaline's effects in comparison with LSD and psilocybin to find ideal therapeutic doses.[4] In the States, Journey Colab, a well-funded* psychedelic pharmaceutical company based in San Francisco, launched a clinical trial in 2022 on mescaline to treat alcohol use disorder. According to their website, mescaline "may provide a less intense and more insightful experience than other psychedelics, allowing for patients to experience a greater degree of mental clarity and connectedness to others."[5]

Mescaline is one of four classic psychedelics, but it has a reputation for being gentler than LSD, psilocybin, and DMT. While the other three tend to take people on wild trips filled with closed-eyed visions and perceptual distortions, mescaline users often describe seeing things *as they are*. Mescaline aids in peering into the depths of physical things, sparking insight into life's ongoing processes of renewal. Contrasting his experience with Greek philosopher Plato's preoccupation with metaphysical "Ideas," Huxley offered one of his most vivid and beautiful passages:

"He [Plato] could never, poor fellow, have seen a bunch of flowers shining with their own inner light and all but quivering under the pressure of the significance with which they were charged; could never have perceived that what rose and iris and carnation so intensely signified was nothing more, and nothing less, than what they were—a transience that was yet eternal life, a perpetual perishing that was at the same time pure Being, a bundle of minute, unique particulars in which, by some unspeakable and yet self-evident paradox, was to be seen the divine source of all existence."[6]

---

* More specifically, Journey Colab has received over $15 million in funding since forming in 2020.

Huxley's spiritual inclinations are evident in his words. Was he describing a vision of the eternal way things *are*, or was he describing his preexisting viewpoints amplified via mescaline? The question of whether psychedelics genuinely occasion mystical insight or extend set, setting, and worldview remains a subject of debate, yet I wonder if getting consumed in this question ends up distancing us from direct experience, tethering us to unconscious resistance against openness to and engagement with the moment.

More than sixty years after he penned them, Huxley's words remind us that there is always more going on now in the present moment than we realize. If we take the time (or perhaps the mescaline) to attune our antennas of awareness to the phenomena of the moment, life's unseen layers manifest through surfaces, revealing their enduring beauty, mystery, and impregnable life force.

I imagine it's this quality that lends mescaline toward healing addiction. For the addict, the substance they are taking meets specific needs, and to strip away the substance cold turkey is to leave them forlorn in their pain. To connect with life in the present moment is to connect with an enduring source of peace, vitality, and equanimity. Perhaps this source is what the addict seeks through their substance use in the first place, and mescaline can reveal its accessibility in all moments, for the fountain of life never runs dry.

Connection

Is healing from trauma as simple as letting go of something painful? It could be, but often, it's not. Sorry, Self-Help Influencers, but when we focus exclusively on "letting go," we often fall into the trap of villainizing parts of ourselves as demons to exorcise rather than wounds to heal. This perpetuates fragmentation, for we define these parts as *not us*. Each time they emerge, we fight to change them and get somewhere other than here, regardless of how futile our efforts prove.

Human beings have a remarkable capacity to section off the aspects of themselves they don't like. These defensive strategies may help us cope temporarily with day-to-day struggles, but they often grow toxically counterproductive to long-term flourishing, disconnecting us from present experience through denial.

In the eyes of Lauren Casalino, a therapist trained in Contemplative Psychotherapy and Buddhist Psychology, disconnection is at the core of suffering.

"Connecting with life, in its many forms, is fundamental at the heart of healing," Casalino told me, adding that "psychedelics can support connection within a framework that is larger than the separate self. Connecting with life *as it is* might be the ultimate, but it depends on where the wound is. If the wound is in relationship, connecting in relationship is part of healing. If the wound is in our capacity to meet life, healing is connecting with our capacity to meet the moment." Casalino believes psychedelics enhance our capacity for connection "with the sense that there is support and guidance in the universe, even if we can't see it or hold it."

There's a helpful notion expressed in Richard Linklater's film *Waking Life*: "Once having said 'yes' to the instant, the affirmation is contagious. It bursts into a chain of affirmations that knows no limit. To say yes to one instant is to say yes to all of existence."[7] Connecting to life is saying yes to the moment, in all its imperfection and glory.

Mindfulness teacher and psychotherapist Tara Brach calls this "radical acceptance." Such acceptance is radical in that we accept our pain as real and valid rather than judging it as a villain blocking entry into a utopian palace of pleasure. In Buddhist teaching, *grasping* is the root of suffering. Pain is unavoidable; suffering stems from the belief that we need *something else* to be happy.

Radical acceptance is not passivity. We can accept the suffering in the world *and* desire to change it. In fact, there's no way we *can* change it without accepting it, for nonacceptance positions our actions on the flimsy plane of denial. Compassion comes not through rejection, but through direct engagement with reality.

This applies equally to the inner world. You can accept your trauma and associated pain while hoping to shift it. Accepting the pain, you engage with it; engaging with it, you connect with its source; connecting with its source, you begin to heal.* Despite MDMA's nickname of ecstasy, its therapeutic use isn't about leaving your pain for a fleeting bliss; it's about opening your heart to your wounds and meeting them with compassion.

---

* Quotes this cheesy are all but destined for plaques and fridge magnets. Should anyone desire to make these, I'll gladly take only 20% of the profits.

Connection comes through authenticity, which is stifled when we deny elements of our inner lives. Recall the ancient Greek maxim of the Oracle of Delphi: *Know thyself.* This includes knowing our capacity for denial. Radical acceptance embraces the denial and that which is denied, revealing connections between inner and outer layers of the present, including those most unnerving to behold.

Meet Your Monsters Like the Deer

In *Medicine Cards: The Discovery of Power Through the Ways of Animals*, Jamie Sams and David Carson's popular divination deck, the section on Deer Medicine relates a story of a demon blocking the way to the lodge of the Great Spirit.[9] All the animals who encounter this demon are too overcome with fear to pass until Deer arrives. The monster assumes its terrible form, and Deer observes it through calm, curious eyes. Confused, the monster grows in terror as Deer beholds it with a nonjudgmental, accepting gaze. Ultimately, the monster is stripped of its power and vanishes, allowing Deer to pass to the lodge of the Great Spirit.

This story expresses an important component of psychedelic use, especially in therapy: when you encounter a monster lurking in the shadows, do not flee it, but turn toward it.* The monster could be a memory, a fear, an unpleasant sensation, or anything you'd rather deny than confront. The more you ignore your demons, the more they end up dominating the trip. Striving to bury the monsters amounts to pushing against a wall; accepting the wall allows it to crumble.

In his "Flight Instructions for Psychedelic Journeys," Johns Hopkins psychedelic therapist Bill Richards wrote, "If the participant is feeling fear, encourage the participant to confront the fear: Look the monster in the eye and move towards it . . . Dig in your heels; ask, 'What are you doing in my mind?' Or, 'What can I learn from you?' Look for the darkest corner in the basement, and shine your light there."[10] When we turn toward a challenging phenomenon instead of resisting, we may discover it has something important to teach us.

---

*   The importance of this component is nullified when the setting feels unsafe, for such lack of safety can contribute to becoming overwhelmed by the monster. Safety and support are important to establish before teatime with the inner demons.

It's well known in horror filmmaking that the buildup is more terrifying than the monster's reveal, for fear of the unknown is greater than fear of tangible realities. Steven Spielberg implemented this in *Jaws*, spending two-thirds of the film *suggesting* the killer shark through gray fins and John Williams' ominous score. When the shark is revealed in full as it eats Robert Shaw, the audience's terror diminishes, for the mechanical monster is nowhere near as frightening as the version their minds had created.

M. Night Shyamalan's film *The Sixth Sense* illustrates this further. In the story, Bruce Willis, playing a psychiatrist, treats distressed young Haley Joel Osment, who is burdened with the ability to see dead people. Osment is terrified of them—no surprise, given they carry the grotesque wounds that took them out. A turning point occurs when Willis instructs Osment to stop fleeing them and instead ask what they want. It turns out the ghosts aren't haunting him; they're seeking closure. Osment's deepest fears are actually messages of distress seeking resolution, and when he shifts his orientation, he finds peace. He even helps Willis, who *[spoiler alert!]*, in a classic Shyamalan twist, has really been *dead all along*.

When we fight monsters in psychedelic journeys, we remain trapped in their influence. By meeting them with nonjudgmental curiosity, we deprive them of power and gain insight into what lies beneath the façade.

The Guide as the Deer

One of many reasons psychedelic therapies require trained facilitators is that if you end up in a dark place with no support to navigate it, you could spiral into a bottomless abyss. A skilled facilitator can help you shift your fear into curiosity, bridging the gap between fear and transformation.

If the client loses the capacity to meet fear like the Deer, the facilitator assumes the role of relating calmly to a client's monsters, reassuring the client of their safety. Therapists must have a strong understanding of the substances they're administering and the realms into which they usher journeyers, for without this knowledge, they risk fearing the client's monsters. Doing so would further convince the client something bad is happening, which wouldn't end well for anyone.

As educator Janis Phelps outlined in her seminal 2017 article on guidelines for training psychedelic guides, facilitators must cultivate a competency of "empathetic, abiding presence." Such presence involves "composure, evenly suspended attention, mindfulness, empathetic listening, 'doing by non-doing,' responding to distress with calmness, and equanimity."[11] This may sound simple, but maintaining such quality of presence requires practice, especially in today's era of infinite distraction residing in our purses and pockets.

As therapists help clients face shadowy unconscious material, clients initiate retrieval of their fragmented parts. The ego's borders expand to include the monster, which had previously sucked up intrapsychic energy through the ego's perpetual effort to keep it submerged.

As it's incorporated into the psyche, the monster often changes forms. Perhaps the angry ogre pounding at the door morphs into a crying child frightened from being left alone in the dark. Perhaps the dementor flying toward you becomes the visualization of a bad habit that drains your life force. Whatever it may be, such transformations often endure, for the clarity of the monster's true form becomes a memory one can access whenever it flares up.

How Do We Measure Healing?

Our contemporary version of the Newtonian-Cartesian paradigm prizes evidenced-based approaches over practices labeled "alternative." To find reliable evidence—or at least *convince* yourself you have—the paradigm requires tools and measurements. In terms of healing, these must extend beyond personal anecdotes; otherwise, every self-help author claiming they hold the key to being awesome would be valid, including the crooks pining for your cash. We view subjectivity as flimsy and unreliable, the opposite of scientific proof. Psychology has thus developed a cornucopia of assessments to measure inner conditions, and positive patterns of results over time are interpreted as evidence of healing.

It can be helpful to track changes and discover patterns, but these assessments can be harmful when regarded with a preexisting inclination toward linearity. Dogmatic linearity will interpret nonlinearity—e.g., a client scoring lower on a depression rating scale after a month of psychotherapy—as "proof" of regression, failing to recognize a client's heavier state could be related to their arriving at a well of sorrow needing attention.

On the other hand, a client's improvement on the scale may not indicate healing, but rather a suppression of symptoms. By these measures, getting a lobotomy and feeling nothing would score better than going through a spiritual crisis on the threshold of transformation. Although assessments are the current standard in psychological research, they are not the ultimate determinant of healing.

This ties into something psychiatrist, researcher, and MAPS therapist Scott Shannon once told me: psychedelic therapies are *evocative* approaches to healing, starkly contrasting the *suppressive* models long dominating the field. As evocation invites expansion, suppressed symptoms are likely to surface. This can feel overwhelming and infuriating, for who seeks therapy to feel worse?

Sixteenth-century Spanish priest San Juan de la Cruz was aware of nonlinearity when he laid out the stages of the Dark Night of the Soul. This essential phase of the spiritual journey is characterized by an intense loneliness amounting to cosmic abandonment, stranding the soul in heart-wrenching hopelessness. To San Juan, such abandonment may be an indication that one is straddling the threshold of a profound breakthrough, so long as they don't succumb to ongoing despair. Assessments score psychological upheavals negatively, but they can be necessary for growth.

The healing journey often requires a terrifying and risky descent to reach the desired conclusion. As depicted in The Tower card of the Tarot, the structures of the ego collapse. Painful as it may be, the fall is necessary for progression into the light of the next card, The Star, emblematic of optimism, balance, and renewed faith.[*]

This notion is essential to an underground LSD therapist I interviewed, whom I'll refer to as Jordan. For over five years, Jordan, a trauma-informed practitioner, has facilitated high-dose LSD journeys—around 400 to 600 micrograms, enough to obliterate one's sense of anything tangible. Jordan explained

---

[*] For anyone seeking a map for their healing journey, the Tarot is an invaluable resource. The twenty-two cards of the Major Arcana chart the soul's progression from outset (The Fool) to wholeness (The Universe), evoking numerous ups, downs, twists, and turns along the way.

that as helpful as MDMA is in healing PTSD, it is less effective than LSD in healing *developmental* trauma of early childhood. Such wounds take hold before one is even conscious, molding their personality into shapes they end up regarding as their essential self.

"It's different than veterans, rape victims, or first responders," Jordan explained. "It's for very early childhood trauma, potentially prenatal birth, which means we have to find ways to reach those early places where the consciousness was formed and experienced trauma. Since they had no chance to process it, that trauma is still stuck in the body."

Jordan has found that high LSD doses facilitate regression into early, traumatized states, opening the opportunity for compassionate contact with repressed material to meet the unmet needs at the core of the wound. "The therapist plays the role of the primary caregiver, usually that of the mother," Jordan said. "Some of my clients, for the first time, experience unconditional love and acceptance."

An LSD dose of this size all but guarantees ego death, ushering people back to preconscious developmental stages. "Very often in the medicine sessions, the clients reexperience their birth or early childhood. They become like vulnerable little babies. From there, the restructuring of the identity begins."

Jordan understands the importance and difficulty of restructuring identity. She requires her clients to commit to a lengthy integration process with her to rebuild new ego structures. "It's normally a two-year process before the client can experience some fundamental shift in their way of being," she said. "The processing and integration create a new way of being, like putting the client together again in a more nourishing constellation. It's like hitting the restart button. I respect the process so much that I introduce extra levels of responsibility and safety."

After the LSD session, Jordan's clients tend to feel worse than before. The ego doesn't always die easily, especially for those unaccustomed to considering their core nature may be different from what they believed. As a result of the lengthy support Jordan provides, her clients undergo rebirth into a healthier identity. "Everybody I have ever worked with went through something like a new evolution, a new development. Each one of them flew away with strong, solid, confident wings. But it takes time."

If you've been suppressing your depression, anxiety, or trauma and decide to amplify it on a psychedelic, there may be no way around contacting the underlying pain. A good therapist will support you through the contact rather than leaving you marooned to figure it out alone, helping you pendulate into the pain and widen your capacity to feel it without becoming overwhelmed.

Suppressive approaches narrow the capacity to feel, promoting defense mechanisms to repress rising difficulties. A skilled therapist helps you integrate the accessed emotions into an expanded identity built on acceptance over avoidance, promoting a cohesive sense of self in place of an endless internal war. It may be difficult to get there, but sometimes, difficulty indicates you're heading in the right direction.

Healing Through Feeling

So much emotional healing relies on feeling things we exert great effort to block. I'm not talking about the blips of pleasure and disappointment we routinely encounter throughout our days. I'm talking about something bigger, like when the perfect song in the perfect moment floods you with memories and emotions, and you're crying without knowing why, unsure whether you want to crawl into a hermit hole or sing like Céline Dion.

Late in the process of writing this book, a generous friend gifted me and my wife some mescaline. I had been intrigued by it for over a decade but never had the chance to try it. We each took 300 milligrams, and after two mild hours, I listened to the Mozart album I'd listened to on repeat while reading philosophy in the Australian sculpture park of my psychedelic initiation. Moments later, I started weeping. The tears continued, and in the pit of my stomach I felt the grief of being so far removed from the innocence, peace, and intellectual exuberance I'd felt so fully in 2009. My mind drifted through memories of childhood friends with whom I had lost contact, and I felt myself pining for the joy we shared playing Nintendo 64 and the excitement we felt shooting bottle rockets on the Fourth of July. In my absorption in work, stress, and fear, I had become alienated from the vitality that animated those days of bliss, and I wept for the pressures of life that push and pull us away from the endless wellspring of exuberance in the deep heart's core.

It was difficult, but the mescaline connected me with love and acceptance. My wife offered support, helping me deepen contact with the void I'd been repressing due to my need to be productive. I did not experience a blissful resolution when the mescaline's effects subsided, but the following day, I noted a sense of peace I had not felt in many months. It was as if something I had been holding left my body with the tears, and I felt closer to the innocence whose loss I had grieved. Life's beauty shone around me once again.

How many moments do we dedicate to feeling *less*? What habits, thought patterns, and substances do we use to filter our emotions and protect ourselves from heartbreak?

Many blame society and capitalism, which offers mirages as solutions while churning the cycles of longing upon which it profits. Perhaps there's validity to this perspective, but these systems work because we participate in them. What gets lost in the blame game is the part around how challenging it is to be human. Much of therapy's work is uncovering ways our systems adapted to survive a hostile world, realizing how these adaptations stifle us, and healing what lies beneath them. Such healing is not about thinking our way out of pain; it is about opening our hearts through walls of protection and feeling all there is to feel. When we turn away from our pain, inner blocks dam the river of emotions, leaving a reservoir trapped inside.

Internal Family Systems

The Internal Family Systems (IFS) therapeutic model conceives of the psyche as a multiplicity of *parts*. As these parts live under the same roof, they operate like a family, complete with the special kinds of conflicts whose roots stretch deeper than anyone can see.

Family therapist Richard Schwartz began developing IFS in the 1980s. It is now taught to therapists and coaches throughout the world, and it's more popular than ever due to how seamlessly it pairs with psychedelic therapy.

Our parts fall into two overarching categories: *protectors* and *exiles*. Protector parts are similar to psychoanalytic defense mechanisms. They take over when something threatening arises, like the pain of a traumatic memory. The protective subcategory of "manager" parts might keep us busy at work to avoid the pain, whereas "firefighter" parts resort to more extreme measures, suppressing pain through harmful behaviors like substance abuse or binge eating. Managers try to maintain regulation in the system, and firefighters react when regulation is disturbed. Both keep parts called exiles sealed away at all costs.

Exiles typically develop at a young age and carry our deepest wounds. If a child's parent, for instance, punished them for crying, the child will develop parts to manage the sadness they feel in order to avoid punishment. But part of them still wants to cry, and this part becomes exiled by the inner system. When something evokes the exile, the protective system takes over to block the individual from having to reexperience the breadth of emotional pain.

Through the lens of parts, we act in ways developed to help us cope with suffering. As there are often better ways of coping than whatever strategies our parts develop, IFS therapy focuses on relieving our parts of the "burdens" they carry and giving them new roles conducive to well-being. Unburdening transpires in connection with the last major concept of IFS, the *Self*. For Schwartz, the Self is our essence, present within us before any part became burdened, accessible no matter how significant our struggles become. When we meet our exiles from a "Self-led" place, we can heal them.

To help people access "Self-energy", Schwartz delineated eight primary qualities of the Self, all of which begin with the letter "C": calmness, connection, compassion, creativity, clarity, curiosity, confidence, and courage. When clients feel centered in one or more of these qualities, IFS therapists recognize them as Self-led, and the unburdening process can ensue.

I spoke to Schwartz about his model and why it pairs so well with psychedelic therapy. "Different psychedelic medicines access different C-words, it seems," Schwartz explained. "With MDMA, you stay in your body and enter a state of utter compassion, calm, and sometimes courage. It's a long, many-hour journey, and a lot of healing work can be done because you're in Self for so long. With ketamine, you're in a unity space of pure Self, and you feel *connected* with everything. People come back with a different perspective about life and death and who they really are, because they get out of the container of their bodies and realize that there is more to who they are. That happens also with psilocybin, which is why it's so useful for end-of-life experiences, because you realize that death is just a transition into a bigger field."

The capacity of psychedelics to connect people to Self is another way of saying they invite the inner healer forward. When I asked Schwartz if this connection was valid, he replied, "Yes. That's all it is. Exactly."

Michael Mithoefer of MAPS was one of the first therapists to recognize the intersection between IFS and psychedelic therapy. He told me about an MDMA session he and his wife Annie facilitated for an Iraq veteran. "At the end of the day, she talked about a part of her that hated her so much. That's why she had to keep the good parts hidden. We asked how she knew this part hated her so much, and she said, 'Because it tells me all the time.' We said, 'Can we talk to that part?' This angry part then came out and said, 'I'm never going to let her get better, asswipe'—that's what the part called me. 'You think you're so smart, but you should have picked a different veteran, because she deserves to suffer forever, and I'm never going to let her get better.' That was the beginning of our work with the angry protector. It was very intense, and it was a long process, but it was ultimately very healing."

A full unburdening process can transpire during a psychedelic session. When this must continue after the effects wear off, IFS can be a tool for integration. Perhaps the psychedelic made you aware of a part of yourself (e.g., an anxious part) that you'd believed defined your identity ("I'm just an anxious person"). Integration occurs through dialoguing with that part from a Self-led perspective. If one then follows the modality's "healing steps," one can understand why the part does what it does, relieve the part of the burdens it carries, and facilitate its positive integration into the psyche. The result will be a reduction in intrapsychic conflict and greater overall balance.

Psychedelics bring the risk of evoking an exiled part the individual is unprepared to encounter. Mithoefer explained, "One of the advantages of MDMA is it can help relax the protectors. People are able to approach their trauma without either emotionally numbing or avoiding it. One of the dangers is the same thing. It'll relax the protectors, and the protectors will feel like they've been bypassed. One of the most important things we teach in our therapy training is to pay special attention not to override protectors. We're never going to push people to go anywhere they're not ready to go or to do anything they're not ready to do."

When relaxed protectors reconstitute after contact with exiles, they may grip the inner wheel with added fervor, rigidifying the psyche through "*backlash*". If backlash occurs, IFS can help people recognize that though they feel worse, they are not necessarily moving backward in their healing. Working with such inner conflict can yield greater understanding of our parts' dynamics. But when the parts of focus are particularly burdened, such as exiles carrying the shame of sexual trauma, it's best to enlist the support of an IFS-trained therapist. Inviting such support into your life after a challenging journey embodies the essential healing component of caring for yourself.

Self-Care

When we get particularly twisted up inside, it is impossible to focus past the unpleasantness. We use tools of distraction like social media and television to reduce the inner conflict's intensity, knowing it's a bandage through which the underlying wound will bleed. But this distraction is different from focusing on important external phenomena, such as one's daily tasks or a loved one after a difficult encounter.

Strife overtakes our emotional bandwidth, and no act of force or intoxication can quite pull us over the hump of inertia. In a sense, one of the most intrusive conditions is excessive indulgence in personal pain, for it facilitates self-absorption to an all-encompassing degree. "You're never so centered on yourself as when you're depressed," wrote Jesuit priest Anthony de Mello in his classic book, *Awareness*. "You're never so ready to forget yourself as when you are happy. Happiness releases you from self. It is suffering and pain, misery, and depression that tie you to the self."[12]

That's not to pass judgment on those who find themselves in a self-indulgent bind. Change is seldom as simple as a sudden choice, despite the message of that annoying song from *Frozen*. The traps of self-indulgence, which can feel irresolvable, are conditions psychedelics can treat, for few of their infinite possible effects garner more agreement than their ability to get people "out of their heads." Self-indulgent booby traps are temporarily released, rekindling the possibility of shifting one's circumstances in propitious directions.

These notions underscore an important point: prioritizing personal healing isn't selfish—and if it is, this form of selfishness isn't *bad*. Many of us have inherited the distorted moral principle that ignoring our inner strife for the sake of helping others is superior to seeking help we need. The most merciless of such burdens implies seeking personal help amounts to *weakness*. While looking beyond yourself can be helpful, it becomes a thorn in the side when it's predicated on denying personal struggles. When we prioritize personal wellness, we strengthen our ability to help others rather than trying to force compassion out of an ongoing struggle raging within.

It's important not to confuse self-care with unhealthy self-indulgence. Pleasurable activities may factor into self-care, but excess pleasure-seeking has destructive consequences. You can delude yourself into thinking binge-watching reality TV while drinking wine and eating ice cream for three months straight after getting fired from your job is self-care, but after a certain point, it's probably not helping. Self-care calls for awareness of what serves your well-being, the most important of which can't be reduced to instant gratification. Perhaps what best supports your happiness and peace is more difficult to choose than transient indulgences. Choosing such things anyway is choosing to respect and nourish your heart. If renewed prioritization of self-care is the only thing that comes from your psychedelic experience, then you have had a successful journey, indeed.

Ecopsychology and the Garden of Eden

The field of ecopsychology developed on the premise that mental illness is rooted in disconnection from nature, one another, and ourselves. The healing that arises through reestablishing these connections is essential to shift the collective patterns churning broken social systems and environmental degradation.

Western culture wires us for disconnection. As children, we are taught to create personas to navigate society, learning behaviors that get rewarded with acceptance and opportunity. As we grow accustomed to presenting our personas to the world, our authenticity stews in doldrums of disconnection, and we don't realize how much turmoil disavowing our essential nature causes. Because culture shames expression of certain parts, we mistake "maturity" for an imagined state wherein our "immature" parts have been eradicated. In reality, our disconnection from our layered facets perpetuates suffering in what the great writer David Foster Wallace called "our tiny skull-sized kingdoms, alone at the center of all creation."[13]

We learn to numb the pain. We simultaneously crave the sense of connection we felt as children and fear the vulnerability such connection requires, romanticizing the past as early days of innocence in the Garden of Eden before the snake of temptation fooled us into banishment. Life becomes a trial of redemption in hope of regaining admittance.

Poetic as it may sound, I consider this a misreading of the Old Testament origin myth. I see the Garden of Eden story not as a linear tale of causality and consequences, but rather as an allegory expressing the enduring human sense of "having had and lost some infinite thing," to quote Wallace again.[14] Rather than expressing hopeless abandon, the myth suggests the titration between primordial connection and burdened isolation, the recurrence of which suggests its acultural inherence.

Maybe the Garden of Eden is less a myth about the beginning of humanity than an evocation of humanity's core wound: loss of innocence and safety, abandonment, and ensuing despair. This wound expresses itself through the mysterious emotion of nostalgia. Nostalgia can become associated with loss and regret, but it can also widen the lens of consciousness to broader processes of life. Although part of us may live in exile, another part resides in the Garden, accessible in all moments no matter how much significance we ascribe to our banishment In lieu of my aforementioned mescaline experience, I believe it has unqiue potential to reconnect us to the Garden of Eternity.

The harms of dogmatic linearity reappear, for even in the religious contexts wherein this myth is typically presented, *eternity* is taught to signify every moment of the infinite forward-moving line of time. Eternity is no such thing. After all, clock-based, chronological time hadn't even been invented when the Garden myth was purportedly written.*

In *Tractatus Logico-Philosophicus*, philosopher Ludwig Wittgenstein followed a progression of propositions as linear and mathematical as one could imagine before concluding eternity exists as an immersive presence that no words, concepts, or logical propositions can describe. The ineffable importance of such a state prompted Wittgenstein's closing assertion: "Whereof we cannot speak, thereof we must remain silent."[14]

A common feature of the mystical experience is a sense of timelessness. As one apprehends profound expansiveness, linear time disappears. William James

---

* The Garden of Eden myth, and the rest of the Torah, is believed to have been written around the 7th century BCE. The first mechanical clocks didn't appear until the 14th century CE.

described the *noetic* quality of mystical experiences, where a felt sense of meaning and value requires no scientific proofs to confirm the apprehended truth as more fundamental than anything previously perceived. The mystic gazes in awe at the *mysterium tremendum*, an immanence whose sublime magnitude causes the soul to tremble, resuscitating the Garden from the depths of forgotten Being. As such, Original Sin refers less to a fundamental, inescapable flaw than the tendency of habits and cravings to keep us ignorant of our ability to apprehend sacredness *right now*, no matter which culture or epoch frames the moment.

Poet William Blake channeled these notions in *Songs of Innocence and Experience*. His poems in the first half express the facets of innocence, while the second half express the turmoil of its aftermath. If we read Blake's book linearly, banishment from the Garden would appear inescapable and dualistic. If we see the book as a mirror of an inherent *yin-yang* panoply of life's possibilities, the songs of innocence and experience coexist in eternity.

Mescaline and the Garden

Mescaline journeys don't take people to strange, otherworldly dimensions as much as connect them to what's in front of them. I imagine Nietzsche would have appreciated it, for the mustachioed German philosopher tore down the religious yearning for a *better place* to point readers' attention toward the bounty of the present. The Garden is not an imagined afterlife; it is all around us, calling for recognition, appreciation, and care.

The evening after my mescaline trip, I went to a Flogging Molly concert. About halfway through the Celtic punk band's set, I noticed my anxiety. Realizing I had been unconsciously fighting it, I welcomed it instead. Nothing changed immediately, but a short while later, the fog of my preoccupations evaporated, and I saw the immanence of my surroundings. Everything was happening now. I was still living, perceiving, and loving the heck out of this precious life. It had been years since I had seen things so clearly, but I felt as if no time had passed at all. Worries, stress, and anxiety had led me to forget how miraculous each moment is, and mescaline's healing magic helped me remember that the Garden of Eternity always was, is, and ever shall be.

Ibogaine and Practical Integration

"People are going back and forth across the doorsill
where the two worlds touch.
The door is round and open.
Don't go back to sleep."

—Rumi, "A Great Wagon"

Like psilocybin and mescaline, ibogaine was isolated in a lab from a plant medicine consumed ceremonially hundreds, if not thousands of years before beakers and Bunsen burners were invented. Its host is neither cacti nor fungi, but a shrub called *Tabernathe iboga* endemic to West-Central Africa.

Ibogaine was first isolated from the shrub in 1900 by French explorer Édouard Landrin, who named the alkaloid and published his extraction method with fellow explorer Jan Dybowski the following year.[1] In the 1930s, it gained popularity in France as a mental and physical stimulant, and in the 1960s, Chilean psychiatrist and psychedelic therapy pioneer Claudio Naranjo studied its therapeutic potential.* The first total synthesis of the compound came in 1966 through Swiss chemist George Büchi at MIT. His timing was bad, given the government-versus-hippie context of the mid1960s. Of all the psychedelics in this book, ibogaine holds the record for shortest gap between synthesis and criminalization with a whopping one year before the

---

* Naranjo referred to ibogaine as an "oneirogen," drawing from the Greek word meaning "dream" due to the rich imagery it evoked. (Source: Jonathan Freedlander, "Ibogaine: A Review of Contemporary Literature," MAPS, accessed January 21, 2024, maps.org/research -archive/html_bak/ibogaine.html.)

US government banned it in 1967, clearing the path for Nixon's Schedule I branding iron in 1970.[2] But sure enough, ibogaine eventually reentered the lab, where it quickly made waves in revival psychedialogues.*

Addiction and Neurodegenerative Disease

Amid its continued illegality in most Western nations, clinics around the world—notably in Mexico—administer ibogaine to individuals suffering from treatment-resistant addiction, particularly to opiates like heroin and fentanyl. While the trip can be long and harrowing, results are often profound. A 2017 study at a clinic in New Zealand, where ibogaine is legal, found twelve of fourteen participants exemplified "sustained reduction and/or cessation of opioid use" after a single ibogaine treatment.[3] Most of these participants were addicted to methadone, a drug ironically prescribed to help people wean off a different substance.

According to testimonies, ibogaine provides lasting relief from craving and withdrawal symptoms. It is theorized to repair the brain's dopamine "reward system," which addiction throws out of whack. As such, it's been labeled a "psychoplastogen," a class of drugs that rapidly and significantly affect the malleability of the brain's interconnectivity.† A landmark UC Davis study from 2018 found that noribogaine, the substance's primary psychoactive metabolite, induced neurogenesis in the brains of rats, promoting growth of new neurons for increased interconnectivity and functionality.‡

---

*   This term, defined as "dialogues about psychedelics," was invented a few seconds ago by your author, who hopes it will catch on.

†   More specifically, ibogaine promotes structural and functional neuroplasticity. Structural neuroplasticity refers to the physical growth of new neurons and repair of damaged ones. Functional neuroplasticity concerns the communication between cells and the brain's capacity to assign damaged areas' functions to undamaged areas. Psychoplastogens like ibogaine—and also ketamine, DMT, and LSD—catalyze both.

‡   More specifically, ibogaine catalyzed neuritogenesis, the phenomenon of *neurite* growth. Neurites are tiny protrusions from developing neurons that become dendrites and axons, which link up with dendrites and axons of other cells to send and receive information. If dendrites and axons are arms, the *dendritic spines* are the hands. Noribogaine was shown to promote dendritic spine density, helping more neurons join the millions of others holding hands and singing "Kumbaya."

The dopamine-repair theory suggests ibogaine specifically targets neurons damaged through addiction. If the theory proves valid, ibogaine holds paradigm-shifting promise in treating not only addiction but neurodegenerative diseases. Currently, most neurodegenerative diseases, like Parkinson's and Alzheimer's, have no known cure—we struggle even to slow them down.

The neurodegenerative application remains speculative. Clinical trials are in their infancy, with one animal study at Columbia University underway. There are, however, anecdotes of individuals suffering from Parkinson's who experience borderline-miraculous reductions in symptoms after taking ibogaine. One example came from a man who called himself "Patient D." At the age of 71, Patient D, a photographer and writer, was diagnosed with Atypical Parkinson's, which differs from Parkinson's through its lack of involuntary tremors amid a common disturbance of motor skills. Two years later, Patient D traveled to a medical center in Rosarito, Mexico, where he took two small ibogaine doses every day for a month.

Within two weeks, Patient D noticed something amazing: he could again use his fingers to pick up objects. By the end of the month, he could even button his shirts. For the first time in years, he could eat independently, climb stairs, and write. After the treatment concluded, he continued taking small doses, and his symptomology continued to improve. His testimony caught the attention of pharmacologist Susanne Cappendijk, and after she presented Patient D's case at the New York Academy of Sciences conference in 2015, ibogaine's neurodegenerative healing potential attracted medical interest.[4]

If ibogaine proves capable of reversing—even slowing—the onset of conditions like Parkinson's, it will provide perhaps the most significant medical psychedelic application, healing a history of helplessness at the knees of some of the most devastating diseases humans face. I hope that happens. For now, we don't know, and so in case anyone is considering self-experimenting with ibogaine, you should know it brings more physical dangers than most psychedelics. Its effects on the cardiovascular system have been linked to numerous unintentional deaths. It reduces heart rate and blood pressure, posing significant risk to people with conditions like hypotension. High ibogaine doses have been correlated with seizures and temporary paralysis.

None of that gets at the psychological risks. Ibogaine has a reputation of being long-lasting and intense, ushering users into a dreamlike state and often keeping them there for more than twenty-four hours. If the dream becomes nightmare, you're going to want someone there to support the journey and its integration.*

Although integration has been mentioned throughout previous chapters, the time has come for a deep dive. Researchers claim integration is the essential component differentiating psychedelic therapy from recreational use, morphing a memorable psychedelic experience whose impact fades over time into a linchpin of enduring transformation. If the psychedelic session is surgery on a broken bone, integration is the physical therapy and shift in habits that continue the healing process and ensure the break doesn't recur. Think, again, of Sam, the retired Navy SEAL. Each time he craved a beer, his integration involved saying, "No." Through this new habit, Sam kept his psychedelic insights alive.

Healing as a Participatory Process

In a culture filled with advertisements for products and programs promising rapid and lasting results with little effort, it's hard not to become hardwired to seek the "magic pill." *Hurry! Act now, before it's too late!* yell the speedy forces of capitalist urgency. We want results, and we want them now—especially when we're paying good money like with psychedelic therapy.

Inevitably, media coverage of psychedelic therapy trials focuses on the "miracle cure" quality of the treatment. Such narratives construct a perception that psychedelic therapy—if not psychedelics themselves—will instantaneously blast your pervasive issues to smithereens and transform you into an awesome, well-adjusted, fulfilled human. These unrealistic expectations block clients' healing processes, for they project what *should* be happening onto what *is* happening. Further, this thin construct sells passivity. People are asked to dish out a few thousand bucks, show up, and then *wow . . . major depressive disorder out the window! Farewell, treatment-resistant PTSD!*

---

* These psychological dangers correspond more with higher doses than the microdoses Patient D was taking. If researchers verify the validity of his claims, people will be able to improve their neurodegenerative conditions without needing to pass through an overwhelming gauntlet of otherworldly imagery.

Unfortunately, it's rarely this simple. While passivity is appropriate for surrendering to the process in psychedelic sessions, integration requires more than showing up at an office and swiping your Visa. Integration is a participatory process, and one's intentional engagement is a critical component of shifting one's conditions in a lasting way. This entails doing the practical, less-alluring-than-tripping work of applying lessons to the daily grind.

Imagine someone—I'll call him Guy—drifting through complex and layered imagery of an ibogaine journey when his "inner critic" chokes out the imagery and scolds, *You're doing drugs, now? You pathetic fool!* Guy notices a sharp and familiar pain in his back, and from his ibogaine-induced vantage point, he senses his critic lives in the back pain. With the help of his therapist, Guy realizes this critic he's unconsciously accepted as a fundamental part of himself sounds strikingly like his fourth-grade basketball coach, Mr. T. A long-forgotten memory materializes. Guy resists, and his back throbs, but the memory breaks through. Guy relives his young, shy self asking for a water break during wind sprints on a sweltering afternoon. Mr. T yells, *Suck it up, fool! Weakness don't belong on my A-team!* As punishment, Mr. T forced Guy to run extra sprints while the team watched, and Guy endured such humiliation he had to find strength he hadn't known he had to force his tears away.

Rather than seeing his back pain as his enemy, Guy hears it communicating an internalized narrative that began with his bullying coach. This narrative forbids Guy from speaking about his pain lest he admit to being the "weak fool" he'd feared he was. Challenging as it is to vocalize this, Guy trusts his therapist and processes the memory. Allowing long-repressed tears to flow with the music's crescendo, Guy feels the cathartic release of recognizing he is more than the harsh voice dominating his inner world. Once all his tears have been shed, Guy is amazed to discover his back pain has disappeared.

What a happy ending! Shifts like this are common in psychedelic therapy, and they're helping psychologists understand the interrelatedness of mind and body. While the media's version might end there, Guy's story continues.

The next week at work, Guy finds himself reveling in the clarity of a psychedelic afterglow, ecstatic his back pain and brutal inner critic have been vanquished. Eating dinner with his partner, Gal, Guy feels uncommon levity.

He's certain his problems are over—until the following week, when Guy wakes up from a sharp pain in his back. He panics. He tries to calm down, but the pain worsens, and panic grows. For the first time since the session, Guy hears the dreaded inner voice: *What did I tell you, fool? You're pathetic!* Guy reminds himself he needn't identify with inner Mr. T, but it doesn't help. Guy's struggle makes Mr. T stronger, and after an hour of sparring, Guy succumbs to hopeless certainty the pain he thought ibogaine cured will never end.

Unfortunately, it's no surprise Guy's symptoms returned. His insights were profound, but he enacted no change in his routine. He didn't actively participate in the process beyond the ibogaine journey, and the familiarity of external conditions reconstituted familiar patterns.

Have you ever returned to your childhood home and found yourself acting like a child? Familiar settings elicit habitual responses. If you don't actively shift at least something in your life, whatever has long interrupted your well-being will almost certainly return. Changes need not be seismic. They call for intentionally and consistently breathing life into the trip's lessons while unpacking what remains to be discovered.

Projecting desire for a rapid, effortless cure-all reduces psychedelic healing to imbibing the right chemical in the right setting. It champions convenience and bypasses the importance of discernment and discipline. While some people undergo lasting transformation after a single psychedelic session, such results usually require dedication. I'm not talking about passive dedication, like religiously streaming the hot new show everyone's buzzing about. Dedication can't come through the self-deception of telling yourself you're committed because you're seeing a therapist occasionally while doing 100% of the things you know hold you back. Transformation lasts when we rewrite the patterns that suck the soul into miserable wormholes. If psychedelic sessions call for letting go of the wheel, integration calls for readjusting our grip to steer along a smoother trajectory.

On the other hand, it's not about flooring the inner Maserati down the open Autobahn. Deep wounds develop over long periods of time, solidified by repeated behaviors and recursive thoughts. These are unlikely to transform overnight. When we rush healing faster than the process calls for, we might as well race the Indianapolis 500 with a flat tire.

Commitment to healing calls for commitment to self-awareness, a dedicated habit of tuning into the inner world through one's method of choice, be it meditation, writing, weightlifting, hiking, or ceremonial magick. It entails engagement in a patient, mindful process of attuning to needs, cultivating self-compassion to meet them, and fostering connection.

When we buy into promises of rapid and painless healing, we set ourselves up to judge our obstacles. Psychedelics can make you conscious of how your pain has influenced things from the shadows, helping you feel emotions you've pushed away. It often takes a long time to feel you have *healed*, and such a result is unlikely to come without intentional integration.

Integration isn't fun, but without it, psychedelic journeys exist in state-specific bubbles with no connection to daily life. English writer, speaker, and Eastern philosophy popularizer Alan Watts famously wrote, "When you get the message, hang up the phone. For psychedelic drugs are simply instruments, like microscopes, telescopes, and telephones. The biologist does not sit with eye permanently glued to the microscope; he goes away and works on what he has seen."[5] Returning repeatedly to psychedelics without integrating is like picking up the phone, hearing the same message, and saying, "Nah." When one no longer feels the need to return to the phone, healing has likely transpired.

The Ferriss Method of Integration

Tim Ferriss has had a massive influence in many fields. He came to prominence with his 2007 bestseller, *The 4-Hour Work Week*, and when he launched his podcast *The Tim Ferriss Show* in 2014, his reach grew significantly, as his podcast became one of the most downloaded programs in the history of the medium.

From the early days of his show, Ferriss promoted psychedelic therapy. Now, he's one of the world's biggest funders of psychedelic research, having put millions of dollars toward MAPS, Johns Hopkins, and other organizations. He speaks openly about how psychedelics and plant medicines have aided his personal healing journey.

"I have had long-term, frequent bouts of depression that almost led me to commit suicide towards the end of college," Ferriss told me. "Many years later, eventually contending with childhood sexual abuse that I experienced from roughly age two to four, I tested many therapeutical approaches, many of which were helpful, but most of which were surface level. Psychedelics, broadly speaking, ended up being a completely life-altering tool that, for the first time, allowed me to grapple with some of these problems at the deepest layers. I was finally able to rewrite some of the dominant stories of my life."

Since Ferriss typically focuses on tools people can use to better their lives, it's no surprise he offered some of the most practical suggestions I'd heard on integration.* "I use the analogy of surgery and rehab," Ferriss said.† "Let's say you're having orthopedic knee reconstruction. If you don't do any rehab, you can end up worse off than you were before. You need to commit to rehab beforehand. You have support structures in place. You ask specialists about how you should prepare and understand the risks involved. If you want a good outcome, you take the rehab extremely seriously."

For athletically inclined folks, he related it to the Olympics. "If you go off the vault at high speed, and you're doing everything perfectly, and you fuck up the landing, you do not get a medal, and you're very likely going to injure yourself. The immediate landing is very important."

Ferriss emphasized that integration begins with preparation. "As soon as you commit to psychedelic-assisted therapy, your journey has begun. You can use that as a catalyst for other things that are beneficial toward the same end as the session itself."

---

*   I have to admit, I was thrilled when Ferriss agreed to an interview. He doesn't do them often. It was particularly meaningful to me because without his promotion of psychedelic therapy, I may never have learned about it in the first place. Through his podcast, he made me aware of Zendo Project, leading me to volunteer at Burning Man two years later. Serendipitously, when I showed up for my first shift at midnight, I got talking to the intensely present volunteer next to me, only to realize it was Ferriss, and we ended up sitting with guests in the same tent for hours. He was an important guide for me as I embarked on this journey, and through the interview, he held no pretension, regarding me with compassion and respect as he spoke from the heart. For readers who have also been influenced by Ferriss, my hour-long video chat with him demonstrated that he's the real deal, and his involvement in psychedelics is clearly rooted far deeper than financial interests.

†   Ferriss mentioned several times that he is not a psychedelic therapist or psychedelic scientist. He offered his perspective as himself, rather than as representative of an overarching institution or body of knowledge.

His preparation advice consisted of two key elements: reading Anthony de Mello's *Awareness* and developing a basic meditation practice.* Together, these help you become "a keener observer of your thoughts and states, so you can begin to differentiate between your thoughts and feelings and the consciousness that observes them."

Ferriss also advised keeping a journal dedicated to your journey, writing in it every day leading up to the journey, and recording impressions from the trip while they're fresh. "I would suggest reviewing your notes on a daily basis for at least the first week, and then every week for a few months afterward," he added.

Another layer of prehab is arranging for as much unoccupied, open time after the session as possible, pushing stress-inducing work tasks to the end of the week. "A lot of people will tell me, 'Tim, I just cannot block out that much time.' My answer is, 'Then maybe you shouldn't have major surgery,' because that answer is *bullshit*. It's a reflection of priorities. We don't *find* time for anything. We *make* time."

Ferriss relayed more specifics through personal experience. "For the first two days, I'll often spend as much time in nature as possible. If you provide the negative space for this, you will find a lot can unfurl, like tea leaves after a few steepings—not always, but frequently. As you're journaling on these things, some of the insights that you come to are just as valuable, if not more valuable, than the insights you had in the psychedelic experience itself."

Aware that psychedelic excitement can obscure their potential for harm, Ferriss added, "I know people who have taken prep and integration seriously and have had one experience that has fundamentally changed their lives. I also know reckless, New-Age folks who do ayahuasca every fucking weekend but can't do their taxes or re-register their car to save their lives. In terms of stability and mental health, the latter group are the same, if not worse, than they were five years before. If you're going to induce massive neural plasticity and you do not take the on and off ramps seriously, you can do a lot of damage to yourself. For that reason, scientists like Roland Griffiths have

---

* He specifically recommended doing the introductory course on the *Waking Up* app created by meditation-enthusiast scientist and author Sam Harris. If this app is obsolete when you're reading this, I'm sure other apps, VR programs, or rooms in the Metaverse can teach you the basics.

metaphorically compared using psychedelics to using nuclear power. This is not a hot stove you simply burn a finger on. These are powerful tools that should be treated with far greater respect."

To summarize in Ferriss-esque bullet points:

- Commit to a psychedelic journey with plenty of time before the date
- Establish support structures
- Read Anthony de Mello's *Awareness*
- Practice mindfulness daily for at least a month beforehand
- Journal often, before and especially after the session
- Block out plenty of open time after the experience, ideally a minimum of 1–2 days
- Spend ample time in nature
- Review your notes often

These simple tools and tactics can make a seismic difference in the value you draw from a psychedelic journey. "If this sounds like a decent amount of work, you're right. It is," he said. "It's sexier to talk about the neon crocodiles that spoke to you in Sanskrit. It's not as sexy to talk about digging the ditches and laying the pipes afterward. The latter is critical."

Nature and Spaciousness

Ferriss spoke to one of the most common pieces of integration advice psychedelic therapists give: spend time in nature. It can sound trite, but if you're willing to take it seriously, you may discover there's a reason this advice is commonly given. Time spent in nature can reconnect us to the spaciousness the psychedelic provided. As Rumi famously wrote, "Out beyond ideas of wrongdoing and rightdoing, there is a field. I'll meet you there." Rumi's field is more expansive than anything to which dualistic categories give rise.

I'm no sociologist, but I'd wager my Nintendo Switch that most city-dwellers feel some degree of longing for spaciousness, as it's more akin to humanity's ancestral birthright than contemporary concrete jungles.

Western capitalist society neither offers spaciousness nor encourages people to find it, unless it's through expensive packages to exotic locations on cruise ships with three all-you-can-eat buffets and a drunk magician. People thus seek healing inside society's mechanistic structures, forgetting the healing potential waiting in less-familiar spaces. Comfortable and important as routine is, primordial *aliveness* can be revived in the rugged and wild unpredictability of the mountains and fields beyond the city's edges.

But many of us are busy, and spacious nature is not always accessible. If the city imprisons us, can we create spaciousness within ourselves without having to escape into nature? Can we feel the spaciousness of the universe in the comfort of our favorite armchair?

> "To see a World in a Grain of Sand
> And a Heaven in a Wild Flower,
> Hold Infinity in the palm of your hand
> And Eternity in an hour . . ."

So wrote William Blake in "Auguries of Innocence," beautifully illustrating the infinite spaciousness within all things. Infinity can be apprehended in the microscopic if one is willing to examine closely. Look no further than LSD for proof, as a few millionths of a gram can transport the mind into visions whose power would render Blake awestruck.

Through patience and commitment, we can cultivate our inner breadth in the face of the greatest pressure. Meditation can lift the weight of the world off our weary backs, launching it over the hills and far away. External spaciousness often helps relax our microcosmic concerns. Many astronauts have recounted their perspectives were forever changed when they saw Earth from outer space and realized how small, beautiful, and situated amid expansiveness our home is.

Or we can get so buried in our roles, responsibilities, fears, and neuroses that we wander through the Painted Desert immersed in worries of having made a mistake on our tax return. There's a famous scene in Stanley Kubrick's *The Shining* where Shelley Duvall stumbles upon the book Jack Nicholson has been writing at the Overlook Hotel. Page after page is filled with the sentence, "All work and no play makes Jack a dull boy." Nicholson took the job as the

Overlook's caretaker to write in the spaciousness of the mountains. But his inner world—and perhaps the spirits and memories occupying the hotel—didn't allow it. Inner density—the opposite of spaciousness—took hold, transforming Nicholson into a raving, axe-swinging loon.*

Psychedelics can curate access to inner spaciousness and corresponding playfulness, even amid the density of city life. Such expansiveness need not impede focus and productivity, both are important components of contemporary life. Creating a yin-yang of focus and space is the name of the psychedelic therapy game. In the space of the non-ordinary state, the therapist can help the client notice an arising image, memory, or sensation. What information and discoveries manifest when the client focuses on it from a spacious perspective? Clients can continue to cultivate this balance through practice, integrating spacious focus into the daily rigamarole.

As dense as life can feel, there's more space than the ego perceives. Quantum physics proved what Blake knew: within each microscopic molecule constructing the physical world exist subatomic particles flittering about in a vast expanse. As solid and dense as matter appears, spaciousness can be discovered beneath the surface.

Loving-Kindness

Plenty of public figures, from life coaches to podcasters quoting Marcus Aurelius, will tell you it's important to meditate, but what does that mean? "Meditation" (like "recreational" and "epic") is a vague term, and the unacquainted may feel so confused about where to begin that it doesn't seem worth trying. There are countless forms of meditation, and one in particular lends itself to psychedelic journeys and integration: metta, better known as "loving-kindness" meditation.

Christopher Germer, a forefront American meditation instructor and mindfulness-based psychotherapist, defined mindfulness as "awareness of present experience, with acceptance."[6] Simple as this definition sounds, it can be challenging to practice. How many aspects of inner and outer life do we struggle to accept?

---

*   Perhaps it's an extreme example, but it's a Stephen King story we're talking about, and King doesn't mess around when Native American burial grounds and creepy ghosts of racist White aristocrats are involved.

Maybe you've been injured. Maybe that injury prevented you from doing what you love, like biking or snowboarding or playing with your kids. Did you accept those limitations? Perhaps. But many of us—myself included—ruminate on how we could have prevented the injury, how life used to be better, and how crummy the discomfort and pain feels.

The pain is one thing; unwillingness to accept the pain turns it into suffering.

Crediting Buddhist teacher Shinzen Young with the formula, Germer defined suffering as pain multiplied by resistance. "That's a way of emphasizing the inevitability of pain in life," Germer told me. "But how we *relate* to pain has an enormous impact on how much we suffer in life. The good news is that when the conditions of our life are bad, it's not hopeless, because we can always change how we relate to our moment-to-moment experience."

The Buddhist concept of "second arrows" illuminates this idea. Say you feel a pain in your wrist like an arrow piercing you. You want the pain to go away. This resistance is a *second* arrow, adding suffering to your pain. In the Buddhist view, pain is inevitable, and suffering is optional. Self-compassion begins with awareness and acceptance of present experience, for such awareness helps us remove second arrows and focus on the first.

Germer emphasized that self-compassion is not self-*improvement*. Self-improvement is fighting to change and fix parts of ourselves we don't like; self-compassion is softening resistances and accepting the parts we believe are flawed.

Healing often requires more than becoming aware of our patterns. Awareness is a stepping stone, but if we are cognizant of our habitual ways of being while continuing to despise them, we will continue to suffer. After awareness comes reframing our relationship to ourselves with compassion and understanding.

This shift can be extraordinarily difficult. Many people learned to dislike themselves at an early age. Particular behaviors were judged, ridiculed, and punished, and they internalized a conclusion that they are "bad." Self-compassion is a practice of shifting such beliefs and recognizing their illusory nature.

"Research has shown self-compassion reduces emotional distress, anxiety, and depression. It improves relationships, enhances the functioning of the body, and improves immune system functioning," Germer explained. "We're discovering self-compassion is an underlying mechanism of positive change in psychotherapy."

No one hates themselves when they're born. Self-loathing is acquired, and self-compassion reconnects us to a birthright that negative self-talk obscures. *Metta* meditation does not end with focusing on the breath. It involves recitations focused on directing compassion toward oneself, and once one develops those capacities, they extend their compassion beyond themselves to encircle the world.

Bridging the Gap

Ibogaine may be powerful, but as with all psychedelics, it is unlikely to do all the work. If it does promote neural growth and repatterning, integration comes through engagement with activities and practices that continue nurturing neurogenesis. The days of scientists erroneously claiming brain cells cannot regrow have ended. In fact, neurogenesis has even been linked to doing new things, like changing an exercise routine, reading a perspective-shifting book, or learning to play an instrument.

The more we view psychedelics as panaceas, the less we place the processes they evoke in the expansive context of life itself. They are one piece of a procedure of transformation. The work of changing familiar habits can be boring and unpleasant, but integration is essential if a profound trip is to become more than a groovy time spent in a galaxy far, far away.

12

5-MeO-DMT and Nonduality

"There is a wealth of information built into us, with miles of intuitive knowledge tucked away in the genetic material in every one of our cells . . . And, without some means of access, there is no way to even begin to guess at the extent and quality of what is there."

—Alexander Shulgin, *PIHKAL: A Chemical Love Story*

5-*methoxy-N,N-dimethyltryptamine*, better known as 5-MeO-DMT, can be found in many plant species, but its most famous host is an amphibian: *Bufo alvarius*, the Sonoran Desert Toad. This toad, when frightened, secretes a venom potent in 5-MeO-DMT to ward off predators. I can neither imagine nor fathom how human beings discovered that collecting the venom, crystallizing it, and smoking the result yielded what is often regarded as the most powerful psychedelic trip in the known universe.

The origins of human consumption of Bufo—one of 5-MeO-DMT's nicknames—remains ambiguous. It's unknown whether the toad's venom has a history of Indigenous consumption, although dubious self-proclaimed shamans like Octavio Rettig[*] claim its use began with Neanderthals one hundred thousand years ago.[1] It's likely that the venom was first discovered in the mid-twentieth century.[†]

---

[*]   I refer to Rettig as "dubious" due to his controversial methods of Bufo facilitation, one of which involves Rettig pouring water into the mouths and nostrils of his intoxicated clients.

[†]   Then again, anthropologists have speculated that Bufo venom was used as a ritual intoxicant in ancient Mesoamerica, for toads featured prominently in the sculptures of the Aztecs, Mayans, and Olmecs—though many maintain their toad of worship was *Bufo marinus*, whose poisonous venom wouldn't even get you high. (Source: Andrew T. Weil and Wade Davis, "Bufo alvarius: a potent hallucinogen of animal origin," Journal of Ethnopharmacology 41, nos. 1–2, (January 1994), 1–8, doi.org/10.1016/0378-8741(94)90051-5.)

One of the earliest documents on Bufo is "Bufo Alvarius: The Psychedelic Toad of the Sonoran Desert," a 17-page pamphlet written by a mysterious individual who called himself "Albert Most." On his *VICE* show, *Hamilton's Pharmacopeia*, documentarian Hamilton Morris uncovered Most's identity as Kenneth Nelson, an independent researcher and environmentalist who'd tracked down the toad in Arizona during his twenty years living on a missile base in Denton, Texas. Decorating the text with iconic illustrations from artist Gail Patterson, Nelson self-published the pamphlet in 1983.

It begins, "Specialized multi-cellular glands concentrated on the neck and limbs of B. alvarius produce a viscous milky-white venom that contains large amounts of the potent hallucinogen, 5-MEO-DMT. When vaporized by heat and taken into the lungs in the form of smoke, its indole-based alkaloid produces an incredibly intense psychedelic experience of incredibly short duration. There is no hangover or harmful effect. On the contrary, a pleasant psychedelic afterglow appears quite regularly after smoking the venom of B. alvarius, the Psychedelic Toad of the Sonoran Desert."[2]

Nelson and Patterson's pamphlet sparked interest in Bufo, and the toad soon attained legendary status in the underground world of interested seekers. The molecule's history, however, precedes the pamphlet, for it was synthesized in 1936 by Japanese chemists Toshio Hoshino and Kenya Shimodaira. In 1959, the molecule was isolated from the seeds used in a South American snuff, revealing its presence in pre-Columbian Indigenous healing rituals.[3] There was even a California-based religious organization founded in 1971 called the Church of the Tree of Life for which Bufo was a sacrament until the church became defunct in the late 1980s. 5-MeO then became available through mail order until the government caught wind of it, and in 2011, 5-MeO-DMT joined the ranks of Schedule I psychedelics. In the years since, Bufo has been the subject of widespread research as a powerful therapeutic agent.

5-MeO-DMT–Assisted Therapy

Rafaelle Lancelotta is a leading researcher on 5-MeO-DMT's therapeutic applications. When I interviewed them in 2019, Lancelotta explained 5-MeO-DMT "can dissolve any ego or sense of self," inducing a sense of "*becoming* everything" rather than *observing* the experience from a removed vantage point. One's perceptual lens zooms out dramatically, transforming the mind into "pure consciousness" and bringing a sense of "inherent belonging to all the energy of the universe."[4] Bufo is characterized less by a visual journey than sensory overload. It can be blissful, overwhelming, or terrifying.

Lancelotta helped establish the foundation for 5-MeO research. In 2018, they co-conducted a survey study of 5-MeO-DMT users in "naturalistic group settings," another term for "not a therapy office." The results, published in 2019, pointed toward Bufo's safety and beneficial outcomes for depression and anxiety,[5] helping generate enthusiasm in the revival. A 2021 study from the Netherlands described as "the first formal prospective clinical study to investigate the safety profile of 5-MeO-DMT and its dose-related effects on states of consciousness" found their synthetic version produced safe and consistent "peak experiences" in volunteers.[6] Likewise, a 2022 study through the Feilding's Beckley Foundation published Phase 1 results demonstrating their intranasally administered molecule was well-tolerated, allowing them to launch Phase 2 studies of 5-MeO-DMT–assisted therapy for treatment-resistant depression and alcohol use disorder.

Like ibogaine and psilocybin, people are offering Bufo-assisted healing in countries where it's legal. Several Mexican clinics offering 5-MeO in retreat-like settings have become popular destinations for military veterans. In 2020, a retired Navy SEAL named "JL" published an article in *Psychedelics Today* about his experience at such a clinic. He'd been suffering from a traumatic brain injury and post-traumatic stress, and after his Bufo retreat, he recounted, "My brain works now, too. It's the strangest thing. Words flow. Thoughts sizzle. Synapses fire and I can discuss, read, think, and elucidate in ways I haven't been able to in at least fifteen years."[7]

JL's trip was funded by Veterans Exploring Treatment Solutions (VETS), a nonprofit founded in 2019 by Marcus Capone, a retired Navy SEAL, and his wife Amber. They were inspired to expand access after Marcus healed his crippling PTSD with ibogaine and 5-MeO-DMT. VETS supports veterans like JL with education, coaching, and funding for psychedelic retreats in countries where the substances are legal.

"These are not drugs," JL reflected. "This is powerful, *powerful* medicine and it has the potential to do enormous good. These are sacraments that require much of you and will bring you what you need and are prepared for."[8]

The Symbiosis of Culture and Worldview

Human history has been populated by thousands of cultures with thousands of unique systems of understanding themselves and the Cosmos, many of which have triumphed over the contemporary West in terms of cultural richness, quality of life, community bonding, and caring treatment of Planet Earth. Still, the West has a tradition of believing it occupies the peak of a historical hierarchy, priding itself as the cultural Übermensch beneath which all non-Western cultures reside.

The West's supreme focus on rationalism and objectivity has factored prominently into its collective disregard for "irrational" states, like those 5-MeO-DMT induces. The West has historically valued one way of seeing things, strictly enforcing a worldview whose supremacy mustn't be broken. When things threaten to break it—such as the strange realities psychedelics seem to reveal—they are aggressively banished. If someone reports feeling "absorbed in timelessness" on 5-MeO-DMT (which tends to obliterate all notions of linear time) and expresses their insight that timelessness is closer to the core of reality than linear temporality, the Western world replies, "You were on drugs. Get a job."

Past → Present → Future time is regarded as a constant, propelling us forward and affecting everyone equally. Never mind that it's been over sixty years since Einstein's Theory of Relativity demonstrated otherwise. Long before mechanical clocks were invented, there were no concepts of hours, minutes, and seconds. Time, measured in relation to the sky and seasons, was understood differently. After all, how different is your relationship with time when you're looking repeatedly at the clock and waiting for the workday to end compared to when you're surfing, kayaking, or gunnin' the Harley down the Pacific Coast Highway?

When I asked Jungian analyst Mackenzie Amara about integration, she evoked the two words the Greeks had for time: *Chronos* and *Kairos*. Chronos refers to the linear, chronological time that structures Euro-American culture. "That's the time of our rational minds," Amara said. "Yesterday's yesterday, tomorrow's tomorrow, and there's twenty-four hours in a day." But the Greeks, recognizing this picture was incomplete, gave the name Kairos to the time of being "in the underworld." Kairos is the time of dreams—and,

I'd speculate, psychedelic trips. Amara described Kairos as "a time of ripeness, a time of everything happening in its season." Chronos is the quantitative time of science, while Kairos is the time of qualitative experience.

Amara argued that a common struggle in psychedelic integration occurs when people attempt to translate their Kairos-time insights into Chronos-time daily life. People strive to apply kernels of wisdom derived from the trip to their lives without realizing the spaces in which those insights arose flow on a different time frame. "Integration means not knowing how long something is going to take," Amara said. "An insight might need to work us around and around until it's ripe, or until our ego is resilient enough to bring it forward."

Imagine you take a psychedelic, and at the peak intensity, you envision yourself at your highest level of fulfillment. You see yourself as happy, peaceful, and at ease as you stand resolutely in a leadership position, offering your gifts to whomever wants to pay attention. Clear as the vision may be, you're probably not going to become that person the next day. Creating those conditions could take months, years, or a lifetime. The desire for immediate deep and lasting transformation falls into a Chronos trap, blocking access to the deep time Kairos process where transformation may occur.

Those who equate time with clocks fail to recognize that things taken as self-evident are seldom so. We are all products of our era, unconsciously influenced by too many factors to count. The current world is no exception, regardless of its electric cars and rocket ships blasting billionaires into space. The boundaries of our worldviews are structured through our culture's language and symbolic systems of meaning. No matter how effectively we convince ourselves we occupy an objective vantage point, baseline conditions relative to our culture are hardwired into our brains.

In his foreword to Hofmann's *LSD: My Problem Child*, Grof argued that one of the major factors contributing to psychedelic criminalization in 1970 was the threat they posed to the linear thinking of "Newtonian-Cartesian science." Models and formulas drawn from Newton and Descartes could not account for the wild inner journeys people were describing, like traveling out of their bodies, communicating with their cells' mitochondria, or "reliving biological birth and memories of prenatal life, encounters with archetypal beings, and visits to mythological realms of different cultures of the world."[9] The nature of such experiences "seriously undermined the metaphysical assumptions concerning priority of matter over consciousness on which Western culture is built."[10] At a deeper level of meaning, psychedelics "threatened the leading myth of the industrial world by showing that true fulfillment does not come from achievement of material goals but from a profound mystical experience."[11]

Grof asserted it was due to these circumstances that "many professionals chose to stay away from this area to preserve their scientific world-view and to protect their common sense and sanity."[12] The scientific establishment's quickness to reject claims that threaten its premises has historically had a nasty way of reinforcing harmful viewpoints on the physical world and cultures who viewed life differently. In these days of social media algorithms designed to feed us information we already agree with, it's important to recognize the destructive consequences of living in an echo chamber, especially when our chambers become so normalized that we can no longer see their walls. As much as the contemporary West adulates science, when we regard it as the ultimate form of knowledge, it can construct as harmful an echo chamber as anything defined by overconfident and unyielding certainty.

Psychedelic Alchemy

In the centuries preceding test tubes and the periodic table, modern chemistry's roots were established through alchemy. These days, alchemy's common associations with witchcraft and fantasy reduces its reputation to an obsolete pseudo-science promulgated by old kooks who thought they could transform rocks into gold. To psychedelic pioneer Ralph Metzner—who, after his work with Leary and Alpert and at Harvard, wrote *The Toad and the Jaguar*, one of the pinnacle texts on 5-MeO-DMT—this viewpoint on alchemy represents a misconception. In a brilliant essay, Metzner pointed out that "the main focus of most alchemical practitioners was healing and what we would nowadays call psychotherapy: the transmutation of the physical and psychic condition of the human being."[13]

Alchemists aimed to transform base metals into gold, the ultimate goal of which was the creation of the "Philosopher's Stone," the key to the elixir of eternal life. To Metzner and many philosophers and occultists who came before him, the stone was a metaphor for psychological and spiritual transformation. Using the metaphor, the "base metal" alchemists sought to transform correlates to the crystallized state of a rigid mind, which modern psychology correlates with numerous ailments including depression, addiction, and OCD. A prevailing view on psychedelic therapy correlates its healing processes with a substance's capacity to break up rigidity of mind, body, and emotion. In this loosening, psychedelics can free people—at least temporarily—from their imprisonment within their fortified minds.

Twentieth-century British-American occultist Israel Regardie wrote that in the rigid mind, "all spontaneity of intellect and feeling is thoroughly eliminated from the realm of possibility. It is a sacrifice which entails the death of all that is creative within. The individual becomes enclosed within an iron cage of his own construction—forged through fear of life."[14] Such psychological *stupefaction* entails "the loss of all that the underlying and dynamic unconscious aspect of the psyche implies—warmth, depth of feeling, inspiration, and ease of life."[15] Stupefaction is the opposite of Aristotle's virtue of *eudaemonia*, often translated as "flourishing." Dogmatic rigidity barricades the free flow of the spirit, stubbornly refusing to budge no matter the pressure.

"It is with this rigidity of consciousness," Regardie wrote, "with this inflexible crystallized condition of mind, that alchemy, like modern psychotherapy, proposes to deal, and, moreover, eradicate."[16]

The alchemical process of disintegrating inflexible rigidity is known as *putrefaction*. Through dissolution, one can "reassemble the fundamental elements of consciousness on an entirely new and healthy basis."[17] If a house stands on an unsteady foundation, it doesn't help to caulk the cracks. Therapeutic methods that target symptoms (e.g., depressed thoughts) while ignoring causes amount to cognitive caulking. The transformation that interested the alchemists involves tearing down the house, restructuring the foundation, and building a new, solid structure conducive to flourishing.

Feilding edited a wonderful compilation of Hofmann's lectures on alchemy alongside alchemical writings of psychedelic thought leaders called *Hofmann's Elixir: LSD and the New Eleusis*. It was evident to Hofmann and Feilding that psychedelics such as LSD induced putrefaction to mirror that of the alchemical elixir. If used in proper contexts, LSD could reliably and safely break down stupefied structures of consciousness, opening the gateways to renewal.

Alchemical imagery can be found throughout Blake's poetry. The title of his Huxley-inspiring work—*The Marriage of Heaven and Hell*—expresses the alchemical notion of *coincidentia oppositorum*, the union of opposites, where seemingly polarized realities are joined in sacred unification. These notions fascinated Jung, who immersed himself in alchemy late in life, writing extensively on its psychological and spiritual implications. He interpreted the alchemical image of the *coniunctio*, the marriage of opposites, as the destination of the individuation process, signifying the psyche's reconstituted wholeness. As we define who we are, we implicitly define who we are *not*. The *not*, however, still lives within us, and the ego battles any desires, fantasies, or visions suggesting our identity may include that against which we have defined ourselves.

"In it [the unconscious] the opposites slumber side by side," Jung wrote. "They are wrenched apart only by the activity of the conscious mind, and the more one-sided and cramped the conscious standpoint is, the more painful or dangerous will be the unconscious reaction."[18]

The *coniunctio* requires the integration of inner opposites. Masculinity is balanced with femininity, light is balanced with dark, and consciousness is balanced with the unconscious in "syzygy," translated from Greek to mean "yoked together." The syzygy is the alchemical wedding, the *coincidentia oppositorum*, the achievement of making the unconscious conscious.

With psychedelics and alchemy, the putrefaction of "cleansing the doors of perception" makes the unconscious conscious. "Consciousness is to be vivified utterly and is not separated from the Unconscious by a sharp and unnatural cleavage or partition from the other levels of the psyche," wrote Regardie. "Thus the contents of the one part . . . have full access of entry into the other, and vice versa."[19] Such unification of opposites hinges on apprehending nonduality.

Nonduality

Nonduality has been a hallmark of spiritual realization since well before "Hallmark" was a greeting card manufacturer or "spiritual" a word. Nonduality refers to the state of consciousness wherein dualisms—or opposites—merge. Familiar dualisms include inner/outer, self/other, good/evil, and life/death. Because these dualisms appear fundamental to existence, they unconsciously structure our beliefs and perspectives.

In the nondual state, the boundaries between categories dissolve. In place of a rigid disposition, fluidity arises, and a sense of oneness holds the torch. Nondual awareness reveals oneness as the fundamental condition of reality, extending beyond the classifications through which we organize our perspectives.

Hinduism offers a nuanced illustration with its distinction between the concepts of *Atman* and *Brahman*. Atman refers to the individual self, whereas Brahman refers to "absolute reality," the highest universal principle. Nondual schools of Hinduism, like Advaita Vedanta, teach that *moksha*— liberation—is attained through recognizing the differentiation between Atman and Brahman has always been illusory. One realizes Atman is Brahman, and one's individual identity corresponds with ultimate, nondual reality.

Through a nondual lens, striving to escape suffering is doomed from the start, for the escape is conceived within the confines of the paradigm from which suffering arises. In other words, dualistic thinking separates us from our nondual essence, and amid the separation, we strive to cross the gap our dualistic thinking creates. Because the gap, like the separation, is essentially an illusion, we build illusions to solve illusory problems created by illusions. As Einstein is often said to have said, "No problem can be solved from the same level of consciousness that created it."

While most, if not all, psychedelics can dissolve rigid mental structures, each one does it in a unique way. In a sense, each psychedelic has a personality and experiential flavor, which plays into the abundance of nicknames and reputations each carries. High doses of psilocybin and LSD are typically regarded as challenging, if not brutal in their dissolution of structures, whereas MDMA and ketamine have a reputation of gently dissolving calcification amid a heightened sense of self-compassion.

At high doses of ketamine, nondual awareness is all but guaranteed. Speaking about his personal ketamine experiences, Schwartz, founder of IFS, told me, "On ketamine, you leave this world, you leave your body, and you enter a non-dual state that, for me, is pure Self. Self isn't something that's just in us. It's more like a field. When we can open space in our body, it can enter us, and there's no separateness. That's what I would enter when I would do ketamine."

As common as nondual states are to ketamine, they're even more common to 5-MeO-DMT. 5-MeO experiences are almost unanimously described as "ego-dissolving" to the extreme. One's sense of identity is obliterated, and consciousness fuses with the Universe-at-Large. Separations and boundaries between the individual self and ultimate reality no longer exist. Such an experience can be profoundly healing.

Presence, Acceptance, and Change

Returning to the experience of Sam, the retired Navy SEAL, I must point out that his psilocybin trip comprised only half of his story. The following day, he was offered 5-MeO-DMT, and his rollercoaster ride with Bufo made psilocybin seem like a carousel. Within seconds of inhaling, he felt like his consciousness had been shot into space. All notions of earthly existence imploded. With no idea what was happening, Sam felt terrified that if he relaxed and allowed it to take him where it wanted, he might die.

"I felt like every individual molecule of my body was floating away, and I was desperately trying to regain control of the situation, so I fought it the entire time," he said.

Sam remained in that space for what seemed like eternity until landing back in his body and asking the facilitator what the *hell* had just happened. He hesitated when he was offered the pipe a second time, but he knew if he didn't accept, he'd regret a missed opportunity. Channeling grit, determination, and courage, he drew an even bigger inhale than before, and again, he was blasted out of his body. The second time was even more excruciating.

Disoriented after returning to Earth, Sam gradually experienced a sense of serenity. He gazed out over a lake, and he realized that in stark contrast to his alcohol-centered life, he felt fully present and engaged with his surroundings. In such presence, he felt grateful to be alive.

As complex as Sam's Bufo journeys were, they resulted in something remarkably simple. The psilocybin and 5-MeO together showed him that life was not something to be numbed. Life was an impermanent, irreplaceable gift to be embraced. This realization was fundamental in his transformation, for whenever an impulse arose to drink, he imagined the lake and reconnected with the peaceful sense of having all he could possibly need.

When we reconnect to a deep sense of gratitude and peace, we realize the external world is not the source of our suffering. Suffering results from inner dynamics fogging up perception's windshield. At some point these dynamics and perceptions became more habitual than brushing your teeth. Although psychedelics take people on wild and wayward journeys, they often deliver them into potent states of well-being. A fresh experience of peace can be all people need to change.

Counterintuitive as it may seem, the process of change in psychedelics and alchemy comes down to a way of engaging with present material and infusing it with intentions and procedures that allow it to change forms. It may get hot and uncomfortable in the alchemy lab, but it's all happening for the sake of transformation. For those whose calcified mental structures refuse to budge from anything else, 5-MeO-DMT can obliterate structures before the mind can form the word "Kaboom!"

5-MeO-DMT is not a "beginner's psychedelic." Its power has caused even the most seasoned psychonauts to tremble. There may be no substance in existence to match its evocation of timelessness and nonduality. It's one thing to ponder these concepts philosophically, and it's quite another to experience them directly. Bufo terrified Pollan in *How to Change Your Mind*, and it fascinated an unlikely pop culture icon in the form of Mike Tyson. The infamous, ear-chomping boxer credited Bufo for his deep healing from years of tremendous pressure to be the baddest dude on the planet. To those called to Bufo, I send you my best wishes, and I hope you create as much safety as possible around the body you are endeavoring to leave behind.

13

DMT: Beholding the Mystery

"The mystery of life isn't a problem to solve,
but a reality to experience."

—Frank Herbert, *Dune*

During act I of most films, a crucial event called the *inciting incident* or *catalyst* sets the story into motion, propelling the protagonist toward their goal. In the *Harry Potter* series, the inciting incident comes through the appearance of mysterious letters addressed to Harry. In *The Big Lebowski*, it occurs as two doofy hitmen break into the Dude's apartment and pee on his rug. In *Alice in Wonderland* and *The Matrix*, it comes via a white rabbit. The inciting incident is a portal into the greater story.

I raise this point because as I see it, the inciting incident of the revival was not Griffiths' 2006 paper, as Pollan and others posit. Griffiths' paper, more accurately, marks the movement from act I to act II. The confoundingly under-reported inciting incident was Strassman's research at the University of New Mexico on *dimethyltryptamine*, the classic psychedelic better known as DMT.

The Search for the Spirit Molecule

DMT is one of the most powerful psychedelics in existence. Perhaps the clearest difference between DMT and the other classic psychedelics is the duration of effects. LSD and mescaline's effects tend to last 8 to 12 hours, and psilocybin's effects clock in at around 6 to 8 hours. Like it's 5-MeO cousin, DMT's effects typically last 30 to 45 minutes. Its shorter duration does not equate to a milder experience. It's more like compressing the potency of a high-dose psilocybin experience into a tenth of the time. Experientially speaking, linear time is irrelevant when dealing with psychedelics, and DMT users regularly report that 20 minutes on the substance feels like a lifetime.

Unlike psilocybin and LSD, DMT is not consumed orally. Recreationally, it is typically smoked or vaporized. In clinical settings like Strassman's, intravenous injection is the standard approach. Its intensity and short duration are common to both routes of administration, but an IV infusion gives clinicians greater control over the dose—and I doubt the Feds would have been thrilled at the thought of people smoking smelly DMT in a hospital.

Strassman was the first American scientist to conduct psychedelic research on human subjects after the first wave ended in 1970. He discovered, cocreated, and documented his achievement of what his first-wave peers thought impossible, catalyzing the second wave in the 1990s, over fifteen years before the Johns Hopkins publication. Strassman led the DMT study for five years, and by the end, he had received approval to study psilocybin and LSD as well. He worked out an effective dose range for psilocybin in a handful of volunteers, information he provided to other sites, including that of Hopkins. The LSD arrived at his lab, but due to various complicated personal and professional factors detailed in *DMT: The Spirit Molecule*, Strassman brought his UNM research to an end.

Unlike most of today's psychedelic researchers, Strassman did not focus on mental health. His scope was broader. He wanted to learn about the subjective effects of this fascinating and bizarre compound to determine if it could be safely administered in research settings and to discover if it was, as he had hypothesized, the elusive "spirit molecule."

"The spirit molecule" was Strassman's term for a biological mediator of spiritual experiences. Strassman knew DMT was both abundant in nature and endogenously produced in the human body. He knew it was the primary psychoactive chemical of the sacred Amazonian plant medicine, ayahuasca. These facts, along with DMT's ease in crossing the blood-brain barrier to attach like a key to important receptors, led Strassman to postulate that DMT may be the spirit molecule he sought.

DMT hardly appeared in first-wave psychedelic research. Little was known about it except that it reliably and rapidly produced powerful journeys to what appeared to be a different dimension. Strassman realized he'd found a research avenue so remarkable he was shocked that few had entered it before him. In case there was any doubt in his pursuit, his first experience with the molecule strengthened his resolve, especially since his facilitator was among history's most legendary psychedelic advocates.

"The first person to supervise my DMT experience was Terence McKenna," Strassman told me. "It was at an Esalen meeting in '87 or '88. I smoked DMT, and I was completely floored, thinking, 'What the hell was that?'"

After a brainstorming session with McKenna the next year, Strassman developed a protocol he hoped would reopen the psychedelic research gates. Six months later, he'd received State approval via a green light from the University of New Mexico, but he still had the "monolithic Federal bureaucracy" to contend with. "I couldn't start the study until I had the drug, but I couldn't get the drug until the FDA agreed it had scientific merit. I couldn't study the drug to certify it was up to FDA standards unless I had a Schedule I permit from the DEA, and the DEA wouldn't give me the Schedule I permit until the FDA had given the provisional acceptance of the study's scientific merit. It was all a roundabout Catch-22."

The Catch-22 continued for two years, but Strassman was tenacious, enduring phone calls, faxes, and dead ends. In 1990, he became the first researcher in decades to receive Federal approval and funding to give a Schedule I psychedelic to humans, sparking the beginning of the revival.

Strassman's Research and the DMT Beings

One would be hard-pressed to overstate the significance of Strassman's work. For five years, he administered intravenous DMT to nearly sixty volunteers. He prescreened participants for physical and psychological red flags, rigorously monitored vitals, and staffed the clinic with medical professionals in case of adverse reactions. And there were adverse reactions, including an instance of frighteningly heightened blood pressure, but nothing proved catastrophic or damaging. In papers published in 1994 and 1995, Strassman concluded DMT could be safely administered to healthy volunteers in a hospital, while not free of adverse effects.

It's difficult to reason why Strassman is commonly overlooked in recent histories of the revival. In the 480 pages of *How to Change Your Mind*, Pollan mentions Strassman's research once, despite calling it a "watershed event." Without clarity, I'm left to speculate one reason is Strassman's discoveries were more bizarre than those of Griffiths, and to change the popular opinion about psychedelics, their weird and disturbing edges must be filtered. A mystical experience shepherding widespread mental health benefits is an easier sell than DMT-induced encounters with "beings" from another dimension, which over half of Strassman's participants reported.

Strassman's subjects described the rapid onset of DMT's effects as "being shot out of a cannon." This lines up with trip reports of recreational users, who commonly reference "blasting off" after taking a series of massive hits from a complicated smoking apparatus. The participants referenced a significant difference between "sub-threshold" DMT trips and those characterized by blasting off and "breaking through." Low doses of 0.2 and 0.3 milligrams per kilogram of body weight proved to be the threshold for attaining a full psychedelic experience. Doses of 0.4 milligrams per kilogram of body weight, however, consistently induced extraordinary experiences that sent participants to another dimension. Such language was not figurative.

Upon returning to their bodies in the hospital room, participants described having had vivid interactions with "beings" in the "other place." They said the beings were conscious, highly intelligent, powerful entities of various forms, shapes, sizes, and activity, and this other place was their home. The beings were usually aware the DMT user had entered their "space", and their responses varied. Some were welcoming hosts who led the DMT voyager on a tour of their world. Others were antagonistic, making the DMT user feel unwelcome and, at its most extreme, meeting their visit with hostility.* Participants all but unanimously intuited they were powerless in comparison to their hosts, and the only option was not to resist.

If this sounds far out, it's because it is. As a scientist, Strassman was perplexed by the strangeness and consistency of such reports. Not only did most participants describe encounters with these beings—they described them with common language and imagery, as if they'd all seen the same thing. Many independently

---

* Perhaps the most unnerving case of the beings' hostility among Strassman's participants came when a man returned to the hospital in disarray, explaining he had just been sexually violated by a crocodile.

reported encountering "jesters" or "clowns" in a "circus-like environment," as well as an "insect-like" and "machine-like" quality to the setting.*

Since participants had no contact with one another, how was this possible? What scientific explanation could account for this phenomenon? If it was to be classified as a simple drug-induced hallucination, wouldn't there be variation in the descriptions?

"I was neither intellectually nor emotionally prepared for the frequency with which contact with beings occurred in our studies, nor the often utterly bizarre nature of these experiences," Strassman wrote in *DMT: The Spirit Molecule.* He struggled to make sense out of the unnervingly consistent reports of the participants. His scientific inclination was to provide interpretations as if the experiences were different than what they seemed to be. Each time he did, the participants resisted, claiming Strassman was trying to "explain away" their visions.

Strassman took an uncomfortable leap. Rather than attempt to explain away the reports using an established theoretical framework, he suspended his disbelief and related to the bizarre stories as if they were real. This thought experiment allowed curiosity to enter, and it deepened the participants' trust in him, making them more comfortable to share the confounding details without fearing they would be reduced to an incongruent model.

In the book's conclusion, Strassman made a valiant attempt at a scientific explanation involving quantum physics, dark matter, and parallel dimensions. Over twenty years post-publication, it remains a fascinating exploration of the possible intersection of physics and spiritual reality.†

How seriously should we take these accounts? Is this other place *real* in the way Florida and Zimbabwe are real? Are these beings as real as my noisy

---

* In his many linguistically rich discourses, McKenna famously referred to these beings as "self-transforming machine elves."

† Those inclined to dig deeper than Strassman's research, limited as it was by the confines of academic science, can find troves of DMT trip reports on internet vaults such as Erowid, DMT-Nexus, and the subreddit r/DMT. Trip reports reference specific locations of the DMT dimension, such as a "threshold" separating the human realm from the other place, with the degree of detail you might expect from a stranger's directions on a pre-GPS road trip. ("Drift until you reach the Big Boy, make a left, and head toward the morphing mandala . . .") Such stories read as if DMT users are traveling to an objective location with specific landmarks consistent from user to user.

neighbors, who are currently partying for the fourth night straight? Or is this all some collective DMT delusion?

Fueling the otherworldly fire, Strassman's subjects described this other place as more fundamentally *real* than the everyday world. A 2020 survey study from Johns Hopkins corroborated this feature: of 2,561 individuals surveyed, each of whom had encountered at least one entity in their personal DMT use, 81% felt their encounter was "more real than reality" as it transpired.[1] The mystery thickens with the knowledge that the human body naturally produces DMT sans exogenous inputs. This fact, combined with the entity encounters, led Strassman to speculate that DMT may be responsible for certain varieties of alien abduction reports. Perhaps extraterrestrial encounters occur when the individual's brain is flooded with DMT, as can happen in states of high distress and pain.*

Scientific theorizing aside, what does this mean?

I doubt humans will ever find an objective answer. Other practices, however, may add validity to the realness of the DMT dimension.

Dream Yoga and Lucid Dreaming

We dream every night, and we have no idea why. Scientific explanations of dreams as the brain's way of processing memories and experiences may be accurate, but do they explain everything? What about the dreams people perceive as inherently meaningful? What about dreams of events or encounters that end up happening the following day?

How about the prophetic importance of dreams in diverse religious traditions, the majority of which believe dreams can be a means through which one can communicate with the Divine? Examples abound in the Old Testament, from Solomon dreaming of God granting him wisdom, riches, and honor to Jacob dreaming of a heavenly ladder. The Islamic tradition began with the angel Gabriel visiting the Prophet Muhammad in what many believe was a dream.[2] In many Native American traditions, dreams facilitate conversation with the Great Spirit, transmitting important information for the community.

---

*   That's not to say alien encounters aren't real. Such a claim would reduce the profundity of the experience to a physiological mechanism. It could be possible that DMT is a key to entering their dimension, which is not governed by physical matter.

The phenomenon of lucid dreaming raises questions. Lucid dreaming is the practice of "waking up" inside a dream to influence the content. Practitioners commonly ascribe spiritual significance to their lucid dreams. Whether lucid dreamers are aware of it or not, a similar practice with spiritual underpinnings can be found in Tibetan Buddhism.

The four lineages of Tibetan Buddhism have practiced and developed the principles of "dream yoga" for centuries. Like lucid dreaming, Tibetan practitioners learn to "wake up" inside their dreams and train their "vision body" to navigate the dream world at will. In Tibetan cosmology, the dream world consists of several bardos, the liminal states of consciousness between death and rebirth. Through dream yoga, one learns to navigate the bardos to prepare for the after-death state, the journey through which determines whether one is liberated from or reincarnated into the cyclical world of *saṃsāra*.

Tibetan masters claim they have the ability to meet up with others in the dream world. Before sleeping, practitioners may agree to meet at a chosen landmark and journey together. They may even wake up with common memories of their shared nocturnal voyages.

I imagine most material scientists would delegitimize these experiences with reductionistic explanations. After all, science has a praxis of squashing thousands of years of culture and tradition if the belief system doesn't fit into its explanatory parameters. But should a material scientist let their imagination stretch and listen to dream yoga anecdotes, they might note similarities to DMT reports: people enter a shared "other world," perceive it to be at least as real as our waking world, and report recurring landmarks. While dream yogis may not talk about entities, they describe a plethora of spiritual beings whose characteristics are vividly documented in *The Tibetan Book of the Dead*. Might dream yogis and DMT voyagers traverse a common immaterial plane?*

Intrigued as I am by dream-DMT parallels, perhaps drawing them confines the DMT experience into unwarranted parameters. When Strassman met his subjects' journeys with psychoanalytic dream interpretations, they shook their heads and told him no dream of theirs had ever been this real.

---

* There's a widespread belief that the brain releases DMT when we dream. Though that would support the dream-DMT connection, this belief has not yet been backed with evidence.

Perhaps they would have been more receptive to dream yoga, which regards the dream world as a real place rather than Freud's "royal road to the unconscious." Regardless, Strassman realized the importance of holding explanations lightly and resisting the tendency to use established models to make sense of such inexplicable experiences. In the world of psychedelics, one can benefit from dropping all frameworks to see things with "beginner's mind."

Beginner's Mind

A cheesy and surprisingly hilarious movie from 1999 called *Blast from the Past* stars Brendan Fraser as thirty-five-year-old Adam, who was born and raised in a fallout shelter that Christopher Walken, his paranoid father, built at the height of the Cold War. When innocent Adam steps outside, he gazes up in awe.

"What is it?" asks a bewildered passerby.

"The sky!" Adam replies.

"The sky? Where?" asks the passerby.

"Up there!" exclaims Adam.

Squinting, the passerby says, "I don't see anything."

"Just look!" Adam cries.

Others look up, searching in vain for whatever has this weirdo so enthused. Only a little girl succeeds, delightedly crying, "I see it, Mommy!"

"I have never in my life seen anything like it before!" Adam says, laughing as he strolls away from the confused crowd.

This moment offers a delightful depiction of the Buddhist concept of "beginner's mind"—a state of perceiving the world as if encountering it for the first time. It is a lens unsullied by concepts or interpretations, clearly seeing the inherent newness of the present, moment by moment.

In all our "knowledge" of the world, we forget there is no such thing as stillness or sameness. Everything is in motion, and everything is changing, from the clouds to the planets to the particles constituting Neil deGrasse Tyson's bottom. The little girl knew what Adam was talking about because she too saw through innocent eyes.

Our world considers anyone crying in delight about the sky to be crazy, all the while considering someone who forgets it's there to be well-adjusted. It's like the great "didactic little parable-ish story" with which David Foster

Wallace opened his Kenyon College commencement speech: "There are these two young fish swimming along and they happen to meet an older fish swimming the other way, who nods at them and says, 'Morning, boys. How's the water?' And the two young fish swim on for a bit, and then eventually one of them looks over at the other and goes, 'What the hell is water?'"[3]

Wallace's point is simple and profound: "the most obvious, important realities are often the ones that are hardest to see and talk about."[4] The consequences of forgetting these realities can be devastating, for their roads lead to isolated absorption into the "rat race" mind of stress, fear, and petty problems. This is the mind of the "sane" person of our world.

Beginner's mind is an antidote. It's a practice that cultivates curiosity, wonder, and playfulness. Beginner's mind doesn't take itself too seriously. It recognizes everything is changing, and we have little idea what's happening. And that's fine.

Psychedelics can reconnect you to beginner's mind. Psilocybin could leave you marveling at a tree blowing in the wind, watching mesmerized as the clouds morph in their gentle flow, causing you to wonder why it's been twenty years since you've *really* watched the clouds when they're up there morphing around every day. DMT could transport you into another dimension, the reality of which undermines all notions of your previously established truth. Rather than needing to find explanations, we can serve ourselves, as Strassman did, by acknowledging the limits of our understanding and surrendering logical frameworks for immersion into the experience's immanence.

Meaning Making

Quite often, the meaning of a psychedelic experience is unclear. After a trip filled with images of ancient civilizations, multicolored patterns of morphing geometry, and a T-Rex eating a wizard on Jupiter, you might be left thinking, "What the hell *was* that?" You may feel disappointed that the visions seem disconnected from the problems you hoped to solve. How does one integrate a trip that makes no sense?

Jung's approach to dreams can be helpful. Unlike Freud, Jung wasn't interested in explaining dream content through an interpretive lens of sexual neurosis. He believed it was more important for people to interpret their dreams, for the meaning they give the content expresses deeper workings of the unconscious.

Imagine a client named John Cleese undergoing a DMT session with his therapist, Wanda. After an hour of lying on the couch and wearing eyeshades, John tells Wanda that the entire time, he felt like he was strapped to a gigantic drill digging furiously into a barren wasteland. Wanda resists the temptation to talk about the brilliant connections her brain has made, reminding herself that her interpretations are probably wrong. She instead asks John what he felt like as it happened. "It was horrid," John says. "I was terrified." Intrigued, Wanda asks, "Do you still feel connected to the terror?" John nods. She invites him to focus on the emotion to the extent he feels comfortable. "What were you afraid was going to happen?" she asks. After a pause, John says, "That I would die."

Who could have known that for John Cleese, a drill digging into a wasteland would evoke his potent fear of death? To deepen the exploration, Wanda might ask, "Do you remember the first time you felt a fear like this?" Maybe nothing comes up, or maybe John recalls a childhood canoe trip when he fell into the water, got stuck on a branch, and thought he was drowning. Now there's a traumatic memory to work with. If no memory arose from Wanda's question, she could inquire about the emotions the wasteland elicited. Perhaps the barrenness strikes John as representing how he's viewed his life of late, void of energy and riddled with isolation. Whatever direction it takes, an open attitude of curiosity will allow John's inner healer to clarify parts of his inner world calling for attention.

If a different client experienced the same image, it would mean something completely different. Perhaps a client named Kevin Kline feels angry, and he realizes it's the anger he feels toward people unconcerned about the degradation of aquatic life. Perhaps a client named Michael Palin feels excitement and intrigue around exploring the subterranean unknown. Objective interpretation is not the goal. The goal is to explore personal meaning based on emotional responses and free associations.

While remaining vague enough to support exploration, Jung created models to make sense of even the most incomprehensible visions. He based them on personal experience: after his split with Freud, Jung experienced a terrifying "descent into the unconscious," a prolonged period filled with visions, fantasies, and nightmares so confounding that Jung thought he had lost his mind.

But he managed to climb out of the underworld by making meaning of it, and that meaning laid the groundwork for his enduringly influential concept of the *collective unconscious*.

The Collective Unconscious

Jung split the unconscious mind into two regions. The personal unconscious, like the Freudian unconscious, consists of memories and impulses related to one's unique life experiences. Beyond the personal's autobiographical limits lies the collective unconscious.

Jung hypothesized the collective unconscious was a species-wide ocean of information accumulated throughout human history. At its foundation exist what Jung termed "archetypes." Archetypes are primordial patterns of energy and thought that human beings express through behaviors, images, and symbols, such as those found in dreams and mythology. They represent varying facets of the inner world, and as they strive for realization, the archetypes guide us along the path of individuation, or becoming our full selves.

Jung named several primary archetypes. The *anima* is the unconscious "feminine" side of the psyche, while the *animus* is the unconscious "masculine" side. The archetype of the *shadow* represents the repressed aspects of the psyche, containing everything seen as "opposite" of the ego. The *Self* is the primary archetype, representing the unified psyche as a whole.[5]

How archetypal patterns manifest in one's personal life is influenced by such factors as one's family system, cultural norms, and unique experiences. Imagine I'm a cynic who believes life has no meaning and humanity is a virus. One of my coworkers, Keanu, is a bubbly, optimistic Christian who only talks about positive stuff. From the moment I met Keanu, I loathed him, and I found myself thinking about how dumb and annoying he is, even dreaming about jousting him on horseback. What I don't realize is that Keanu represents my shadow: he embodies the positive, joyful qualities I have disowned in myself, because my ego judges them as foolish. The archetype of the shadow filters through personal imagery—Keanu—and generates an egoic struggle. Quite possibly, Keanu, who has shadowed all I represent, is having a similar experience.

If the collective unconscious is a blueprint of potential experience, the personal unconscious filters that blueprint into recognizable forms intuited by the conscious ego. By nature of their transpersonal qualities, psychedelics can take people beyond their personal unconscious toward the common language of collective archetypes.

"By elucidating the underlying metaphoric structures—which have been variously referred to as archetypes, deep structures, or primordial images—we are uncovering something of humanity's common language," wrote Metzner in *The Unfolding Self: Varieties of Transformative Experience.* "The language of symbols is this common language. It is the language we still use and understand—in dreams, in poetry and art, in the visions and voices that tell us of the sacred and the mystery."[6]

To ground these abstractions, Jung frequently turned to mythology.

Mythology as Expression of the Unconscious

Why are characters, situations, and lessons of myths shared by and relevant to countless people across cultures and time? Why do the stories of Adam and Eve, Noah, and Jonah's trials in the belly of the whale resonate with so many? Why do worldwide academics continue studying stories from *The Arabian Nights*? Why do Marvel movies make billions of dollars in numerous nations?

Through a Jungian lens, these stories express collective archetypes eternally animating the unconscious from its source. Communicated through narrative content specific to each culture—e.g., the heroism of Achilles, the treachery of Hades—archetypes express broad patterns common to humanity—e.g., the call toward heroism (Achilles), the temptation toward deception (Hades). Mythology parallels the relationship between the personal and collective unconscious: the broad patterns of the collective filter through the culturally specific imagery and story structure of the personal.

Because the collective unconscious is abstract, its expressions through stories leave room for interpretation. That's why mythology can seem so bizarre, with no clear-cut, Disney-style meaning. Like dreams and psychedelic experiences, myths may have no objective meaning unto themselves; rather, we make meaning of them, relating to symbols based on which archetypes are knocking on our mind's door.

As Freud demonstrated with his unwavering adherence to the Oedipal myth as an expression of an essential structural truth of the unconscious, people easily become dogmatic with mythology, using stories like mathematical equations to present an interpretation as an absolute. For example, in the Garden of Eden story, entire religious lineages have interpreted Eve's temptation by the snake through a chauvinist lens, using the myth as "proof" to claim ridiculous absolutes like "women are the cause of men's problems." Such an absurd assertion comes from mistaking personal interpretation for a collective absolute, when really the interpreter cannot see beyond their own misogynistic walls.

When mythology becomes dogma, problems result. Like a Zen koan, mythology invites engagement with symbols to stir ongoing reflection and offer direction through life's ongoing challenges. Dogmatic interpretation blocks alternate perspectives, betraying the fluidity of the collective unconscious by crystallizing the ego against engagement with the archetypes. This drives a hefty wedge between identity and wholeness.

Every myth is filtered through its culture's values and belief systems, lending an important historical context to each story. Nevertheless, myths provide inner signposts along the abstract journey of development. With their aid, we can make meaning from our wildest, most abstract psychedelic experiences, recognizing that while the images seen behind eyeshades are uniquely personal, they express something fundamental to humanity.

The Monomyth

Joseph Campbell's concept of the monomyth, better known as "the Hero's Journey," has been so widely referenced that it may have earned a permanent seat at the Round Table of Eyeball-Rolling Clichés. As common as it is to hear people reference this journey, it's not often acknowledged that the monomyth is rooted in Jung's ideas.

Campbell became fascinated with how cultures having no contact with one another expressed common patterns in their myths. Many, for instance, featured a "call to adventure." King Arthur's arrival at a mysterious fountain initiates his quest for the Holy Grail. Theseus, upon learning that young Athenians are being sent to the Labyrinth of Crete to be sacrificed to the

Minotaur, realizes he must slay the beast. Archetypal heroes typically seek what Campbell named the "Ultimate Boon," a prize whose achievement brings the hero and/or their community heightened power and healing, often of a spiritual nature, such as the Grail's endowment of everlasting life.

Campbell hypothesized mythology follows unconscious archetypal structures nonspecific to place, people, or era. Echoing Jung, he believed the mythological expression of archetypes offered guidance on the individual's search for meaning and fulfillment. In his most famous book, *The Hero with a Thousand Faces*, he aimed to synthesize mythology's archetypal code by delineating patterns in global examples of recurring characters, themes, and story beats. His synthesis resulted in a sequence of stages that collectively comprise the Hero's Journey.

The Hero's Journey was more than a catchy structure for fireside storytelling. To Campbell, it mirrored the process of individuation, symbolizing the ego's voyage into the unconscious to unite its light and shadow in wholeness. The hero represents the ego, the journey represents the path toward wholeness, and the ultimate boon represents the *Self*, the archetype of integration and fulfillment.[*]

While Campbell pinpoints over a dozen stages, the monomyth follows four primary beats: Hero departs from ordinary world (consciousness), crosses threshold into special world (unconscious), faces trials and enemies (shadow), and returns with ultimate boon to ordinary world (wholeness). The journey into the unconscious is fraught with danger, but the reward of restoring balance calls the ego to challenge and expand its confines.

Psychedelic experiences mirror the Hero's Journey. When someone takes a psychedelic, they are choosing to venture into the unpredictable territory of the unconscious. The journey may be filled with trials, but the journeyer accepts the risk in hope of returning with something valuable. The valuable discovery could be insight, repressed memories, mystical attunement, or countless other possibilities. As discoveries happen in the depths of the special psychedelic world, the return home—and the trials it brings—is the integration.

---

[*] I hate to make things more confusing, but this Jungian Self is different from the Internal Family Systems Self. The Self attained in the ultimate boon, the apotheosis of the Hero's Journey, is the completion of a process of restoration. In Internal Family Systems, the Self is a fundamental essence accessible in all moments, requiring no journey to access.

If you find yourself struggling to make sense of things, consider reading about the Hero's Journey and asking yourself, "Which stage am I in?" Such questions can help you view your story as a personal chronicle of an ancient tale, endowing you with a map to connect your struggles to an enduring process of human development. Perhaps you'll discover that the images from your non-ordinary adventure correspond to those found in the myths and dreams of cultures with which you have had no contact. Over-saturated as the Hero's Journey has become, its essence holds great power in helping people see past the limits of their ordinary worlds.

Stan Grof's Cartography of the Psyche

I believe Stanislav Grof is the greatest thinker in Western psychedelic history. As he was influenced by Jung and friends with Campbell, it's high time for me to explain why he holds such a lofty position.

Grof's training in psychoanalysis predisposed him toward seeing psychedelics as keys to the unconscious. As he facilitated hundreds of high-dose LSD sessions, however, he realized psychoanalysis could not account for the experiences of his clients unless he reduced them to illusions or psychoses. Like Campbell, Grof used the frameworks of archetypes and the collective unconscious to organize his clients' seemingly chaotic and untethered experiences into categories that suggested meaning without dogmatically ascribing it. Unlike Campbell, Grof's categories followed a biological process every human experiences: being born.

Grof was struck by how often clients reported womb-like imagery and memories of being born. He theorized that the fundamental trauma of being born is stored in everyone's unconscious. His conception of birth followed four sequential stages, each of which housed a plethora of possible emotions, images, and ways of being and perceiving. All LSD experiences fit into one of four "Basic Perinatal Matrices" Grof detailed.

BPM I: being in the womb; bliss, unity, comfort, and tranquility

BPM II: beginning of birth process; terror, chaos, hopelessness in the face of something vast and powerful

BPM III: movement through the uterus; constriction, pressure, sense of dying

BPM IV: being born; release, catharsis, sense of rebirth

One's LSD experiences of these four matrices can take a multitude of forms. They may be animated with personal content, such as a client feeling like their work is suffocating them (BPM III). They may take a transpersonal, archetypal form, as in a vision of being trapped in a hell-like inferno (BPM II) or drifting through a primordial ocean of bliss (BPM I).

In the world of film, Ridley Scott's film *Alien* expresses BPM II, for the crew is trapped in a claustrophobic environment, pursued by an unknown powerful force threatening the well-being of their recent hyper-sleep.[*] In the climax of Kubrick's *2001: A Space Odyssey*, Dave travels through a vortex of light, terrified under the force of intense pressure (BPM III) before being reincarnated as a Star Baby, tranquilly in utero of space (BPM I).

Campbell believed Grof had discovered the biological underpinning of the monomyth: its main stages of status quo comfort, movement into trial and fear, and renewal could all be reduced to the four perinatal matrices. In this sense, the experience of being born sets up the archetypal conditions for all experiences to come.

That Grof found a way to categorize the incomprehensibly vast reaches of thousands of LSD trips and connect those categories to a fundamental human experience blows my mind. Several of his books—*Realms of the Human Unconscious, LSD Psychotherapy,* and *The Way of the Psychonaut*—provide so many examples of each category that anyone struggling to understand their psychedelic journeys may find not only meaning but even descriptions of exactly what they saw or felt.

For Grof, recognizing the prenatal and perinatal roots was an important step, but healing came through resolving one's birth trauma during and after the psychedelic session. For people stuck in BPM II or BPM III, for instance, Grof often took a somatic approach, guiding meditation and breathwork to mobilize the painful emotions stuck at the roots of their physiology and bringing the process to completion, thereby allowing relaxation in the peace of being released from the pressure.

---

[*] Grof was fascinated with the Swiss artist H. R. Giger, who designed the iconic sets and the creature in Scott's film. Connections between *Alien* and birth trauma are underscored by the fact that the creature is incubated in poor John Hurt's body via its face-hugging kin and subsequently birthed out his chest.

Grof's basic perinatal matrices were a remarkable contribution to psychedelic research and the field of psychology as a whole. His insight, compassion, and understanding of LSD were so great that Hofmann named him the "godfather of LSD." It's a testament to his towering intellect and enormous heart that the BPMs are but one of several significant concepts he formulated. If Freud and Jung represented the first two essential developments in the history of psychoanalysis, Grof ushered the model through its next evolutionary leap. In my humble estimation, Stan Grof is the greatest psychologist of the latter half of the twenty-first century, and I hope more people realize that as the West continues to integrate psychedelics into its culture.

DMTx

Again, do these frameworks help us understand DMT? Can transpersonal, archetypal explanations account for the entities? Or are these models too *psychological*, blaspheming the reality of the dimensions to which DMT affords access? I suppose it's up to the individual voyager to decide. Be that as it may, one project in particular has the potential to shed light on these ambiguities, for it fearlessly turns toward the DMT world with curiosity as its guide.

The revival's most far-out application of DMT is The Extended-State DMT program, also known as "DMTx." I first heard about DMTx at a Red Rocks concert from a dedicated psychonaut who was looking to be a participant. He described it as the ultimate trip: several people simultaneously receive a steady supply of intravenous DMT for hours, allowing them to sustain the often-brief peak DMT state. As thirty minutes on DMT can feel like eternity, I can't compute what several hours would correspond to in DMT time.

Daniel McQueen, a psychedelic therapist and innovator of cannabis-assisted therapy, has spearheaded the project. His inspiration came from the work of Strassman and neurobiologist Andrew Gallimore, who discovered a procedure using an intravenous drip to keep people safely in the peak DMT state for extended periods. McQueen and his team believe their project can bring back important information to better humanity.

"There are therapeutic applications at lower doses, but I'm more interested in what I call scientific or creative problem solving," McQueen said. "What if we can create a protocol that puts a scientist into the experience, and the DMT elicits a process with their expertise and brain content so that they can come up with a solution to what we would consider an unsolvable problem? Scientific technology and psychedelics are intertwined, so I think it would be possible to protocol the seemingly random eureka moment, and I think we can create a reliable process to do advanced scientific problem solving."

Countless DMT users report receiving "downloads" from their hosts. Descriptions frequently portray the entities as highly evolved spiritual beings with advanced technology they wish to share with humanity. Others say they are as interested in learning about humans as psychonauts are in learning about them. They communicate telepathically and perform procedures that many voyagers intuitively sense facilitate an "upgrade" to their spirit. Some users claim that these beings are architects of human life on Earth, structuring fundamental laws too extraordinary for people ordinarily to perceive. It's all too sci-fi to be regarded as paganism.

If the psychedelic trip parallels the Hero's Journey, it's most apparent in the DMTx project. Those who partake are indeed crossing the threshold into an unknown world. Their intention to return with boons that could not have arisen from the confines of the status quo appear to be more than a hopeful dream.

"We just completed our first DMTx expedition, and it was stellar," McQueen updated me a year after our interview. "Everything we considered possible is truly possible. And we're just scratching the surface of it."

DMT's Ambiguous Future in the Revival

While DMT hasn't made a big splash in the mental health world yet, there's growing interest in its therapeutic potential. The 2020 Johns Hopkins survey study, for example, found that 89% of survey respondents attributed persisting positive changes in well-being and life satisfaction to their DMT experience. Similar percentages noted improvement in social relationships, mood, and general attitude about life. Only about 5% reported negative changes in the same domains.[7]

In 2021, a London-based Phase 1 trial on DMT-assisted therapy for major depressive disorder demonstrated safety in volunteers. The placebo-controlled second Phase is the world's first regulated trial of DMT-assisted therapy, and if the results are as significant as the researchers hope, DMT could join psilocybin and ketamine as a therapeutic adjunct to treat depression.[8]

I didn't get around to asking Strassman for his opinion on DMT's mental health applications. I doubt he'd have expressed much optimism. One of the reasons he shut down his research was that as profound and life-changing as participants initially declared their trips to be, very few exhibited radical long-term changes in their lives. Many took away a new appreciation for life, and some proclaimed specific changes they'd realized they had to make, but a few months later, their enthusiasm had faded.

Then again, Strassman's protocol didn't include integration therapy. Perhaps more formal follow-up and integration would have yielded long-term changes. Or maybe DMT's power can induce excitement and amazement, but the world to which it delivers people soon feels too far removed from the everyday world to make any shifts. There's no absolute, of course, as the Johns Hopkins survey study suggested a vast majority of users got better.

Strassman's research was indeed, as Pollan suggested, a watershed event, and its influence deserves more recognition than it often attracts. Had Pollan presented Strassman's research as the genesis of the revival, perhaps his audience would not have embraced psychedelic research with the fervor they did. As mentioned, mystical experiences are more palatable than interdimensional voyages to the domain of morally ambiguous humanoids. They would have, however, received a more complete picture of the revival. Strange as this revised origin story may be, it is more telling of the general reaches of psychedelic states than the media's therapeutic stories suggest. As lovely as it is to regard psychedelics as a mental health panacea, their mysterious, unsettling potential endures.

The more I learn about these compounds, the more they evoke a mystery defying explanation. As much as I find this to be the case with psychedelics, it's even truer regarding Indigenous uses of plant medicines, whose roots reach thousands of years deeper than those of psychedelic therapy.

IV

INDIGENOUS ROOTS
OF THE REVIVAL

14

Deconstructing Shamanism down the Amanita Rabbit Hole

> "'I can't explain myself, I'm afraid, sir,' said
> Alice, 'because I'm not myself, you see.'
> 'I don't see,' said the Caterpillar.
> 'I'm afraid I can't put it more clearly,' Alice replied very
> politely, 'for I can't understand it myself to begin with; and
> being so many different sizes in a day is very confusing.'"
>
> —Lewis Carroll, *Alice's Adventures in Wonderland*

Thus far, I have focused on psychedelics in Western culture. Concluding the narrative within Western boundaries, however, mistakes a few tributaries for the great river of humanity's relationship with psychedelics. The revival may be a breakthrough for the West, but to many cultures it's no more than the minions of materialism claiming discovery of things known for longer than the mind can comprehend. LSD was discovered in 1938. The use of plant medicines for healing purposes dates to around 3000 BCE, if not earlier.

Broadly, the category of "plant medicines" includes all organisms of the plant and fungal worlds known to have healing properties. In a narrower sense more relevant to this book, the term refers to a subset of plants and fungi containing naturally occurring psychoactive compounds and having a history of human consumption in sacred, ceremonial contexts. This subset includes cacti, vines, shrubs, leaves, roots, flowers, bark, and mushrooms, among other hosts. Other than ketamine and MDMA, the psychedelics discussed thus far were synthesized after scientists discovered their chemical structure in natural organisms.

While the West continues to research plant medicines, none have factored into psychedelic science to the same extent as their synthetic derivatives. When lab-based science focuses on plant medicines, the research often divorces the plant from the cultural context in which it has been consumed, eliminating what may be learned from communities who understand the substances beyond what information a microscope or brain map can provide. Given this, I've demoted science to a lower degree of consideration in these chapters, as most of what it could offer would amount to glossing over what's important.

I focus on four plant medicines that occupy unique positions in the revival:

1. *Ayahuasca*, a brew made from a vine and a DMT-containing leaf found in the Amazon rainforest, consumed ceremonially by cultures of South and Central America

2. *Peyote*, a mescaline-containing cactus endemic to regions of Mexico and Texas, long held as sacred in numerous tribes and currently a sacrament of the Native American Church

3. *Iboga*, a shrub native to West-Central Africa, the ibogaine-containing root bark of which has been imbibed ceremonially by several West African cultures

4. *Amanita muscaria*, the famous red-and-white toadstool boasting a vast and influential history, whose calming effects are generating renewed interest

This list of plant medicines is far from exhaustive. It excludes important medicines such as *San Pedro*—also called *huachuma*, another mescaline-containing cactus held as sacred to cultures near the Andes Mountains; *Datura stramonium*—also called *jimsonweed*, a flower whose intense physical and psychoactive effects were important to rituals of Algonquin tribes and the Aztecs of Mesoamerica; and *Salvia divinorum*—a member of the sage family whose name translates to "sage of the diviners," used for divinatory purposes among the Mazatec in Mexico.[1] If this book could be a thousand pages, plant medicines would receive the attention they deserve.*

Recognizing the Revival's Indigenous Roots

Jamilah R. George received a master of divinity degree from Yale University and the Yale Institute of Sacred Music. She is now a PhD candidate at the University of Connecticut, and part of her research and clinical work investigates the efficacy of psychedelic-assisted therapies for a range of psychological disorders and associated health outcomes in ethnoracial minoritized communities. Jamilah's "upbringing and education were informed by Afrocentric values and practices," whereby she "grew up doing years of West African drum and dance, was exposed to plant medicine at home, and learned the importance of being in community." These experiences inspired her curiosity and respect for community-based traditions, including the plant medicine lineages the revival often obscures.

"This work almost always pays homage to white, male researchers from the 1950s and 1960s," George told me. "While they've made incredible contributions, there's a privilege of the synthesized aspect of these medicines and less of an homage to the plants, the soil, and the sweat, bravery, and desperation for healing that so many Indigenous communities engaged in to heal their bodies and their land."

She continued, "When we only focus on Hofmann and Huxley, for example, we invisiblize the importance of these other communities and their histories, practices, and rituals, which further dissociates the potential of this work from where it came from. When we do that, it wipes out civilizations, many of whom gave their lives so that we can differentiate between a plant that will heal you and a plant that could kill you."

There is a call in the revival for more efforts to give back to Indigenous stewards. This Indigenous reciprocity can take many forms, from financial support of communities to greater representation of Indigenous healers in psychedelic conferences. It hinges on recognizing and honoring cultures whose people have

---

* Psilocybin mushrooms are also an important plant medicine, but since they've been discussed at length, I'm focusing on others in these chapters.

developed relationships with plant medicines for millennia, often in the face of life-threatening oppression. If the preceding chapters laid out the facets of the revival, these next chapters follow the story toward its roots, revealing psychedelic therapy less as a novel discovery than a young culture coming around to important practices it had previously been too naïve to recognize.

What Westerners Call "Shamanism"

The widespread history of plant medicine consumption is often categorized under the umbrella term "shamanism." While this term can be academically helpful, it carries a breadth of issues that must be addressed before delving into the plants themselves.

"Shamanism" is a word coined by Western anthropologists to combine diverse cultural practices into a singular category. Most of the individuals the West has described as "shamans" would not use the term themselves. In Native American Church peyote rituals, for example, the facilitator is often called the "Roadman" or "Medicine Man." The Shipibo people of the Amazon basin call the leaders of their ayahuasca ceremonies *onanyabo*, while separate lineages from Columbia name their facilitators *taitas* and *maimas*. María Sabina was known to the Mazatec as a *curandera*.

Referring to all these individuals as shamans would be like calling leaders of every religion "priests" and assuming they were all essentially the same. It's important to hold the term "shaman" lightly. While there are commonalities between traditions, differences in rituals, intentions, mythologies, symbolism, and general worldviews abound. Ascribing sameness across the spectrum undermines the uniqueness of each tradition.

The term "shaman" comes from the Russian word *šamán*, which derives from the word *samān* spoken by Tungusic people native to Siberia. Its introduction to the West occurred in the late seventeenth century when Dutch traveler Nicolaes Witsen published a book on his journeys with the Indigenous peoples of Siberia. English use came through a translation of the work of German merchant and traveler Adam Brand, who wrote about Siberian shamans in 1698. Gradually, English vernacular adopted "shamanism" to describe an array of global practices bearing some degree of similarity to the "spirit journeys" of the Siberian shamans referenced in the seventeenth-century texts.

In his book *Pharmakon*, psychedelic writer and ceremonial magician Julian Vayne wrote that Western ethnographers' use of the term has resulted in those labeled shamans being "generalized out of many specific societies."[2] Vayne added, "This figure has become the convenient peg upon which all manner of quasi-new-age nonsense has been hung."[3] Western projection of a simple-minded view onto diverse, complicated traditions resulted in a distinction between the "quasi-new-age nonsense" sometimes presented as shamanism and "traditional shamanism."

On traditional shamanism, anthropologist Shelly Beth Braun wrote, "The status of the shaman, the techniques used, the means for altering one's consciousness, and the problems addressed vary with political, social, economic, and environmental context."[4] Reducing shamanism to one category eliminates these layered factors. As stated by Piers Vitebsky, who in the 1980s became the first Westerner in decades to live long-term with the Evens people of Siberia, "Shamanism is scattered and fragmented and should perhaps not be called an '-ism' at all."[5] My ensuing uses of "shaman" and "shamanism" in reference to traditional practices come with these stipulations.

Commonalities Between Traditions

Amid his appreciation of the differences between shamanic cultures, Vitebsky conceded, "There are astounding similarities, which are not easy to explain, between shamanic ideas and practices as far apart as the Arctic, Amazonia and Borneo, even though these societies have probably never had any contact with one another." While the shaman's role assumes numerous forms, Vitebsky noted the shaman commonly "works in partnership with spirits."[6] Shamans do so by inducing an altered state of consciousness to enter the "spirit world." Cultures use various methods to catalyze the trance state—e.g., drumming, fasting, dancing, and, of course, consuming sacred plants. Whatever the method, the culture regards the spirit world as real and more fundamental to life than the world of everyday existence.

Once the veil is permeable, the shaman cultivates relationships with specific spirits, summoning their aid for a variety of purposes often related to individual, cultural, or universal healing. Given such responsibilities, Vayne described the traditional shaman as a "technician of the sacred."

Their techniques include "transgressing or dissolving of the boundaries between human body and animal body, between heaven and hell, between subject and object, between the symbolic and the real."[7] Traditional shamans, travelers between worlds, are individuals of unique power and cultural influence, living both apart from and connected to their communities, revered for the skills they develop over a lifetime of devotion.

Vitebsky spoke to several core elements of what he called the "shamanic worldview": "Being chosen by spirits, taught by them to enter trance and to fly with one's soul to other worlds in the sky or clamber through dangerous crevasses into the terror of subterranean worlds; being stripped of one's flesh, reduced to a skeleton . . . and then reassembled and reborn; gaining the power to combat spirits and heal their victims, to kill enemies and save one's own people from disease and starvation—these are features of shamanic religions which occur in many parts of the world.

"At the same time," he continued, "shamans live ordinary lives, hunting, cooking, gardening and doing household chores like everyone else. When shamans talk of other worlds, they do not mean that these are disconnected from this world. Rather, these worlds represent the true nature of things and the true causes of events in this world."[8]

Consolidating his analysis, Vitebsky wrote, "Shamans are at once doctors, priests, social workers and mystics. They have been called madmen and madwomen, were frequently persecuted throughout history, dismissed in the 1960s as a 'desiccated' and 'insipid' figment of the anthropologist's imagination, and are now so fashionable that they inspire both intense academic debate and the naming of pop groups . . . The shaman seems to be all things to all people."[9]

White Elephant

It's time to address the elephant in the text: I'm a White person of the Western world writing about traditional shamanism. I can write about the "Western mindset" from myriad perspectives, but in the end, it's akin to theorizing about consciousness: thoughts on the subject are inescapably realized within the subject's confines. Writing about the Western perspective doesn't exempt me from its influence at conscious and unconscious levels.

As a result, my understanding of plant medicines and their traditional uses is significantly inferior to my understanding of Western psychedelics and therapies. If I read a thousand books on the subject, every person raised in a plant medicine tradition would still know multitudes more about their significance, for understanding a culture and its medicines doesn't come through anthropological observations or theories. Unless I take a significant life detour and seek initiation into a traditional lineage, plant medicines will remain more a mystery to me than psychedelics synthesized in the culture that conditioned my perspective.*

I say this not to demean myself but to express that as a Western-minded person, I feel a responsibility to maintain cultural humility on plant medicines rather than acting like an expert because I'm writing a book. I hold enormous respect and curiosity toward these medicines, cultures, and traditions. I've learned enough to recognize their depth of wisdom about the natural world, the human heart, and the spiritual nature of the Universe. Still, my words will be filtered through unconscious influences of a Western lens. They don't convey comprehensive truth on the subject matter; rather, they express the work of a student in a foreign school who can only learn by unlearning much of what he's been taught. To segue into the first plant medicine of focus, I'll add that in learning about plant medicines, I find myself tumbling down a rabbit hole.

Amanita Muscaria

Amanita muscaria, the recognizable red-and-white toadstool also known as the fly agaric, presents an intriguing rabbit hole to those who stumble upon it. Perhaps that fact led Charles Dodgson—better known as Lewis Carroll—to create the exploratory metaphor in *Alice's Adventures in Wonderland*. It's no secret trippy mushrooms play a central role in Carroll's classic novel. After following a tardy white rabbit through its subterranean portal to Wonderland, young Alice encounters a hookah-smoking Caterpillar sitting on a toadstool. The Caterpillar tells her one side will make her grow taller while the other will make her grow shorter. Alice wonders, "'One side of *what*? The other side of *what*?'" The Caterpillar replies, "'Of the mushroom,'" responding "just as if she had asked it aloud."[10]

---

*   And that's saying a lot, because psychedelics are among the most mysterious and impossible-to-understand things in existence. I will never understand everything about them, but I can understand their role in Western culture more than that of any plant medicine.

Sure enough, as Alice nibbles the fungus, she undergoes tremendous alterations in size, furthering the rabbit hole's confounding of who she thought she was.

Thanks in large part to Jefferson Airplane's hippie anthem "White Rabbit," which interprets Alice's story as a drug-induced voyage beyond the confines of parental control, Carroll's book became associated with psychedelics in the 1960s. It's popularly assumed Carroll's trips inspired the story, but there's no clear-cut evidence. Nevertheless, a common theory interprets the size-shifting mushroom to be based on *Amanita muscaria*.

In his article "Mushrooms in Wonderland," psychedelic historian Mike Jay offered a theory supporting the *Amanita* connection. A few days before writing Alice's story, Carroll reportedly visited a library which held a recently released book on drugs called *The Seven Sisters of Sleep*. The library's copy remained largely intact over the next century and a half; however, the chapter on the fly agaric had been cut out. This excised chapter contained a noteworthy description of the mushroom's effects: "Erroneous impressions of size and distance are common occurrences." Jay theorized this influenced Alice's mushroom-induced changes in size.[11]

One hundred eighteen years later, the world was introduced to another beloved character, who became famous for growing in size after consuming what appeared to be *Amanita muscaria*: Super Mario, the enthusiastic Italian plumber of the classic Nintendo games. I can't quantify the amount of childhood joy Mario brought me and my friends as we bopped his head on mystery blocks and chased the elusive red-and-white toadstools that magically appeared. Shigeru Miyamoto, the legendary creator of *Super Mario Bros.* and *The Legend of Zelda*,* has maintained ambiguity on Mario's psychedelic connection despite stating that "there has always somehow been a relationship between mushrooms and magical realms."[12]

---

* If I could connect *The Legend of Zelda* to psychedelics, I assure you I would take that opportunity to nerd out hardcore on how incredible the *Zelda* games are. But I'm afraid I can't, so I'll leave it to this footnote to share that one of the most joyous capitalist delights of my life came when Santa Claus gifted me the gold cartridge of *Ocarina of Time* in 1998. I believe my appreciation for adventure, wonder, and heroic quests has deep roots in that beautiful game, which epitomizes my personal version of nostalgia. And to ensure this footnote isn't completely inconsequential, I'll add that it contains a hidden bit of jolly old foreshadowing of what awaits down the *Amanita* rabbit hole.

Amanita muscaria imagery extends far beyond pop culture. If you attend a psychedelic conference, you'll find it on laptop stickers, T-shirts, and other swag. It could be considered a mascot of psychedelics, making it safe to claim that though psilocybin would get the award for "Most Widely Consumed Psychedelic Mushroom" in the West, the fly agaric would clobber its psilocybin-containing relatives in the contest of "Most Recognizable Psychoactive Fungus." That's a curious thing, for it's extraordinarily rare to meet anyone—including the most fervent of psychonauts—who has imbibed or wants to imbibe *Amanita muscaria*.

The Fly Agaric's Effects

Popular as the *Amanita* image may be, the mushroom's effects have a bad reputation. The fly agaric is known to produce stomach cramps, muscle spasms, dizziness, and vomiting. It has a reputation for inducing terrifying trips. Paul Stamets, the aforementioned "celebrity mycologist," offered a firsthand report on *The Joe Rogan Experience*. Stamets has a gruff and chompy voice that sounds like what I imagine mushrooms would sound like if they could talk. He grew wide-eyed when *Amanita muscaria* came up, sharing that when he took it with a friend, he looked up to find his friend foaming at the mouth. Without going into detail, Stamets indicated it was not a pleasant ride.[*]

Reputation aside, sparks of interest in *Amanita muscaria*'s healing properties are appearing in the West. One of its most vocal internet enthusiasts calls herself "Amanita Dreamer." In the first of hundreds of videos she's shared, Amanita Dreamer detailed her lifelong struggle with anxiety and panic attacks related to her autism diagnosis. After no therapeutic or meditative

---

[*] I haven't met Stamets personally. I have, however, urinated beside him on three occasions. Each instance took place in 2019 during the Psychedelic Science Summit in Austin, Texas, where he was a keynote speaker. I was there for two days, and it became a consistent thing that when I entered the bathroom, I either found Stamets already there or noticed him appear in my peripherals after I had initiated bladder release. During the third encounter, Stamets and I were the only two people in the bathroom, and I considered breaking the awkward silence with a joke about mushrooms, which could have gone a number of directions. Alas, my reservations prevailed, and now my memories of Stamets involve no personal interaction amid a weirdly vulnerable situation I'm certain he doesn't remember and probably didn't even notice happening. I'm not sure what this triplet of synchronized urination means, but it felt significant at the time. My best guess is it has something to do with Stamets being a funny guy, or maybe he also drinks coffee and has to pee more frequently than ideal.

interventions helped, she became addicted to Klonopin. The powerful benzodiazepine helped her anxiety but snuffed her life force, leaving her unable to think clearly. After years living in perpetual fog, she realized she had to get off the benzo and restore her sense of self.

Tapering off benzodiazepines is a brutal process. Amanita Dreamer spent two-and-a-half years attempting to get off them. Each time, debilitating anxiety took hold, bringing muscle spasms and other nasty physical symptoms. No Western medicine could help. In the throes of misery, she took a walk through the woods and stumbled upon *Amanita muscaria*.

When she researched it, she read it was poisonous enough to kill you. When she dug deeper, she discovered it had roots in shamanic lineages of Siberia and at particular doses can have calming, benzo-like effects. When she found that a boiling process eliminated the toxins, she brought the mushroom home, prepared it, and took a strong dose. Like Alice, she felt "a little loose and larger," and she fell asleep without realizing it. When she awoke, she felt "ready to conquer the world."[13]

The next night, she repeated the process. The following evening, she decided to toss her Klonopin and hasn't renewed her prescription since. She continued to take *Amanita muscaria* on an as-needed basis, and it consistently eased her anxiety without the negative side effects of benzos.

"I'm not telling you to do this," Amanita Dreamer added as a disclaimer. "I'm telling you what happened to me." With all the negativity surrounding the mushroom, she felt called to share her story of its healing powers with the Western world that had passed it off as unworthy of interest. She concluded her testimony saying, "This mushroom has saved my life."

I'm not telling you to try the fly agaric. But if you think you might, it's important to know it's not like psilocybin, which can be picked and eaten with no processing. Safe consumption of *Amanita muscaria* requires drying the caps, mixing them together, simmering them in water, and straining the liquid into a tea.[14] This kills the poisonous *ibotenic acid*, eliminating the main culprit behind the stomach cramps and vomiting.

You may be surprised to learn that the recipe I'm providing is not for an illegal substance. *Amanita muscaria* is legal in many countries, including the United States—with the exception of Louisiana, which passed a weird law in 2005 banning it for all but decorative uses. In 2022, a Canadian company called Psyched Wellness even began selling and shipping a lab-tested *Amanita muscaria* tincture. They advertised the tincture as "detoxified and safe for consumption," claiming it "may help to reduce stress, ease muscular tension, and promote restorative sleep." No lawbreaking was required.

One of the few scientific publications on *Amanita muscaria* suggest these reports may not be farfetched. In 2020, a team of Bulgarian researchers at the Medical University of Sofia gathered all the facts they could find on the mushroom's "morphology, chemical content, toxicological and pharmacological characteristics and usage from ancient times to present-day's opportunities."[15] The historical information combined with the mushroom's chemical composition suggested "that *A. muscaria* offers a great versatility of beneficial effects in cell protection and especially in neuroprotection, cardio protection, hepatoprotection, inflammation process, oxidative stress, and may even contribute to development of new drugs."[16] In line with previous examples, this conclusion suggests Western science has a lot to learn by appreciating the value of traditional wisdom rather than continuing a legacy of perceived superiority over "archaic" forms of knowledge.

History of Amanita Muscaria Use

Several cultures used *Amanita muscaria* for healing and divinatory purposes thousands of years ago. It was consumed by inhabitants of Siberia and Kamchatka—both part of present-day Russia—and by the Vikings, who may have taken it before battle, to enrich their mead, or both.[17] *Amanita* imagery was found on rock paintings in an Algerian cave dating to 3500 BCE depicting "dancing figures, holding mushrooms in their hands."[18] Similar imagery found in Central America spawned theories that Mayans and Aztecs used the fly agaric.

It may have held a hallowed role in ancient India. The Vedas, ancient India's sacred texts written in the second millennium BCE, reference a sacramental drink called *soma*. Different translations of the Vedic Sanskrit cast different light on the powers the drink imparted. Ralph T. H. Griffith's translation of the third verse of hymn 8.48 of the *Rig Veda* reads: "We have drunk the soma; we have become immortal; we have gone to the light; we have found the gods."[19] A thousand or so years later, soma appeared in chapter 9, verse 20 of the *Bhagavad Gita*, as Lord Krishna tells Prince Arjuna that those who drink it "free themselves from evil and attain the vast heaven of the gods."[20] Although the Vedas contain details of the drink's recipe, *soma's* organic source is a mystery lost to time—except to R. Gordon Wasson, who presented an argument in 1968 that the sacred drink was a hallucinogenic inebriant made from *Amanita muscaria*. Wasson cited parallels between Vedic descriptions and the practices of Siberian shamans, who had consumed the fly agaric mushroom for centuries, if not millennia.[*21] While the academic world ignored Wasson (a precursor to his fate a decade later with the ergot-Eleusis theory he cocreated), the theory remains alive today.

As these stories indicate, *Amanita muscaria* grows in many places. It was once restricted to the Northern Hemisphere, but as humans transported it south of the equator, the fungus began to grow in the Southern Hemisphere as well. It primarily grows in coniferous and deciduous woodlands, where it forms mycorrhizal relationships with numerous species of trees. Historically, it has tended to link up with birch and pine.[†] Because it can now be found on every continent but Antarctica, *Amanita muscaria* is classified as a "cosmopolitan species." And since past interpretations proclaiming mycorrhizal relationships were harmful to root structures have been proved wrong, I'll conclude my anthropomorphizing of the red-and-white toadstool by saying *Amanita muscaria* seems to be pals with Vikings, Siberians, Mesoamericans, and many international denizens of the plant world.

The fly agaric's widespread consumption across Siberia accounts for its most well-founded historical use. In western Siberia, consumption was restricted to shamans, who used it to enter trance-like states. In the east, the Koryak people regarded it as a "sacred gift" from the first shaman, known as Big Raven, who ate the mushroom—called *wapaq* by the Koryaks—and

---

*   After all that stuff about the drawbacks of using the term *shaman*, I figured I ought to reiterate that the term was originally derived from a term Siberian shamans used for themselves.

†   Mycorrhizal relationships are the points of intersection between fungal mycelium and the root structures of plants. When these relationships become widespread, they create a vast subterranean network of interspecies communication. It's really trippy. Source: "Retracing the Roots of Fungal Symbioses," Joint Genome Institute, February 23, 2015, jgi.doe.gov ./retracing-roots-fungal-symbioses/.

became extraordinarily strong. Big Raven's experience prompted a desire to share it with his people.[22]

The folklore associated with *Amanita muscaria* dovetails into another narrative. This dubious origin story, which has my vote for the most delightful psychedelic theory in existence, centers on a figure more popular than Alice or Mario: Mr. Kris Kringle, Father Christmas, the one and only Santa Claus.

Shaman Santa, Giver of Mushrooms

According to the theory, the myth of the jolly, present-delivering, sleigh-riding fellow dressed in red-and-white garb stems directly from *Amanita muscaria*. The character of Santa is said to derive from shamans of ancient Siberia. During annual midwinter festivals, a shaman would harvest the red-and-white mushrooms, gather them in a sack, and visit the yurts housing his clan members. To avoid bringing snow into the yurts' warmth, the shaman would descend through the smoke hole atop the yurts—a.k.a. chimney—and share his bag of magical gifts before continuing to the next abode.[23]

Shaman Santa theorists purport that these Siberians were reindeer herders who had close relationships with the animals. Some say the reindeer would pull the shaman and his mushrooms from yurt to yurt on a sled. But the *real* closeness was cultivated by means of the shaman drinking the reindeer's pee. Taste wasn't his motivation. The shaman drank it because reindeer were known to chomp wild *Amanita muscaria*. Since the animals' organs filtered the fly agaric's toxins, their urine was potent with its psychoactive properties, allowing the shaman to travel out of his body on a magical trance ride over the yurts and far away.[24]

If this theory is true, the joy quotient of the known Universe expands permanently. That the theory exists at all pushes the quotient's edge, at least for me. Regardless of whether the original Santa Claus was a mushroom-giving Siberian shaman, *Amanita muscaria* sings a unique melody in the song of psychedelic history, a melody becoming audible once again, beckoning people toward its rabbit hole of stories, visions, and healing.

How Deep Is the Rabbit Hole?

For those who don't want to wait for science to catch up with ancient knowledge, it isn't difficult to find *Amanita muscaria*, especially these days when companies like Psyched Wellness make its accessibility simpler and tastier than slugging reindeer pee. Still, there are negative physical effects of unprepared use which, at high doses, could result in death. *Amanita muscaria* may have numerous healing properties, but their nature appears to be more confounding than those of Western psychedelics.

Novel as its reappearance in the West may seem, no known psychoactive fungus or plant has factored into human history in as widespread or mysterious of a way as the fly agaric mushroom. For some time, the cosmopolitan toadstool has been the most common plant or fungal image representative of the psychedelic rabbit hole. And yet, while all popular psychedelics and plant medicines have been illegal in the US for decades, *Amanita muscaria* has somehow eluded Uncle Sam's stern eye to continue its thousands of years of traveling, growing, and captivating a peculiar facet of human interest irreducible to any specific time or culture. Should you follow the white rabbit down *Amanita muscaria's* Hole of Wonderland Weirdness, remember that, as Alice discovered, it may upend your concepts of what is real and what is imagined in this wild world wherein this mysterious mushroom thrives.

15

Iboga and the Single Story

"Classifications, typologies, labels, and other organizational tools help
us wade through complex cultural contexts and specificities . . . Yet, if
not subject to renewal . . . they can become static mechanisms that
constrain and obscure the wealth of changing and seemingly anomalous
factors that are essential features of dynamic cultural realities."

—Dunja Hersak, "Power Objects:
On the Transient Nature of Classifications"

The plant medicine *iboga* comes from the root bark of the *Tabernathe iboga*
shrub. Among practitioners of the spiritual discipline of Bwiti in West-
Central Africa, it has been consumed ceremonially for centuries, if not millennia.[1]
As with many plant medicines, its precise origins of use are unknown.

It wasn't until the nineteenth century that the West became aware of
iboga. It appeared in the writings of French and Belgian explorers such as
Henri Ernest Baillon, who gave *Tabernathe iboga* its name. Griffon du Bellay,
a French naval surgeon who traveled the region of Gabon in the mid-1800s,
wrote, "Taken in small quantities, it is an aphrodisiac and stimulant of the
(central) nervous system; warriors and hunters make considerable use of it in
order to stay awake during their night vigils."[2]

It has been estimated that five percent of Gabon's 2.3 million people have
been initiated into Bwiti, and practitioners span roughly fifty different ethnic communities.[3] Bwiti practitioners do not limit use to the small quantities
du Bellay described. In traditional high doses, practitioners undergo powerful
journeys into an otherworldly realm where the spirits of their ancestors reside.

Iboga's Ceremonial Use

As with most plant medicine traditions, Bwiti practitioners prepare for at least a month before an iboga ceremony. Their preparation consists of dieting, fasting, meditating, spending time in nature, and centering on intentions for the journey.

To the Bwiti, iboga opens a gateway to communication with the dead. People can contact their ancestors, from whom they may receive wisdom and insight into who they are. Within three-walled temple structures, ceremonies are conducted with fire, music, and dance.[4] Many people who undergo an initiation ceremony have direct encounters with death.[5] But details of the ceremonies are sparse. Like several other plant medicine traditions, the Bwiti kept their practice close to the heart, for secrecy was essential in the face of opposition from colonial missionary campaigns.

Uwe Maas and Süster Strubelt, two Westerners who were initiated through traditional Bwiti ceremonies, wrote a detailed report on their experiences in Gabon. "The Iboga healing ceremony induces a near-death experience and is performed to cure serious mental or psychosomatic diseases, but people also undergo initiation rites for reasons of spiritual or personal development."[6]

Strubelt continued, "I was fitted out with ritual weapons and protective objects for the encounters in the spiritual world."[7] When the effects took hold, she recalled, "I had a typical out-of-body experience in which I experienced myself as a football-sized spiritual being moving through visionary spaces."[8] At the same time, she maintained contact with the external world and could describe her visions as they were happening.

The morning after, as she "began to return back to life,"[9] Strubelt was met with singing and physical work as some of the people present moved her joints. She was then instructed to dance, after which she was given a ritual bath in a river. She was left mostly alone for a period, meant "to mark the beginning of a new phase of my life."[10] Then, "the ceremony came to an end with a dance celebration where I was admitted into the community of the initiated and simultaneously released into my real life."[11]

Strubelt wrote about the significance of near-death experiences, which she understood the iboga ceremony to facilitate. She referenced the work of

C. P. Flynn in 1984, who interviewed twenty-one people who'd had a near-death experience. "Nearly all of them were less afraid of death and more likely to believe in life after death," Strubelt wrote. "Most of them also believed in a deeper meaning of life and had the impression of feeling the presence of God. Interest in material things had dropped whereas tolerance, empathy, sensitivity, understanding and acceptance of other people had increased. In addition, most of those interviewed were less dependent on the opinions of others."[12]

The purpose of iboga ceremonies contrasts with Western psychedelic healing approaches. "According to the traditional healer Antoine Makondo," Strubelt wrote, "the initiation should not be considered as a direct form of healing but as a method to broaden one's self-concept. It would allow you to see the world with different eyes and to see and resolve problems in a new and better way. It should be a step towards a new spiritual vision of the world."[13] In this sense, the iboga ceremony is a rite of passage into a more mature developmental level of the culture's spiritual tradition.

Music is essential to Bwiti iboga rituals. "To the Mitsogho, continuous musical support from musicians playing the mouth bow and the harp, accompanying percussions and singing is essential for the initiation process," Strubelt added.[14] "Music is the 'life-line' that reaches from this life to the hereafter and serves as a means of locomotion in visionary space."[15]

She observed that lyrics only accompanied the music when the individual was returning to Earth. "There are no human voices in the spiritual world, that is why the person to be initiated is guided there by instrumental music. On the long way back to this life, however, he is welcomed by songs located between spiritual and earthly communication. The lyrics are only understandable to initiated people."[16] Music was so integral to her visions that she questioned, "Is music a kind of medicine that provokes specific physiological reactions, which promote trance states?"[17]

The profundity of the music and the Bwiti's understanding of its role in facilitating other-worldly journeys led Strubelt and Maas to conclude, "We believe that many procedures in Bwiti are based on neuropsychological knowledge, although it is not yet proven by international science, because international science has hardly made efforts to investigate these subjects. We think it could be useful for pharmacological and musical science to formulate hypotheses on the basis of the knowledge contained in traditional medicine."[18] If anyone carries out such research, perhaps they will continue the trend of Western science "proving" what people more in tune with the elements and the spirit have known for a long time.

Western Interest in Iboga

More than any other plant medicine or psychedelic, iboga has piqued Western interest in its potential to heal people suffering from heavy addictions. Many have claimed one treatment with iboga or ibogaine cured them of a long-term addiction when all other methods failed. Thillen Naidoo, who grew up in the township of Chatsworth in South Africa, credited one dose as having cured him of a fifteen-year addiction to crack cocaine.[19] Reaching sobriety on iboga or its derivative may entail a rough ride.

An iboga experience often lasts for forty-eight hours, and it has a reputation of being grueling. Psychiatrist and psychedelic medicine advocate Dan Engle described it as "the most arduous psychedelic experience I had ever endured up to that point."[20] A beloved psychedelic writer named Teafaerie wrote that iboga "totally schooled me, healed me, cracked me up, pissed me off, gobsmacked me with beauty, shocked me to the core, redeemed my most closely held mythos, and then fundamentally reoriented my entire reality grid." Teafaerie echoed the claims of many others in referencing iboga's facilitation of a lengthy "life review," which came in the form of "thousands of photo-realistic screenshots" from her past.

"Here were all of the most pivotal moments in my personal history, and each thumbnail seemed like the best possible picture that could ever have been taken of that particular scene," Teafaerie wrote. Such vivid revisiting of one's most significant experiences can be brutal—Teafaerie described it as "absolutely merciless."[21] But for Teafaerie and many others, it can facilitate healing of extraordinary depth.

Of the fifty-ish people I interviewed, somatic practitioner and self-described "Social Imagineer" Camille Barton is the only one who described a personal iboga experience. Barton was drawn to iboga for many reasons, a prominent one of which was a desire to connect with their African heritage; their mother was born in Nigeria, not far from Gabon. Barton offered a refreshing revision on the "iboga is relentlessly brutal" narrative. "For me, it felt very loving," they shared. "I felt very held."

Barton was told that the effects would be rich in visual imagery, but their journey was overtly sensory, leading them to recognize iboga, like other psychedelics and plant medicines, affects different people in different ways. "Iboga has an association in the West as this really scary and intense thing," they reflected. "For those who haven't done much shadow work or tending to their deeper wounds, it can be a bit like a smack in the face. But for people who have been in relationship to that work, it can feel very loving and nourishing." Barton's testimony expressed a larger trend in plant medicines: the truth is often far more complex than common narratives suggest.

Fractals of Variation Beneath the Single Story

For Bwiti practitioners of Gabon, a leader of a sacred iboga ceremony is called a *nganga* (plural: *banganga*). While many other societies of Africa and the African diaspora who speak the common language of Kikongo use the same term for their spiritual healers, few have traditionally used iboga, for the shrub is indigenous to Central Africa's tropical forests far beyond their reach. This demonstrates the nuance that shamanic practices can contain, varying even within an interconnected lineage.

Here's a clearer example. Dunja Hersak has carried out a decade's worth of ethnographic field research in several African regions since 1977. In a brilliant article she wrote for *African Arts* in 2022, she deconstructed the academic world's homogenized and simplistic interpretation of the rituals, customs, and beliefs of the vast Kikongo-speaking region extending from southern Gabon to northern Angola.[22] Hersak recognized that scholarship on the region's art has for decades assumed a "single stories" approach, categorizing the production and ritual use of various "power objects" in accordance with a unified cultural narrative. This narrative categorizes all such power objects as *nkisi*, the Kikongo term for the magical figures banganga concoct with secret animal, vegetal, or mineral "empowering ingredients." Aided by the *nkisi*, *banganga* facilitate communication with "common spirits of the dead" called *bakisi*.[23]

Hersak noted that in the "northwestern Equatorial Atlantic sector of the Kongo world," the term *nkisi* refers to "the domain of *nature* spirits, which are environmental and territorial entities,"[24] while magical power objects are referred to as *nkosi*. *Nkosi* draw their power not from familiar spirits of the dead, but from "enslaved human spirits that become agents of sorcery."[25] The single stories approach common to Western academia overlooks such differences, embellishing a false narrative and reinforcing it without question.

Hersak elaborated on nuanced differences between regional traditions, recounting discoveries from her field work in the Kwilu province of the Republic of Congo. Of particular interest was an architectural structure called a *mwanza*, "where male and female practitioners perform both visionary and therapeutic cult activities" and "varied sources of power may be concentrated, displayed, and performed." An important source of power is a mystical auxiliary known as the *chinkoko*, a "so-called nocturnal animal" *banganga* create through an "imaginary surgery" Hersak described as "transmutation with the head of a human grafted on to the body of an animal." For *banganga*, the *chinkoko* is a source of extraordinary power, providing its master "extrahuman capacities" to protect the community and, in some cases, bring healing and transformation to those afflicted by curses.[26]

Although iboga was not consumed during the practices Hersak observed in the Kwilu province, she noted the influence of Gabonese Bwiti iboga rituals through a dance called the *liboka*, a term that derives from iboga. This observation supported her recognition of the dynamic nature of cultural practices of the Kikongo-speaking region.[27] The region's rituals, techniques, and relationships to sacred objects evolved as their technicians drew from distinct lineages and neighboring traditions, all the while learning from the ceaseless cycles of change churning the wheels of history.

Dynamism and nuance are squelched beneath the weighty imposition of the word "shamanic" onto all practices of West-Central African cultures. How many significant details are erased when this categorical imposition is extended to encompass all cultures seen through Western society's scuffed-up goggles as similar?

In her 2009 TED talk, Nigerian writer Chimamanda Ngozi Adichie said to create a single story is to "show a people as one thing, as only one thing, over and over again." With enough repetition, "that is what they become."

Adichie added a wise maxim on the role of power in writing a single story: "Power is the ability not just to tell the story of another person, but to make it the definitive story of that person."[28]

From the Roman Empire's sacking of Eleusis to the multinational European colonization of North and South America, the Western world is rooted in imperialist histories of enforcing a single story onto entire nations as a mechanism of control. Those who resisted the story's imposition were not typically met with respect for their autonomy as authors of their own stories. This was true for the many Native Americans who fought against the US and Canadian "boarding schools" built to enforce assimilation into Western ideologies. Given that the Americas' colonialist history is intertwined with militant suppression of plant medicine use, these historical narratives are important to bear in mind. A lack of awareness combined with unquestioning abstraction of cultural complexities into the single story of "shamanism" may pave the road for repetition of past trends that descendants of the oppressors often prefer to ignore as much as descendants of the oppressed are incapable of forgetting. With these complexities, it comes as little surprise that among the many Western individuals with New Age ideologies who call themselves shamans, a pattern of harm has emerged in the psychedelic underground.

The Perils of the New Age

These days, "New Age" isn't typically a flattering designation. In academia, it's a death sentence for legitimacy. It tends to refer to a wishy-washy, illogical, dreamy disposition with a propensity toward using any number of "folk remedies" for healing, claiming historical precedence that often doesn't exist, and reducing life's complexities to bumper sticker slogans. Sometimes, such outright dismissal is a shame, for many things labeled New Age have merit, despite science's quickness to label them hogwash.* At the very least, it can be helpful to call "consensus reality" into question, which New Age thinking unanimously does. But New Age ideologies can go so far as to become absurd, and its boundaries know no limit.

---

* I wish scientists would use the term "hogwash" more often. It's far more enjoyable than "unscientific," and it gets the same point across.

I was exposed to New Age philosophy in 2012 while traveling around the Mayan ruins of Tikal in Guatemala about six months before the Mayan Calendar's purported apocalypse of December '12. I benefited from the visualization meditations, the studies in Hermetic philosophy, and the breathing patterns my teacher said could remove blocks in my chakras to promote a balanced flow of energy. But some drifters I met who'd drunk gallons of the New Age Kool-Aid were, for lack of a better term, annoying. Their vernacular was so far out that it made no sense—and that's coming from a guy willing to get a good deal more irrational than those abiding the standard dictates of Western materialism. They'd frequently explain my problems in incomprehensible terms. I'd mention a mild headache, and they'd say something like, "That's a disruption to your energy flow in your Crown Chakra, which makes sense since Mercury is in retrograde and Venus is in Scorpio, which are of course in trine, and since your Venus is in Aquarius, there's more conflict than usual, especially as the energies are heightened due to the prophecy, which is really a Great Awakening for light beings who have prepared—so call on your ancestors to deliver a mantra, and chant it for two hours a day while visualizing pink light and invoking the elements of the Four Corners, laying rose quartz on your belly button and mugwort on your pineal gland with a liquid diet for the current moon cycle so the interdimensional beings can penetrate the veil and invoke sacred geometry to transmute the energy into unity consciousness. That will take care of your headache."

I'd say, "Actually, the guy who read my birth chart yesterday said my Venus is in Pisces."

They'd nod and continue, "That makes sense, because Pisces, a water sign, relates to the blockage of your third house . . ." To these individuals, everything made sense because their terms of sense-making were vague enough to encompass everything. Most important, they always *knew more than you.*

---

*   Don't take my critique of New Age thinking as a dig at astrology in general. I think skilled astrologers can offer enormous insight. I also know that some New Age people think they know more about astrology than they do, and they use words they don't understand to act like know-it-alls and say things that would even have a *People* magazine astrologer responding, "That makes no sense."

As it turns out, psychedelics and plant medicines attract such perspectives. If explain-it-all-as-energy philosophies help people heal with psychedelics, that's fine by me. What's not fine is when zealous New Agers decide they are shamans after "the mushrooms showed them the way," administer plant medicines to naïve seekers, and harm them through their ineptitude and self-delusion. These charlatans have infiltrated North, South, and Central America—and I imagine Europe and Asia as well—where they charge people yacht-loads of cash to administer plant medicines about which they know nothing, opting instead to dance around with rattles and drums, chant sounds they've made up on the spot, and violate numerous ethical standards of proper care. There are ongoing reports of such pseudo-shamans sexually and physically abusing their unsuspecting clients, and since they operate outside the oversight of the law, they do so without repercussion.

Seekers somehow find these practitioners, and when they participate in their ceremonies, they enter powerful non-ordinary states in unsafe environments, for these pseudo-shamans lack or ignore cultural and historical foundation and do not understand the realms where they are abandoning people to navigate an otherworld. While this occupation can arise from cruel motivations, it can also stem from ignorance about the complex history of traditional shamanic work and all it implicitly excludes.

Neo-Shamanism

Except for rare cases wherein Western individuals have been initiated into a specific lineage, the Western trend of "shamanic practitioners" is categorically distinct from traditional shamanism. Shamanic practitioners of the West typically practice some form of "neo-shamanism." Self-appointed shamans who seek power and financial gain through fraudulent claims of connection to traditional lineages occupy the category of "pseudo-shamans" or "plastic shamans."

Neo-shamanism is a Western practice that uses techniques of various shamanic traditions for psychotherapeutic and growth-oriented purposes. Two of the most influential figures in neo-shamanism's development were anthropologists Carlos Castaneda and Michael Harner.[29]

Castaneda is known for his series of books chronicling his apprenticeship under the enigmatic Don Juan Matus, a Yaqui "sorcerer" from Sonora, Mexico. His series began in 1968 with *The Teachings of Don Juan: A Yaqui*

Way of Knowledge, which Castaneda presented as an autobiographical account of his journeys to study Mexico's medicinal plants for his graduate thesis at UCLA. His travels led him to Don Juan, a *brujo* ("medicine man," "witch," or "sorcerer") said to possess "secret knowledge." Castaneda focused on the psychedelic plants with which Don Juan worked: peyote (*Mescalito*), Datura (*yerba del diablo*), and psilocybin-containing mushrooms (*humito*), chronicling his trips through the non-ordinary states they induced with rich verbosity and endearing characterization of the Yaqui *brujo*.

Although his autobiographical claims have been largely debunked and his tales are generally considered fiction, Castaneda's books became massive bestsellers in the 1960s and '70s, popularizing the concept of the "native shaman" and generating widespread interest in shamanic use of plant medicines. In Shelly Beth Braun's words, Castaneda ushered neo-shamanism "into the open arms of a jumbled American counter-culture experimenting with psychoactive drugs, Eastern philosophies, free love, and, in general, acting out against the mundane materiality of modernity as manifest in U.S. society."[30] As much as Castaneda influenced neo-shamanism's development, his influence was neither as vast nor as lasting as that of Michael Harner.

Core Shamanism

In the 1980s, beginning with his popular book, *The Way of the Shaman: A Guide to Power and Healing*, Harner distilled what he considered to be universal tenets of shamanism into a system of practices aimed toward personal development. When he began teaching classes on his system, which he named "Core Shamanism," neo-shamanism spread to a broad audience.*

On Harner's work, traditionally initiated shamanic teacher and author Itzhak Beery told me, "It's a synthesis of ideas and principles of traditional shamanism mostly from Siberia and Mongolia. Michael Harner, who was a Ph.D., created a whole system that's very much what you'd expect in academia.

---

* I wonder if Core Shamanism's popularity resulted from its filling a cultural void left over from the 1960s, providing a path for Western seekers desiring a primordial spiritual connection absent in Western values and mainstream religions. After all, Harner presented Core Shamanism's tenets as rooted in the Stone Age, and the hippie counterculture believed that through psychedelics, they were connecting to humanity's birthright, the essence of which Western Culture veiled.

That system works, but it's not the whole truth and not the way many other Indigenous cultures practice or believe in."

The Foundation for Shamanic Studies, which Harner started with his wife Sharon, continues to offer a breadth of Core Shamanism trainings ranging from two-day workshops to multi-year certificate programs. Since tuition costs are not published on the website, I assume they are expensive. And presumably because detailed explanations of Core Shamanism's tenets would lessen the demand for training, the website offers vague definitions, devoting far more space to testimonials of students expressing how the training fundamentally bettered their lives.[31]

I'm left to speculate based on testimonials, vague descriptions, and *The Way of the Shaman* that teachings in Core Shamanism include inducing trance states through methods like drumming and imaginative journeying into a spirit world, meeting and building a relationship with spirit allies and "power animals," retrieving fragmented parts of the soul, and integrating those parts into a present state of alignment with the forces of the Universe. Core Shamanism does not appear to emphasize or teach traditional methods of plant medicine use for visionary journeying. As website copy emphasizes a cultural extrapolation of "universal principles," I doubt Harner's trainings teach about any specific traditional lineages in depth, preferring instead to perpetuate a view that at their core, traditional lineages and practices are essentially the same.

"I never met a shaman who had a certificate," Beery said. "With Michael Harner, everybody has certificates. That kind of a program created entitlement of white people who are doing this work. They think that they do the real thing." Despite Harner's conviction that his system's universality belonged to no culture, he has been accused of appropriating traditional ways of life for personal gain and watering down complex realities to invent a neo-shamanic formula that speaks to the Western mindset.*

---

* Harner and others have made efforts to delineate Core Shamanism from neo-shamanism. Anthropologist Joan Townsend argued, "Core Shamanism is a conservative, purist approach to shamanism," while neo-shamanism relies on "metaphorical images and idealized concepts of shamanism, which are often joined with beliefs and diverse rituals that have little to do with traditional shamanism." Despite such arguments, Core Shamanism continues to be associated with neo-shamanism and New Age appropriation of traditional practices. (Source: "Core Shamanism," The Foundation for Shamanic Studies, accessed January 15, 2024, shamanism.org/workshops/coreshamanism.html)

Beery illustrated how watered-down entitlement can manifest. "I had a participant on a trip I organized for Brazil who was a professor of shamanism at a university in the U.S. He came to the shamans in Brazil, took off his clothes, and started dancing with a leaf on his loins and making noises, imitating the natives. They were angry and offended and asked him, 'What are you doing?' He laughed and said, 'I'm doing shamanism.' They said, 'That's not shamanism,' and this man said, 'You can't tell *me*—I'm a *PhD* in shamanism!' He was telling the shamans in Brazil, whom he came to learn from, that they were not shamans and didn't know what they were talking about!" Needless to say, he was banned from ever coming back.

To Beery, the biggest difference between Core Shamanism and traditional shamanism—and the main factor at play for this university professor—comes down to worldview. "In the West, we try to understand everything with our minds, our intellects. This is our sickness. We have to see the shamanic work is understanding from your heart. The mind is only one part."

It is impossible to understand traditional shamanism through a Western lens, for its reducing valve of rationality filters out essential depths of significance behind traditional practices. To learn about traditional shamanism, people of Western conditioning would benefit less from intellectual synthesis than from following Yoda's advice to Luke Skywalker on the planet Dagobah: "You must *unlearn* what you have learned." Unlearning what we think we know opens space for the heart to guide into nonlinear depths that the rational mind habitually rejects through its limited faculties of judgment.

16

Ayahuasca and the Spirit World

"This coming psychedelic renaissance has its roots in both the
laboratory and jungle. It is both scientific and shamanic."

—Don Lattin, *Changing Our Minds*

When it comes to Western unlearning, no plant medicine has been
more influential than the visionary tea derived from the *Banisteriopsis
caapi* vine and the leaves of the *Psychotria viridis* shrub native to the Amazon
rainforest. This tea has many names. Natives of Columbia and Ecuador call
their brew *yagé*. In Brazil, the medicine is *caapi*, *uni*, and *nixi pãe*. But the most
well-known name is used by cultures of the Peruvian Amazon: *ayahuasca*, a
Quechuan word commonly translated as "vine of the soul."

Ayahuasca

Although ayahuasca is the name given to the *Banisteriopsis caapi* vine, the
plant medicine is more than the vine. The decoction comes from combining
the vine with the leaves of *Psychotria viridis*, a shrub-like plant also known as
chacruna. Chacruna leaves contain ayahuasca's most powerful psychoactive
alkaloid: DMT.

Approximately one hundred Indigenous groups from Peru, Columbia,
Ecuador, Brazil, Bolivia, and Venezuela have historically drunk the brew.[1]
Specific recipes vary between cultures, but the ayahuasca vine and chacruna
leaves are typically the primary ingredients. A complex, multi-day process
of boiling the plants extracts key psychoactive molecules to create a brown,
chunky mixture. Though many describe its taste as indescribably gross, those

who force it down consistently report profound journeys into a different dimension where physical, emotional, mental, and spiritual healing occurs.

The chacruna leaves are essential for their naturally occurring DMT. If one were simply to extract the alkaloid from the leaves the resulting brew would produce no psychoactive effects. The human gastrointestinal system contains *monoamine oxidase enzymes*, which rapidly degrade orally consumed DMT and prevent its metabolization. The ayahuasca vine is essential because it contains *harmala alkaloids*—β-carbolines—that work as monoamine oxidase *inhibitors* (MAOIs). The vine's MAOIs interrupt the GI tract's degradation of the DMT molecules extracted from the chacruna leaves, allowing the tryptamine to enter the bloodstream and produce the psychedelic effects.

Motivations and contexts for ayahuasca use vary between cultures. Intentions can be as simple as social bonding or as complex as interfacing with a spiritual reality to cure an illness.[2] Regardless, many of these cultures drink ayahuasca in ceremonial settings for healing purposes. Exactly how long this has been going on remains a mystery. While websites and blogs written by individuals selling their "shamanic" services commonly contend Amazonian cultures have consumed ayahuasca for at least five thousand years, some anthropologists suggest its origins date back only a few centuries.[3] Ethnopharmacologist, writer, and researcher Dennis McKenna—younger brother of the late-great Terence—wrote, "About all that can be stated with certainty is that it [ayahuasca] was already spread among numerous indigenous tribes throughout the Amazon Basin by the time ayahuasca came to the attention of Western ethnographers in the mid-nineteenth century."[4]

A particularly evocative aspect of ayahuasca's history concerns the mystery of the brew's inspiration. On the surface, chacruna leaves and ayahuasca vines have no clear, causal relationship—if I'm strolling through the Amazon with my cargo shorts, fanny pack, and DSLR camera, I may notice a vine growing nearby and an unremarkable leaf growing in a different place down the buggy trail. How did humans figure out that combining these plants via a complex brewing process yielded profound, sacred visions?

The answers some lineages have provided won't satisfy the material scientist, for their explanations ring the bells of myth. Of one of the most common explanations, McKenna wrote, "Mestizo ayahuasqueros in Peru will, to this day, tell you that this knowledge comes directly from the 'plant teachers.'"[5] In other words, they received instructions from the spirits of the plants.

Hearing this, a material scientist would scratch his head and scowl, grumbling, "Not possible. Plants don't have consciousness! That's a silly superstition!"

Perhaps this scientist hasn't learned that some contemporary biologists have concluded that plants and fungi may indeed have consciousness. At the very least, plants can communicate complicated messages based on information gathered from the environment, demonstrating what science journalist Linda Geddes described as "anticipatory, goal-directed, flexible behaviour."[6] Intricate, underground systems of plant and fungal interconnectivity called mycorrhizal networks can be found in forests, jungles, and other densely vegetated areas, and the complicated signals that different species send to one another through the connection points between roots and mycelium have lent mycorrhizal networks the nickname of the Wood-Wide Web. Through this organic internet, plants can share important resources like sugar and nitrogen with one another. Additionally, plants under threat can send others warnings to raise their defensive responses. These discoveries have raised fascinating questions, including, as *New Yorker* writer Robert Macfarlane phrased it, "whether a forest might be better imagined as a single superorganism, rather than a grouping of independent individualistic ones."[7]

The skeptical scientist might respond, "That doesn't explain plants communicating with *people*, let alone teaching them how to make an illegal *drug*." Be that as it may, why does this scientist default toward imposing his explanatory framework onto people who are far more connected to the mystery? Why would he veer toward judgment instead of trying to understand and respect a different worldview?

I suppose many scientists find comfort in rational explanations. But it turns out the non-scientific qualities of ayahuasca appeal to countless people from Western cultures. Often, these individuals have become disillusioned with a diagnostic, linear approach to medicine, and they take ayahuasca in search of a depth of healing Western approaches cannot offer. The 2000s have seen such a significant rise in Westerners flocking to the Amazon to take part in traditional ayahuasca ceremonies that reference is commonly made to an "ayahuasca boom." The conditions these seekers hope the brew might heal appear to be limitless, ranging from depression and addiction to cancer and other terminal illnesses. As Indigenous cultures often teach, physical ailments typically have emotional, mental, and spiritual causes. Unlike pharmaceutical medications, ayahuasca delves into these abstract layers.

Ayahuasca's Effects

People who take ayahuasca report being flooded with otherworldly visions. This may indicate the closest point of connection between ayahuasca and synthesized DMT, where other-dimensional visions may as well be regarded as an essential feature. In both routes of DMT administration, people intuit the "other world" they enter to be more significant and causal than the default plane of waking consciousness. They feel certain that the substance provided a deeper understanding of unseen realities underpinning existence. Yet while DMT users describe humanoid entities occupying a mechanical realm, ayahuasca imagery tends to be more organic, filled with colorful, vine-like threads, mysterious snakes, and stealthy jaguars slinking through the darkness.

Common descriptions of ayahuasca's healing mechanisms are sure to weird out rationally minded folks. Ayahuasca makes people "purge," typically through vomit and/or diarrhea, and this purging is the body's way of releasing nasty stuff it's holding. This can include underlying causes of chronic illnesses and emotional complexes surrounding repressed trauma. While purging can be painful, it is often regarded as a sacred, spiritual cleansing of inner muck and grime.

As far as I'm aware, medical doctors don't typically equate barfing with healing the soul. Distinct from Western models as it may be, ayahuasca's popularity continues to rise, and occupants of remote regions of the Amazon have become accustomed to backpack-wearing, patchouli-smelling gringos showing up with wallets full of cash, asking for directions in broken Spanish to off-the-path villages in the jungle where ayahuasca is brewed.

Impacts of Ayahuasca Tourism

Ayahuasca's surge in popularity has created an industry of ayahuasca tourism. The demand from mostly affluent White people has prompted the establishment of countless ayahuasca healing centers throughout South and Central America. Other centers can be found in Mexico, several islands of the Caribbean, numerous European countries, and even Florida.

At some centers, Elders native to the region facilitate ceremonies traditional to their lineage. Others are led by plastic shamans looking to cash in on the trend. Some plastic shamans are gringos, and some are Native Amazonians who realized all they had to do was learn a basic ayahuasca recipe and claim membership to a shamanic lineage to make a lot of money. Phony centers often claim to offer "traditional ayahuasca ceremonies," for they know this language speaks to the seekers' idealized visions of Indigenous healing. The truth is, no generalized "traditional ayahuasca ceremony" exists, for the medicine's use varies significantly between cultures.

Beery, who has been initiated into two shamanic lineages, had much insight on the subject. "Many people serving ayahuasca are practically glorified bartenders without the deep experience necessary. For the Pixoto tribe, it takes *four years* of monthly drinking to become an ayahuasquero. How many people in the West are doing that? They go to Peru for two weeks, and they start shipping and giving the drink. They don't know how to create and hold a sacred space, and they don't 'see' energies. Most importantly, they don't provide integration into the everyday afterward."

Charlatan shamans present a danger to ayahuasca tourists. Therapist and writer Gemini Adams, who spent eighteen months living at, working in, and visiting healing centers in Peru, wrote several stories she'd either heard or witnessed firsthand. She once "watched a 'shaman'—who claimed to be of Peruvian lineage and to have studied the plants with his grandfather's guidance for twenty years—have absolutely no clue as to what to do with the woman who screamed and screamed during his ceremony, eventually resorting to locking her in a separate room." One of Adams's clients told her that "after drinking ayahuasca for the second time, he'd gone into a state that the staff seemed unable to handle, resulting in four of them pinning him down, breaking two of his ribs in the process." Adams referenced another plastic shaman "whose hands were known to be creeping into private spaces during his ceremonies, who, when asked to leave, threatened to bring 'dano'—illness from black magic—on the retreat owners and guests."[8]

These anecdotes begin to reveal the dark side of ayahuasca tourism. It has become extremely difficult to ensure one is traveling to an ethical center rather than some phony's money-making scheme.

Ayahuasca tourism has raised issues of conservation. "It takes five years for an ayahuasca vine to grow and be harvested," Beery said. "How big are the vats the fake shamans are using to cook? Do they plant enough ayahuasca for commercial use? Or are they going deeper into the Amazon and cutting more because they are lazy?"

Beery has been involved with Amazonian ayahuasca for long enough to understand the natural and cultural degradation its popularity is causing. "The cost of every cup of ayahuasca is the destruction of Indigenous societies. The shaman gets rich, but the whole village community is broken down because suddenly, you have castes. You have a shaman with a Rolex and a tourist motorboat, and you have the other poor people, which is something these villages never had before."

While ayahuasca is undoubtedly helping people around the world heal, the impact of its globalization casts a dark shadow over its popularity. "If you ask me, ayahuasca is wonderful, but it's also a destructive force of the Amazon," Beery added. "Nobody talks about that, because in the same way the shamans are greedy for our money, we in the Western world are greedy for authentic spiritual experiences. We're getting a shot of a little meaning or personal growth, but in the same way, we are helping destroy the jungle and the Indigenous societies' old traditions." Dark as it may be, ayahuasca tourism only scratches the surface of the shadows the powerful brew can evoke.

Battling Dark Spirits

The mainstream narrative of the West frames psychedelics as isolated molecules that work like medicines—you take it, you do therapy with it, and you heal. In plant medicine cultures, one may take a plant medicine to heal, but the process is not so straightforward. The medicine is not regarded as an isolated molecule, but as a teacher that opens people to a "spirit world."

There, guides and ancestors heal afflictions—but they are not alone. Benevolent spirits coexist with dark spirits that feed on fear and vulnerability. In some traditions, certain ailments and illnesses are understood as dark spirits burrowing in the body and feeding like leeches off life energy. The ethos of universal surrender psychedelic therapists teach may be the right approach with substances like MDMA and ketamine, but it does not apply to all plant medicines, and believing it can and does get people into trouble.

Let's imagine an entrepreneur named Fred travels to Peru because he heard a podcast where a supplement company's CEO explained how ayahuasca helped him optimize his life. Fred's in for a surprise when the *maloca* ceiling becomes a hellish vortex sucking him into a decaying fortress filled with bile-spewing demons. Fred realizes life optimization isn't as simple as drinking a magical brew, throwing up a few times, and following an immaterial jaguar. When it's too late to turn back, Fred has no clue what to do.

That's because Fred's culture provided no framework to understand such visions. He'd trusted the scientists claiming such realms were fairy tales. Fred's cultural indoctrination made him extraordinarily naïve about the complexities of reality and consciousness that plant medicines reveal.

Perhaps the *ayahuasqueros* take their roles seriously and come to Fred's aid with a cleansing ritual to protect him from the dark spirits. Unfortunately, it doesn't always work out that way, despite how much Fred learned about the inner healer. If Fred read an article explaining that psychedelic healing comes through surrendering, he might mistakenly surrender to the evil spirits, allowing them to take residence in his body and leaving Fred incapable of returning to everyday life in the States. His friends may tell him none of it was real, but Fred knows in his bones that it was more real than anything he had ever experienced.

When I asked Beery what someone should do if they encounter an evil spirit on ayahuasca, he didn't advise surrendering. He emphasized the opposite: "You *fight* it!"

During an ayahuasca ceremony, Beery once heard a spirit whispering at him to follow. The spirit appeared to be Jesus, and it told him that if he followed, he would gain riches, power, and gratification. When Beery expressed that he was "willing to give my life but not to surrender," the spirit transformed into a demon and tried to overtake him. Fortunately, Beery's training had prepared him.

"We started fighting," he said. "In that moment, I thought, 'The only thing I can do is to send him light.' From my heart, I sent a beam of strong light into his heart. It took all my energy, but slowly, he disappeared."

Beery's encounter didn't end there. "From this light I sent, a man showed up. He said, 'I am from the village near you. I grew up near Nazareth.' He was moving forward with light around him, and he said, 'These forces are using me, but this is not my teaching. These are the evil spirits using me to control the world.' That was very powerful to experience."

A pop culture illustration can be found in the second season of the TV series, *Stranger Things*. Young Will Byers is suffering from horrible visions of a malevolent entity called the "Mind Flayer" trying to possess him. His mother's boyfriend, the ever-naïve Bob (Sean Astin), tells Will that instead of fleeing the entity, he should face it and yell, "Go away!" Will takes Astin's advice, and it doesn't work. The Mind Flayer seizes the opening and possesses Will's body, feeding off his vulnerability, fear, and energy. Astin underestimated the dark reality Will was facing, mistakenly interpreting an autonomous evil spirit as an illusory projection of the mind.

As I listened to Beery's story about the dark, shapeshifting spirit he encountered, I noted connections to Jesus Christ's final temptation. As he hung on the cross to die, Jesus was approached by Satan, who promised him riches and power if he revoked his faith in God. Like the dark spirit, Satan beckoned his subject to follow. But Jesus resisted the temptation, reaffirming his connection to the Divine. Satan gained no power over him, and Jesus accomplished his redemptive mission.

Such stories are not unique to Christianity. In Buddhist lore, Siddhartha Gautama faced the temptation of *Mara*, a malicious entity who tried to seduce him with sensory pleasure as he meditated beneath the bodhi tree. Mara sought to keep humans trapped in the cycle of suffering and reincarnation, but Siddhartha, paralleling Jesus's redemption, overcame the spirit's temptation to awaken as the Buddha.

Beyond this redemptive arc, the phenomenon of spirit possession appears in most major religions. In Jewish folklore, a *dybbuk* is a malicious, dislocated spirit of a dead person that roams in search of a host body to possess. In Islamic theology, *shayatin* are evil spirits known as *ifrits*, which whisper to the soul to tempt people to follow their baser impulses.

When viewed through the lens of traditional shamanism, stories of encounters with dark spirits are not reducible to mythology. They are instructional tales teaching how to navigate a spirit world that has existed alongside the material plane ever since the material plane came to be. Whether or not these stories encompass accurate historical accounts is beside the point.

I find it hypocritical that Christian colonists from Europe derided the Indigenous peoples' plant medicine use and spirituality as "devil worship" and "paganism" because of their belief in and engagement with spirits. Christian theology is built on a hierarchy of spirits called "angels" and "archangels," many of whom have specific names, personalities, and gifts to bestow. Visions and encounters with "cherubs" are regarded with the utmost significance, for these spirits are harbingers of God's grace, connecting the material world to the immaterial reality of Heaven. Benevolent spirits are contrasted with the malevolent demons controlled by Satan. The Bible suggests that Satan once resided in Heaven, where, according to the Book of Isaiah, he sought power over God.[9] The Book of Revelation chronicles a war in Heaven, where Satan, taking the form of a dragon, led a band of angels in battle against those led by Archangel Michael. Michael prevailed, casting Satan and his followers out of Heaven.[10] Revelation and the Book of Job suggest Satan and his minions were sent from Heaven down to Earth, where they were fated forevermore to roam.[11]

I'm no Biblical scholar, but that sounds an awful lot like evil spirits roaming the material plane since the beginning of time. I'm not saying all religions are essentially the same, but maybe a long history of focusing on differences has veiled connective tissue between widespread spiritual traditions, and perhaps science's excessive focus on the material world gradually eclipsed realities toward which the connections pointed. In case that needs a little more fleshing out, Saint Paul wrote to the Corinthians that Satan "masquerades as an angel of light."[12] Sounds suspiciously like the sinister spirit Beery encountered, doesn't it?

So . . . What *Are* These Dark Spirits?

There's no straightforward answer—how could there be? Different traditions understand them differently. And if they are real, it appears the spirits themselves differ across geographical regions.

The mythology of the Algonquin people features the *Wendigo*, a bipedal, hooved beast of the woods that possesses people with hunger and greed so insatiable as to turn them into murderers and cannibals.[13] It's no coincidence the Algonquin people resided in the heavily wooded areas of present-day northeastern United States and Eastern Canada. According to some tales, the Wendigo was a lost hunter whose extreme winter hunger drove him to cannibalism; other stories chronicle the beast's origins as a warrior who made a deal with the Devil.

Similar spirits have been detailed in other wooded settings. The Algonquins' neighboring Iroquois tribes told stories of the *Stone Coat*, a demon who hunts and eats humans. Colombian folklore features the *Patasola*, a female entity who seduces male hunters deep into the jungle, where she transforms into a pale, one-legged monster, and feasts on the hunter's flesh. A nearly identical spirit appears as the *Sayona* in Venezuela and the *Tunda* in the Colombian Pacific. Centuries later, in modern storytelling, a camouflaging "demon who makes trophies of man" faced off against Arnold Schwarzenegger in the Central American jungles of the blood-pumping classic *Predator*. Although the Predator doesn't eat flesh, that ugly mofo can't get enough of ripping it right off its buff and sweaty targets. These human-consuming demons appear in heavily wooded areas, suggesting connections between geography and the spirit's characteristics.

Is that because topography affects the human imagination in acultural ways? Or is it because people in touch with the spirit world tap into the same realities?

Beyond cannibalistic entities of the woods, numerous evil spirits throughout the world share the common characteristic of an unappeasable appetite for human vitality. The *Sluagh* were among the most feared entities in pre-Christian Ireland. They didn't feed on human flesh, preferring human souls. They flew like ravens across the sky, approaching from the west and seeking sustenance through whomever they could find in their restless, cursed existence.[14] Legend tells that St. Patrick was tormented by the *Sluagh* during his lengthy period of fasting and prayer on top of Croagh Patrick, Ireland's Holy

Mountain, where he successfully drove them away. Still, the *Sluagh* survived the transition into Irish Catholic mythology, transforming from birds into unrepentant, decrepit souls of dead sinners who shared their avian ancestors' appetite for human vitality.[15] Homeowners in the Irish countryside sealed their west-facing windows to protect themselves from the demons' onslaughts.[16]

Similar spirits called "vengeful ghosts" appear in many mythologies. These spirits of deceased people wander the earth with an appetite for revenge. In Japanese folklore, the *Funayūrei* ghosts haunt the sea, channeling their malevolence by causing boats to sink.[17] In Chinese tradition, the *mogwai* are vengeful, demonic spirits of the dead who inflict harm on humans, especially those who caused them suffering during their lives.[18] The *hungry ghosts* of Buddhist mythology are less vengeful than tormented with eternal dissatisfaction and insatiability, doomed to roam in helpless pursuit of appeasement.[19] These souls of the deceased are trapped, unable to reincarnate or pass on due to unresolved trauma, pain, and loss. Some portrayals of hungry ghosts depict them with pity and compassion, while others regard them as malevolent entities seeking to possess the living by latching onto humans' baser impulses for fleeting satisfaction.

Hungarian-Canadian physician Gabor Maté has become an international spokesperson on addiction, developmental trauma, and ayahuasca's potential to help Westerners heal these afflictions. Maté evoked the concept of the hungry ghosts to describe the people suffering from crippling addictions whom he spent decades treating in Vancouver's Downtown Eastside. Like the tortured ghosts, those of us caught in the violent throes of addiction "constantly seek something outside ourselves to curb an insatiable yearning for relief or fulfillment."[20]

Although the object of craving and means to grasp it differ between spirits, many share a thread of insatiable desire, the dominion of which is invariably entangled with eternal suffering. Regarding the dark spirits of the ayahuasca world, Berry told me, "Their goal is to feed on dark and heavy energy, like fear. In essence, it is about sucking that energy and letting the person who has it die, because the goal of negative energy is to stop the flow of life."

A mind vulnerable to evil spirits is ruled by scarcity, a sense of never being or having enough. Dark spirits cultivate envy, competitiveness, possessiveness, jealousy, and wrath. Perhaps Dante knew this when he structured the descent through the nine circles of the Inferno on the Seven Deadly Sins in *The Divine Comedy*. If there's a common characteristic to be found in the evil spirits across cultures and religions, it is their commitment to preserve themselves through the devastation of life.

The Economic Incentive to Feed the Dark Spirits

If one is willing to suspend disbelief and imagine these spirits are real, one might recognize that the Western capitalist ethos benefits less from healing that on which dark spirits feed than from *cultivating* it. There's an economic incentive in fostering a scarcity mindset: people who believe they need something they don't have are easier to manipulate into forking over their paychecks.

In the markets of self-help and biohacking, programs and products are often advertised as the missing piece that will fill the void the consumer has felt for as long as they can remember. But every product ultimately falls short, and the consumer continues seeking the next thing, and the next thing, and so on down the endless chain of insatiable yearning exploited for profit. Why would anyone buy anything but basic necessities if they knew they had everything they needed? Fulfillment and satisfaction are dangerous emotions to the capitalist ethos unless they're presented as a mirage money alone may manifest.[*]

---

[*] Speaking of mirages, have you ever been to Las Vegas? The Vegas Strip is the apocalyptic epitome of cultivating and exploiting a scarcity mentality for profit. If I were an entity in the US, I would definitely hang out there. My wife and I realized this when, inspired by Hunter S. Thompson, we took LSD and tripped through the Strip. The dazzling façade revealed itself, and we saw that the whole damn town operates on cultivating scarcity by selling fantasies of satisfaction. Gamble here, make millions! Go to this strip club, feel happy! The Strip is such a dirty, hot, weird environment built on an illusion that if you "play your cards right," you will have the greatest night of your life, when the truth is closer to a bunch of cigar-chomping crooks inviting you into their home, taking your wallet, dropkicking you to the curb, and wiping their asses with your money. Each neon sign points only to itself: a carnival display of cheap bulbs. Las Vegas does everything it can to make you salivate while flooding you with promises to satiate your saliva's yearnings, none of which amount to more than a cold corn dog and an under-boozed slushy. Once my wife and I saw the façade, we realized we didn't have to play into it. We had the joy of being together, and it gave us deeper fulfillment than any VIP lounge or limo ride could come close to offering. Laughing at the absurdity of it all, we had the time of our lives doing nothing you're "supposed" to in Vegas (with the exception of LSD). No dark spirit could penetrate our protective shield of satisfaction, and our love deepened through the contrast. That's why I asked her to marry me when we returned to our secret spot outside The Mirage a year later.

Inner emptiness cannot be filled by anything external. Think of Charles Foster Kane (Orson Welles) in *Citizen Kane*, who built an empire of possessions but died alone and sad. With his dying breath, Welles yearned for "Rosebud," his beloved childhood sled that represented the innocent satisfaction he'd spent his life trying and failing to reclaim through material gain. Kane didn't lack possessions; he lacked connection. Such lack drives distorted patterns in an endless cycle of want that cannot end until the underlying need is recognized and met.

If dark spirits are real, then capitalism creates plenty of optimal conditions for them to flourish. At its worst, capitalism promotes alienation and profits off ensuing desperation. I doubt these trends are reducible to capitalism. Capitalism is the convenient board on which to peg complaints. As George Orwell depicts in *Animal Farm*, his greatest work,* no system built on utopian dreams can furlough the will of piggish greed.

How the Dark Spirits Get In

If Western readers will continue suspending disbelief for a moment, there's a question of where these dark spirits came from in the first place. According to Beery, "They were always here. It is the other side of life."

From this vantage point, dark spirits are integral to life's balance. Dualism, as expressed in the *yin-yang*, is an essential property of the Universe.

"They come to people with cracks in their energy field's protective shield," Beery said. "When you experience a trauma or sudden fear, it cracks the shield, and negative energy enters into you. That attracts other negative spirits, which are fed by it. They go down deep into your tissue, bones, and organs.

---

* Perhaps you did a double take to check that I indeed described *Animal Farm* and not *Nineteen Eighty-Four* as Orwell's finest. I know dogmatic rigidity causes problems and all, but I will argue until my dying day that *Animal Farm* triumphs over *Nineteen Eighty-Four* on every metric of literary value. Orwell's allegorical approach rendered *Animal Farm* timeless, whereas *Nineteen Eighty-Four* has become a reference point for people who like to imagine a government of mass surveillance and repressive control remains but a fiction. The US was already far beyond *Nineteen Eighty-Four* (minus the rat torture device) when Edward Snowden leaked thousands of NSA documents in 2013, but high school teachers around the country still teach the novel as a "thought experiment" for what "could go wrong." It's historical fiction at best, a chronic yawn at worst. *Animal Farm* will never cease to delight, and *Nineteen Eighty-Four* will never cease to age terribly.

That's where you get sick. The role of the healer, the shaman, is to clear that energy field and ensure the shield is repaired and solid again."

I don't know how traditional shamans do this. All I know is it takes many years to develop the skills, which are learned from deep wells of tradition. If these spirits are real, do psychedelics make people more vulnerable to their entry just as plant medicines do? Are psychedelic therapists equipped to protect their clients and cleanse their cracked shields? Or is the Western world tampering with realities of heavy consequence about which they know basically nothing?

Regardless, even therapists who don't believe in autonomous spirits roaming like ethereal leeches in search of human hosts recognize that for psychedelic treatment to be effective, the therapist must clear themselves of impulses toward manipulation and power as much as possible. Otherwise, they may usher darkness into their clients' experiences, unconsciously perpetuating harm instead of healing and edging toward the moral depravity of those known as "dark shamans."

Shamanic Warfare

During their apprenticeship in navigating the spirit world, a shaman turns dark by choosing to work in partnership with dark spirits. Beery said he once hosted a dark shaman from Ecuador in his home, and the shaman, under the influence of ayahuasca, told Beery he would send spirits to kill his enemy for a hundred dollars. As shamans lead with protective intentions, dark shamans follow negative intentions to harm others for personal gain.

The concept of "black magic" is more than a Brothers Grimm plot device. Troves of texts contain complex spells of ill-intent, and psychedelics, being *non-specific* amplifiers, can theoretically enhance the power of any ceremonial intention. Albertus Magnus, an influential German philosopher of the Middle Ages, wrote in 1250 AD that *necromancers*—people engaged in a particular type of black magic—used the psychoactive plant *henbane* to invoke demons and the souls of the dead.

Now that thousands of White people have ventured to the Amazon, the internet is filled with countless ayahuasca tales. While many of these accounts involve profound healing, others are quite freaky. More than a few

Yanks have found themselves exposed to the reality of "shamanic warfare." This warfare involves neither nukes nor drones, but entities and bad blood.

Traditional shamans build relationships with helper spirits to protect their communities and support their intentions. Dark shamans use negative intentions to pollute and harm the ceremonial spaces of other shamans, perhaps to drive them away from an area they want to control. They work in cahoots with hostile, malevolent spirits and send them to attack victims. According to Vitebsky, their intentions can be as extreme as directing spirits to "eat the victim's soul."[21] Shamans and the participants in their ceremonies become vulnerable to attacks when a plant medicine lifts the veil between worlds. Traditional shamans develop the skills to block such attacks and maintain a safe container.

I think Western culture knows this stuff is real at some level of awareness, for many of its most beloved stories tell the same tale. In *Star Wars*, the Jedi—Skywalker, Kenobi, Windu—are, like shamans, protectors of balance and harmony, while the Sith—Vader, Maul, Plagueis—have turned to the "dark side" for power and control. Rip on the three prequels all you want, but they show how Anakin's turn to the dark side was fueled by the trauma of his mother getting murdered in cold blood, igniting fires of fear which sensed from the start, Master Yoda did.

The same goes for Voldemort from the *Harry Potter* series, whose childhood trauma and lack of connection to any family or love prompted him to split his soul into several pieces and control a band of Death Eaters with fear. Like Skywalker, Harry Potter undergoes training in the ancient magical—or shamanic—arts to overcome the threatening darkness with light. Both Skywalker and Potter must wrestle with the darkness within their hearts, face great temptation to succumb, and overcome the temptation to prevail. Cliché as it may sound, Dumbledore taught Harry that he had access to a power not even Voldemort's darkest curse could penetrate—the protective magic of love.

A Lesson for the West

Plant medicines have unique powers to open people to extraordinary realms that mustn't be taken lightly. It is too common of a story for unprepared people to take ayahuasca and become overwhelmed, terrified, and abandoned, fated to return to a culture incapable of helping them understand what they witnessed. In such a state, people can essentially "lose their minds," and the Western diagnostic system will at best label them psychotic or schizophrenic, at worst confine them to sterile rooms among others whose visions don't fit into the culture's materialistic, linear paradigm.

Without developing an appreciation for psychedelics' potential to unlock realities similar to those of plant medicines like ayahuasca, Western therapists may find themselves unprepared to support people navigating realms beyond their autobiographical selves. A mantra of "trust the medicine" can fail to guide through the astounding realities to which plant medicines grant access. In the excitement of psychedelic healing potential, we must not forget their potential for harm and take seriously our responsibility to train practitioners to protect people from threats in the darkness.

17

Peyote and Reciprocity

"If you want to be a shaman, watch a thousand
sunrises and a thousand sunsets."

—Don José Matsuwa, Huichol *mara'akame*

While origins of most plant medicines like ayahuasca remain speculative, archaeological evidence has proved that one psychoactive cactus
has been ceremonially consumed by Indigenous people of North America for
well over five thousand years. Today, the Native American Church (NAC)
regards this cactus as a sacrament, and many members consume it with their
communities for healing. As such, the *Lophophora williamsii* cactus, better
known as *peyote*, is the plant medicine with the longest known history of
human consumption.[1]

Mescaline is abundant in peyote's characteristic "buttons," the common
term for the disk-shaped body of the mature, spineless cactus. Buttons picked
for ceremonies are typically dried and chewed or brewed into a tea. When
harvested correctly, the plant regenerates new buttons, expressing the boun-
tiful nature of the Earth that peyote-using cultures revere with gratitude.

Numerous Indigenous tribes of North America have historically engaged
in sacred peyote "meetings." Traditionally, these ceremonies take place in a
tipi or hogan, a sacred Navajo dwelling whose entrance faces the rising sun.
Meetings begin in the evening and last through the night, following structured rituals layered with cultural meaning. Ceremonial plants like cedar and
tobacco factor prominently, and prayers are offered as the latter is smoked and laid
down. Through the night, community members ingest peyote—served as a

powder, tea, or mush—many times. Through the medicine and ceremony, many connect with their ancestors for healing and guidance.

My friend Danny Vandever, a Navajo—or Diné, the word the Navajo use for themselves—told me about his grandfather, a code talker in World War II who became a medicine man in the Native American Church. After the war, he was having problems, physically and mentally. He found the Native American Church, and he used to say it saved him.

"The peyote plays a role in helping diagnose yourself, helping to broaden and expand your understanding of the universe," Danny shared. "Whenever my grandfather would host meetings, it was said to get the bad out of you and make that connection to the spiritual world. It was always treated as medicine, something not to be abused."

Throughout the night, the community sits in a circle around a fire, which directs the ritual's focus on the elements. "The fire is like the heart of the Hogan, but it's also used to do your readings and diagnosis as well," Danny explained. Everything is symbolic. When I interviewed Debi Roan, educator and holder of the Navajo lineage, she explained, "The fire chief constantly feeds that fire, so the ash grows. Once the ash gets put forward, a bar of sand is sculpted in a moon shape. That represents your road of life. Right in the middle of the road of life, you have a groove that represents a highway. Right in the middle of that, at the V-point of the fire and on top of the mound of sand altar, you put the grandfather peyote."[2]

A drum filled partially with water is passed around the circle along with a rattle for community members to sing songs of prayer and ancestral connection. Traditionally, everyone sits up throughout the night, requiring self-sacrificial discipline that honors the medicine and promotes inner strength.

"It's really tough to sit up all night, listening to the songs and the prayers," Roan explained. "You're thinking about all of these things throughout the night, sitting on your knees on the ground or on a pillow. That's how I was raised, and that's how I respect medicine."[3]

Danny remembered the same rule. "One of my first memories of peyote ceremony is getting in trouble for falling asleep. I remember being woken up towards the end of it when the tobacco was passed around. I woke up to a cloud of smoke in the hogan, and I had to smoke some of that."

When morning comes, prayers of gratitude meet the rising sun, and the community shares a meal. "Everybody is fed before they go home," Roan said. "They drink coffee, making sure they are safe on their journey home. You take that whole day to recuperate and to rest. My mom says, 'Don't go to sleep until nightfall, so you have all the blessings of the day to go on.'"[4]

Peyote's effects have long informed Native American cultures' spirituality, which forms a perspectival centerpiece permeating all facets of a way of life. As with many plant medicine traditions, the ceremony is an essential component of the medicine. To take a plant medicine with no traditional ceremony would dilute its healing power. Healing in a peyote meeting cannot be reduced to consuming a psychoactive cactus.

The Spirit of the Medicine

If you stroll through a college campus in the US, you're likely to hear some shirtless dude with a backward hat and ping pong ball in hand talking about "tripping." It is possible when this person took mushrooms at the big frat party last night, he was "tripping balls," perhaps even "freaking out." If instead you overhear a peyote roadman speaking about the cactus, you might hear him describing its unique *spirit*. In traditional contexts, taking a plant medicine is not about having a wild time but about entering the medicine spirit's world, which most traditions regard as more real than the day-to-day world.

The spirits of specific medicines are typically interwoven with the features of the natural world where the community resides. For the Shipibo drinkers of ayahuasca in the Amazon, jaguars and serpents are powerful spirits whose apparition signifies something important—serpent spirits, for instance, are sometimes believed to clear negative energy and purify the heart.[5] For many North American cultures, the Great Spirit infuses all matter, and peyote deepens one's capacity to communicate with and offer prayers to the unique spirits animating all things. Connecting to the spirit world is connecting with the essence of life, and kinship with this essence is central to living in harmonious balance.

In the Lakota tradition, visions from the spirit world have brought powerful messages to important leaders. In the early 1930s, Black Elk, an Oglala Lakota medicine man, told American writer John Neihardt the story of how the famous Lakota war chief Crazy Horse, Black Elk's cousin, got his name. Black Elk's son translated his father's Lakota words into English, which Neihardt transcribed:

"Crazy Horse dreamed and went into the world where there is nothing but the spirits of all things. That is the real world that is behind this one, and everything we see here is something like a shadow from that one. He was on his horse in that world, and the horse and himself on it and the trees and the grass and the stones and everything were made of spirit, and nothing was hard, and everything seemed to float. His horse was standing still there, and yet it danced around like a horse made only of shadow, and that is how he got his name . . . It was this vision that gave him his great power, for when he went into a fight, he had only to think of that world to be in it again so that he could go through anything and not be hurt."[6]

Bolstered by the power he'd received from his vision, Crazy Horse led roughly fifteen hundred Lakota and Cheyenne people in the Great Sioux War of 1876. His leadership was central in their legendary defeat of the US Army's 7th Cavalry Regiment during Lt. Colonel George Armstrong Custer's raid of their encampment along the Little Bighorn River, which came to be known as Custer's Last Stand.

As Crazy Horse's vision didn't come from peyote, you might question its relevance. This question arises because a distinction between a "peyote vision" and "non-peyote vision" only matters to the categorically driven Western mind. In the Lakota perspective, a vision is a message from the spirit world, regardless of catalyst. Crazy Horse's vision contributes to understanding peyote because it broadens understanding of a way of life in which peyote factors centrally. The medicine, spiritual worldview, and customs cannot be separated.

Plant Consciousness

Many traditions believe plant medicines have autonomous consciousness distinct from that of humans. In the revival, it's common to hear this perspective reflected through statements like, "The mushrooms showed me [insert lesson]" or "The mushrooms told me to tell you [insert advice]" in which the mushrooms are given the pronoun "they." Another person might say, "Ayahuasca told me to quit my job," referring to the brew's spirit as "she," for ayahuasca's spirit is commonly regarded as feminine. Ayahuasca is sometimes called "Grandmother," while the masculine spirit of peyote is sometimes called "Grandfather." Each medicine has a unique spirit, and plant medicine traditions emphasize respecting that spirit's autonomy.

Narratives framing the revival rarely include this kind of language. You're more likely to come across terms like "functional connectivity" and "modulation" than "spirits" and "messages." Science doesn't typically approve of such language, and the Western world is not prepared to integrate it. Would psychedelics gain mainstream approval if renowned experts talk about accessing a spiritual dimension to communicate with a plant's consciousness? No chance. The esoteric verbiage of scientific academia garners mainstream approval, even if no one understands it. And even if scientists took Indigenous views seriously, how might they study the consciousness of a plant medicine? Their gadgets couldn't go there, especially given their enduring inability to study human consciousness beyond a physical level.*

Scientific disregard does not eliminate the question. Do plant medicines possess consciousness? If so, what does this teach us about consciousness in general? Does an individual plant consciousness have an agenda? If so, what—or whom—do their agendas serve? Scientists will chase their tails attempting to answer any of these questions. They might consider having a discussion with a member of the Native American Church, who may know more than they do about such matters.

More Differences Between Neo- and Traditional Shamanism

Traditional shamanic practices like peyote meetings can focus on individual healing, but this healing typically occurs in group ceremonies uniting the community. One person's ailment may be regarded as the community's sickness rather than something the individual needs to deal with personally. The communal bonding that transpires inside a Lakota tipi during an all-night peyote meeting strengthens interpersonal connections grounded in a shared worldview.

---

* When philosopher Daniel Dennett reads this sentence, I imagine he'll exclaim, "Consciousness is physical, you idiot!" In response, I'd say, "How about you try these mushrooms, and then we can continue our discussion?"

On the other hand, neo-shamanism, according to Shelly Beth Braun, "is focused on the individual rather than the community." Individuals "can learn neo-shamanic tools and techniques solely for personal use, not in service to others."[7] Despite focusing on humanity's inherent connection to nature and spirit, neo-shamanic practices usually aim toward self-improvement and personal healing.

Traditional shamans like the peyote roadman undergo lengthy apprenticeships that may continue throughout their life. They don't take a two-year course to get certified. Initiatory rites are common to traditional shamanism, while no such requirement exists for Core Shamanism practitioners. In some cultures, shamans are determined at birth,[8] while neo-shamans may ascribe themselves the title for any reason they choose.

Lastly, traditional shamans do not exclusively occupy the "love-and-light" world on which many neo-shamanic practitioners—especially the plastic variety—focus. Traditional shamans are acquainted with the world of darkness and respect its power, for they know it poses an ever-present threat to stability.

"Even though the shaman enters trance under controlled conditions, his or her 'mastery' of the spirits remains highly precarious," wrote Vitebsky. "The shaman's profession is considered psychically very dangerous and there is a constant risk of insanity or death."[9]

Amid traditional shamans' unique techniques to aid journeys through the spirit world is a humble recognition that the forces of that world act according to their own agenda. These forces can overpower even the most advanced practitioners. Imagining love and light may not help during a battle with dark spirits intent on overcoming the shaman's vulnerable, trance-induced mind. If it does help, then it's because these imaginings have been practiced with greater discipline than plastic shamans care to mimic.

Vitebsky summarized the distinction between traditional shamanism and neo-shamanism: "Shamanism is not a single, unified religion but a cross-cultural form of religious sensibility and practice . . . There is no doctrine, no world shamanic church, no holy book as a point of reference, no priests with the authority to tell us what is and what is not correct."[10] Western culture's lack of an established shamanic tradition casts a barren pall over neo-shamanism in comparison with the numerous shamanic cultures its material ethos has long eschewed.

Peyote's Effects

Descriptions of peyote experiences are less likely to include visions of an "other world" than clear perception of *this* world. Things don't tend to transform into other things as much as reveal their spiritual essence.

Descriptions are unlikely to come from Native Americans, for they have historically kept their understanding of the cactus close to home. To many cultures, peyote is a sacred medicine provided by the Great Spirit to connect them to their ancestors, traditions, communities, and land. With the use of peyote, boundaries separating the ordinary world and the spirit world become permeable, and with the help of the spirits, community members focus on living in harmonious balance with nature, recognizing their interconnectivity with all things.

White people who have experimented with peyote are often more eager to describe its effects. In his book *Peyote Dreams*, French writer Charles Duits described his 1965 peyote experience as revealing things "in their nakedness," continuing, "Appearance no longer concealed essence but expressed it."[11] Having taken the cactus with scientific skepticism, Duits was amazed to discover that "far from veiling reality, peyote unveils it, and, because the sensation that accompanies this unveiling is glorious, it can legitimately be called a revelation."[12]

His words are reminiscent of Huxley's descriptions of his mescaline visions in *The Doors of Perception*. Both writers traced the dualism between appearance and essence to Plato, who abstracted the essence of things into an eternal realm of Forms. For Duits and Huxley, peyote and mescaline revealed this distinction as illusory, consequently casting suspicion over the history of Western philosophy built on Plato's foundational work.

These men had no cultural relationship with the cactus. They were outside observers subjecting a new experience to theoretical frameworks rooted in Western philosophy and theology. Indigenous members of tribes grounded in long histories of peyote use would describe its effects not in terms of Greek philosophers but in terms of a worldview distinct from Western models of conceptualizing existence.

For Danny and his community, peyote helps restore Hózhó, the Navajo philosophy of balance and harmony in life. "You don't want to be overwhelmed with bad things, but even with too much good, you need the bad to balance it out. That's the basis of Navajo culture—you have to walk this fine line. And if you're able to on a day-to-day basis, you'll be able to live a life into old age. Peyote and the NAC is figuring out this pathway of how you live your life."

The gap between Western and Indigenous ways of viewing peyote factors centrally in the lengthy history of conflict surrounding *Lophophora williamsii*. As trends of this conflict are expressing anew today, peyote has become one of the most controversial subjects of the revival.

Decriminalize Nature

In 2018, a political campaign called Decriminalize Nature—or Decrim for short—made headlines by passing a measure in Santa Cruz, California, that decriminalized possession of several plant medicines. By decriminalizing these plants, the measure did not *legalize* them; rather, it relegated the plants to a bottom-of-the-list priority for law enforcement.* Decriminalization is often presented as a step toward legalization, and so when Santa Cruz's list of decriminalized plant medicines included psilocybin mushrooms, ayahuasca, iboga, and peyote, psychedelic enthusiasts rejoiced in victory for the liberty to choose what one can legally imbibe.

The rejoicing did not extend to all cultures. In communities the measures neglected to recognize, members of the Native American Church were not happy. The NAC already had legal access to peyote—and it wasn't easy for them to get it. The legacy of conflict between Native Americans who held peyote as a ceremonial sacrament and regulatory bodies who assumed the authority to block its use began more than a century before the United States became a nation. Recognizing the role of the cactus in the history of colonial repression of the Native American way of life is essential to understand the controversy Decriminalize Nature provoked in 2018, which, here in 2024, has yet to reach a resolution.

---

* In the case of Decrim Nature, this applies to possession but not to sales. That means if you are selling mushrooms in a city where they are decriminalized, you are still a dealer of a Schedule I substance, and you can be prosecuted to the full extent of the laws governing such activities.

Suppression of Peyote in North America

The European Christians who colonized North America saw peyote as threatening. Their writings tended to equate use of the cactus—or, as the Spanish called it, the *raiz diabolica*, translated as "diabolical root"[13]—with devil worship and paganism. In 1620, the Mexican Inquisition outlawed peyote use, declaring it a "heretical perversity . . . opposed to the purity and integrity of our Holy Catholic Faith."[14] Jesuit missionary Andrés Pérez de Ribas forbade and punished peyote use in Mexico, declaring its "heathen rituals and superstitions" were aimed at contacting evil spirits through "diabolic fantasies."[15] In the cactus, the Mexican Inquisition "plainly perceived the suggestion and intervention of the Devil, the real author of this vice,"[16] condemning it as "an act of superstition . . . opposed to the purity and integrity of our Holy Catholic Faith."[17]

Thus began centuries of persecution of a ritual that dramatically predated European arrival on the continent. In the wake of sixteenth-century conquistadors torching the Mayan codices to erase their worldview from history, the British and Spanish colonists knew the best way to conquer a nation is to separate them from their culture. Destroy their identity and system of meaning, and the infrastructure collapses.

The late nineteenth century was an important time in the conflict between the US Government and peyotism, the term for the peyote-based religion of Indigenous tribes. During that time, the US forced numerous tribes onto reservations in the Indian Territory. Though it originally encompassed all land West of the Mississippi River, the Indian Territory gradually shrank as the colonists spread their settlements. By 1890, it had been reduced to what is now Oklahoma.[18] Children were removed from their homes and sent to boarding schools built with a mission to assimilate Native Americans into Western culture. Amid the dark history of European arrival on their land, the late 1900s were among the bleakest years for Indigenous peoples across the continent.

Recognizing the threat to their way of life, tribes of the Southwest reconnected with the peyote cactus their ancestors had consumed sacramentally. Through visions and messages from the spirit world, they realized the cactus would keep them connected to their identity and values amid colonial efforts of enforced eradication. No act of hostility could sever the spiritual roots peyote restored.

Due to the interconnectivity opened by the railroads, peyotism spread beyond the lands of the Southwest. Independent tribes throughout the nation unified in reclaiming and sharing ancient practices to maintain their way of life amid systematic oppression. One of those practices was peyotism, and the other was an ancestral ceremony called the Ghost Dance.

During the solar eclipse on New Year's Day of 1889, a Paiute religious leader named Wovoka fell asleep, whereupon he "was taken up to the other world."[19] Wovoka had a vision of God and a peaceful land where the dead were alive and well.

"After showing him all," wrote anthropologist James Mooney after interviewing Wovoka, "God told him he must go back and tell his people they must be good and love one another, have no quarreling, and live in peace with the whites."[20] Wovoka then received the vision of the Ghost Dance, and God told him that by "performing this dance at intervals, for five consecutive days each time, they would secure this happiness to themselves."[21]

Due to the exuberance of the Ghost Dance's practice in large communities, the US perceived it as more overtly threatening than peyotism. In 1890, the dance's history reached a tragic conclusion in what came to be called the Wounded Knee Massacre. The US Army, fearing the Ghost Dance would inspire an armed uprising among the Lakota, attempted to arrest Chief Sitting Bull on the Standing Rock Reservation. Sitting Bull's refusal to comply resulted in an officer shooting the Lakota chief in the head.

Fearful of more violence, Sitting Bull's community fled to the Cheyenne River Reservation to join Chief Spotted Elk, who then led them to seek shelter with Red Cloud, leader of the Oglala Lakota, on the Pine Ridge Reservation. The three hundred and fifty Lakota never arrived, as the US 7th Cavalry Regiment intercepted them and forced them five miles west to Wounded Knee Creek. The next day, as the US disarmed the band, Black Coyote, a deaf Lakota man who spoke no English, held onto his rifle. A cascade of altercations ensued, and the 7th Cavalry opened fire, killing nearly three hundred Lakota men, women, and children.* The devastation to the Lakota could never be adequately expressed, and twenty US soldiers involved in the massacre were awarded the Medal of Honor. Wovoka's vision of peace had reached a horrific conclusion.

As the US aimed to neutralize the Ghost Dance, peyote ceremonies continued in secret. Having had their tipis taken from them, the Lakota held ceremonies inside army tents and dug pits to hide their fires from the Bureau of Indian Affairs.[21] In the years preceding and following Wounded Knee, peyote spread through the tribes forced into the Indian Territory, and a common ritual was established to preserve the Native American way. Key figures like Quanah Parker, the last chief of the Comanche nation, played pivotal roles in warding off government attempts to squelch peyotism. Parker's skills as a diplomat even convinced one of peyote's staunchest opponents, Superintendent Charles Shell, to try the cactus himself. Contrary to the devilish paganism he anticipated, Shell found himself having thoughts "along the line of honor, integrity, and brotherly love."[22] His experience prompted him to shift his oppressive position.†

Still, the government continued to suppress peyote use. The tribes' recognition of the threat deepened their unification, yielding the intertribal unification movement of Pan-Indianism and the formal establishment of the Native American Church in 1918. The protections the NAC sought were unstable, and government raids of ceremonies and arrests for peyote possession continued through subsequent decades.

At long last, the battle between the Native American Church and the US Government concluded in 1994, when Bill "Didn't-Inhale" Clinton signed the American Indian Religious Freedom Act Amendments. The amendments

---

*   Historians continue to debate the specific events prompting the massacre. Some contend that Black Coyote was restrained, and in the process, his rifle fired, prompting several Lakota to recover their rifles and shoot as the 7th Calvary shot back. Others claim a medicine man named Yellow Bird began performing the Ghost Dance in an effort to protect the Lakota band from the bullets. Regardless, the undeniable fact of the tragic conclusion remains.

†   Parker's diplomatic skills were likely informed by his mother, Cynthia Ann Parker, a White woman who had assimilated into Comanche culture after being captured when she was nine and living with them for twenty-four years. When Texas Rangers who believed they were saving her tried to "free" her, she fervently resisted. When the Rangers succeeded, she mourned the loss of her Comanche culture for the rest of her days.

declared that "the use, possession, or transportation of peyote by an Indian for bona fide traditional ceremonial purposes in connection with the practice of a traditional Indian religion is lawful, and shall not be prohibited by the United States, or any State." After centuries of conflict, the Native American Church had earned legal protection to use peyote in religious ceremonies.

For the next twenty-four years, the NAC conducted ceremonies in peace, relatively free of harassment from European descendants. Then, in 2018, Decrim's Santa Cruz measure passed, empowering non-Native people to consume peyote for any reason they saw fit. With this long and violent history in mind, it comes as no shock that the measure did not spread rejoicing through the Native American Church, nor did the ensuing measures spreading peyote decriminalization to several more US cities.

Peyote in the Revival

Dawn Davis, a member of the Shoshone-Bannock tribes, is among the many NAC members who took issue with Decrim's efforts. Peyote has been a part of her life since she was a child on the Fort Hall Indian Reservation of Idaho, where she resides today. Davis wrote her dissertation at the University of Idaho on peyote conservation, and she remains committed to spreading awareness of peyote's history to broaden recognition of its unique status.

Davis told me when Decriminalize Nature passed their Santa Cruz measure in 2018, they hadn't consulted the Native American Church. If they had, there would have been pushback, for the measure offered no new rights to NAC members. The measure's promotion of the "unalienable human right to develop our own relationship with nature"[23] did not benefit the NAC; it benefited every person who is not a member.

Davis saw another major problem. Peyote is endangered in the wild, and it can take more than a decade for a new cactus to mature into its full medicinal potential. Peyote grows in a small region of southern Texas and northern Mexico, and after Castaneda spread interest in the cactus with his *Don Juan* books in the late 1960s, non-Indigenous people began seeking it. A friend told me an acquaintance of his father once traveled into the Texas desert and returned three days later with two trash bags full of peyote buttons—thousands of years of collective growth, foraged by one person to trip out and distribute at will.

What many peyote poachers don't know—or don't care about—is there is a right and wrong way to harvest peyote. Members of peyote-using cultures learn to harvest the buttons without destroying the root structure of the cactus, allowing regeneration. Ignorant poachers, on the other hand, often yank it all out, obliterating roots and any chance of rejuvenation.

Davis believes Decrim's measures empower poachers' convictions of a fundamental right to pluck peyote out of the ground. Many NAC members regard this as a betrayal of the plant's scarcity and sacredness. Their reverence for the cactus is evident in its ceremonial harvesting. Indigenous cultures don't pick peyote and consume it in isolation to serve any desire the harvester may have. Among the *Wixárica*—called the Huichol—people of Mexico, designated groups called *xukuricate* harvest peyote during a sacred pilgrimage to the land where it grows.[24] Along the way, the *xukuricate* observe ritualistic customs to honor the cactus and connect the harvest to their spiritual lineage. When they return, the *Mara'akame*—the *Wixárica* term for what the West would label "shaman"—leads all-night ceremonies of praying, chanting, singing, and dancing.[25]

To protect peyote from the potential ramifications of decriminalization, the Indigenous Peyote Conservation Initiative (IPCI), a nonprofit led by influential members of the NAC, has called for the removal of peyote from all Decrim initiatives. Although some Decrim chapters—which have organized in over fifty US cities[26]—obliged, others resisted, claiming no group or ethnicity has sovereignty over anything that grows in the earth. Debate churns over peyote's future—IPCI focuses on conservation while Decrim calls for a consolidated effort to repopulate the gardens of Texas.

The issue became so complex that it yielded conflict within Decriminalize Nature as a whole. Ideological strife led chapters in D.C., Seattle, and several Massachusetts towns to break away from the parent organization. Some took issue with Decrim's leaders requiring them to sign statements mandating inclusion of peyote on lists of decriminalized substances in order to continue using the organization's influential name. Further criticism of Decrim's position on peyote came from Bia Labate, executive director of the Chacruna

Institute for Psychedelic Plant Medicines, an organization through which she and cofounder Clancy Cavnar lead advocacy for Indigenous reciprocity. Labate wrote, "In sectors of the decriminalization movement, there appears to be an underlying ideology that what is 'nature' belongs to everybody. This idea seems very appealing to affluent New Age, White or mestizo psychedelic activists, and indeed, it's a very nice philosophy in theory, but it's extremely problematic and simply not accurate; just ask Native Americans."[27]

Turning Closer to the Source

Immersed in these debates as I became, I recognized internet scrolling could never provide as much insight as speaking with Native Americans affected by Decrim's measures. Although leaders of various tribes are often hesitant to discuss these matters with White people, I was fortunate to have a Lakota leader of IPCI agree to an interview. He is well known in the psychedelic world, for he has chosen to speak about the conflict and educate non-Indigenous people on the issues surrounding Western peyote harvest and use. As I would discover, his presence, wisdom, and generosity were of equal power to his name: Sandor Iron Rope.

Crossing the Threshold

"The Great Spirit is everywhere; He hears whatever is in our minds and
our hearts, and it is not necessary to speak to Him in a loud voice."

—Black Elk, Lakota medicine man

When I reached out to Sandor Iron Rope, he agreed to speak on the phone to begin developing a relationship. During our thirty-minute conversation, we discussed the Lakota peoples' reluctance to interact with White people. After having been misrepresented in past publications, he felt a particular reluctance to speak with writers, but he and his community had decided outreach was important for education on issues White people don't often understand. I emphasized my commitment to represent his perspective with respect and care, and Sandor agreed to sit for an interview.

As we exchanged emails, I felt a curious call to conduct the interview in person. With the fifty people I'd previously interviewed, a video-chat sufficed. With Sandor, my curiosity surpassed what technology offered. I was interested not only in his thoughts, but his way of life, and driving from Colorado to his home in South Dakota felt like an expression of gratitude and respect. When Sandor expressed willingness, we scheduled a weekend visit.

The fates intervened. I caught a nasty cold a few days before, and since I didn't want to infect him or his community, I stayed home. When the next opportunity arose a few months later, I drove through Wyoming late in winter and got caught in the most brutal snowstorm I'd ever encountered on the road. My '98 RAV4 may as well have been riding on skis, and the danger prompted me to pull over and fight the punishing wind that stripped feeling from my fingers as I fastened chains around my tires. I wondered if this was a trial to endure, especially since my first attempt had been thwarted. When I contacted Sandor and explained my dilemma, he wisely advised me to turn back.

Maybe the Universe was informing me that my desire to drive to his home wasn't significant after all? Regardless, the desire remained, and we scheduled a final attempt. Sandor instructed me to bring tobacco and a gift for his community, and after purchasing both, I hit the road. In my heart, I knew it wouldn't be a simple journey.

The challenges began two hundred miles shy of my destination. The rural darkness of the Wyoming night obscured the vastness surrounding the unlit state highway. All I could see was the thin strip of grass bordering the miniscule shoulder, and it wasn't long before my headlights shone on a herd of deer grazing along the strip. With one wrong movement, I'd collide with them, possibly totaling my car in the freezing expanse void of cell phone signals. More deer appeared every mile. Herds of six or more stood on both sides of the road with hooves on the pavement. The further I drove, the bigger the herds became, until each featured one or more bucks boasting intimidating antlers, staring at me with scorn.

After two hours of white-knuckled steering, the deer stopped appearing. As I neared my destination, a truck sped past me. Two massive antlers rose from the bed.

The deer felt meaningful in a way I didn't understand. I sensed I was journeying along a slippery edge separating two worlds. My conviction grew the morning of the interview, when the sign for one of the final roads leading to Sandor's property read "Deerfield."

Sandor greeted me with a gentleness that contrasted with his imposing physicality. He introduced me to his daughter as his two grandchildren, no older than three, ran over to me and looked up with curious eyes. Their innocence spread warmth through my heart.

As Sandor stepped outside, his granddaughter handed me a small object—a Teenage Mutant Ninja Turtle action figure. The turtle's sword-wielding arm had broken off, and I realized she was asking me to fix it. I struggled to screw it in, eventually getting it to stick. She asked where her grandfather had gone, and as she led me outside to find him, the turtle's arm fell off. She handed it back to me, and her mother took her to the house, leaving me with the broken pieces.

Sandor appeared around a corner and led me across his property to the sweat lodge and firepit he'd built for ceremonies. He wrapped tobacco in yellow rolling paper and smoked contemplatively, and the interview began with him telling me that one normal day in March of 2018, as he was driving with his family through an alley in Rapid City, he was shot five times, twice in the head and three in his right arm, in a random act of violence.

"I saw lightning when the first one hit, and I heard thunder when the second one hit," he said. "Within a split second, my spirit was gone."

A spiritual being appeared. Without words, the being informed him he would be okay. It showed him the car—now situated in a ditch after having struck a light pole—in which Sandor and his wife bled profusely. His son pulled his sister out of the car, and officers and paramedics who'd heard the shots arrived promptly and put Sandor in an ambulance.

As his consciousness flickered in the hospital, his nephew gave him peyote. "You have to talk to it [peyote] and tell it things," he explained. "It rejuvenates your perspective on your surroundings. It helps you control yourself and your body a little more. It awakens all of your senses so you can help yourself heal."

Remarkably, Sandor survived, although fragments of the shattered bullets remain in his body. "The doctor said, 'Mr. Iron Rope, you might have heard this already, but you're pretty hard-headed. This time, it's a good thing,'" Sandor shared with a laugh.

The shooting gave him a new perspective on his life and mission to carry on the peyote lineage from which he came. "*Wakȟáŋ Tȟáŋka*—Creator God, the Great Mystery—has a different plan for me. I rejuvenated myself through many ceremonies to go back out in public. I didn't want to be in public. Mental health has always been a concern in Indian Country. We've been survivors of historical trauma. My dad and grandpa were in boarding schools, you know? Disruption of a way of life. Why? They said, 'We needed to *civilize* you.' That civilization disrupted the Indigenous communities who live in unison with nature, and what did it get us? It got us to where we are now, with this imbalance of climate change."

---

*   Wakȟáŋ Tȟáŋka, sometimes spelled Wakan Tanka, is an important Lakota word usually translated as "Great Spirit," the sacred, mysterious, universal force living in all things.

Peyote has factored prominently in Sandor's bloodline. "My dad was a peyote man, and my grandpa was, too, both sides of my family," he said. "In the beginning, it was a healing ceremony for a lot of issues and health concerns going on in Indian Country, trying to get accustomed to reservation life."

I asked him if peyote helps his community heal their collective trauma.

"It helps because it offers a different perspective. Everybody has a different time frame for healing. In my healing and in my mind, everybody was a threat. So, I stayed away from public. To integrate back into public was a challenge. When there's a lot of loud and aggressive people, staying close to Spirit or prayer is my best bet."

I'd learned about Sandor when I heard him speak at a large psychedelic conference in 2019. The crowded event was challenging for him, but his new lease on life guided the way. "The Creator of Life allowed me to stay alive for a purpose. I had to embrace this reason that I'm alive, and I had to speak about our life, mental health, and medicines. This psychedelic movement says, 'We want everybody to be free,' but there's a way to do it. There's this *shamanism*, this 'I want to administer plant medicines to everybody that needs healing.' You might not even be authorized to administer medicine. You go to Indigenous communities, and you see an elderly man, a medicine person—how many years did it take for him to do that? But everybody says, 'I went to a four-year course, and I'm certified to administer medicine.' No. There's more to it than that. You have to be careful because you can hurt someone or hurt yourself."

A missing ingredient in this Western mentality is reciprocity. "People have to learn to take care of nature and be in unison with the natural world. You can't just *take*. Before you take a plant, you make an offering. You tell this plant what you need and why you need it. Certain people are authorized to do that in Indigenous communities. A medicine person talks to the trees, because the tree is a life force that we *respect*. Making offerings to nature before you take is important for this movement to understand. Why do you want to take our medicine and not understand our perspective? The mentality of colonialism and the Western world is to *take* it. What's changed over a hundred years? Nothing."

I was surprised that Sandor didn't declare non-Indigenous people should be barred from peyote. His point was that if people are interested in it, they shouldn't take it as if they are entitled to do so—they should learn about his culture's perspective, prioritizing understanding, relationships, and reciprocity over feeding personal desire.

"There are adopted people in Indigenous communities, and that happened because there was a rightful relationship, trust was established, and they nurtured that community in some way. Then, they were invited in and accepted as an outsider. But nobody wants to do that. They want to take the medicine and take off."

With these issues raised, I asked about his thoughts on Decriminalize Nature. He puffed tobacco thoughtfully and said, "It started off on a good foot with the intent to decriminalize some plants that were classified as harmful drugs. Even our sacred peyote is classified as a Schedule I hallucinogen in the Controlled Substances Act of 1970. But the Decrim movement was naïve about Indigenous communities. There was no prior consent to the inclusiveness of peyote. You have to understand Indigenous communities within the United States' Indian policy. Then, you understand why we feel how we feel. Our grandmas and grandpas were hunted by Texas Rangers who said, 'A good Indian is a dead Indian.' When you come from that, you'll have a little bit of understanding of what we're saying. We were a part of nature, and our life was disrupted. They said, 'We're going to civilize and teach you, because your way is no good.' No. You got it all wrong. Your way's no good. You disrupted thousands of children, took them out of their homes, and sent them to boarding school. Somebody's got to be responsible for these children. There is a spiritual answer for that."

He continued, "When you come from this kind of a history, you understand the issue with Decrim Nature. There's a point to it, but Indigenous communities were not given any consent to it. Grandmas and grandpas fought hard before this current policy to protect peyote from the United States, which was freed from Great Britain for religious freedom—but they are oppressing the Indigenous caretakers of the land? How ironic. Decrim Nature had a good perspective initially, but they're naïve in thinking that nobody was connected to some of these sacred plants. They don't want to reference the original people in the United States. So, I gave up talking to them, I gave up hope for them, and I gave up respect for them."

In Sandor's eyes, Decrim—and much of the psychedelic movement—overlooks essential components of healing with plant medicines by focusing excessively on the chemicals.

"They're not factoring in the caretaking of the medicine, the sustainable cultivation, or the process of obtaining the medicine. People want to take these medicines, but what is your goal? What are you trying to heal from? In Indigenous communities, there's a *container* in how we heal. The elements of fire, earth, wind, water—they're always here. But people just want to explore. What are you trying to escape? Where are your elderly people, your medicine people? These Indigenous communities surpass your PhDs with their natural education. The University of the Universe is right here."

Through all he shared, I sensed Sandor's grounding in compassion for humanity. Compassion need not be soft and gentle. Sometimes, fierceness and challenge are necessary. "I'm not out there sharing just because I want to share," he said. "I'm trying to get people to respect themselves. That means relearning about yourself, your nature, and what you're doing. If you want to understand the plant medicines, understand the people and how they're viewed and used. They're viewed in a natural world perspective, and they're not overharvested. They're given back."

Sandor had told me to bring tobacco and a gift because by interviewing him, I was taking something—his perspective. It would be selfish to give nothing in return.

"It's not about *I want*," he said. "You give something, then you receive. Take the natural spring water, give an offering, and say, 'Thank you.'"

Historically, this principle of reciprocity guided Indigenous communities in harvesting peyote. When they took a mature button,* they offered a prayer. But the US Government's involvement led to licensed distributors controlling access, and the exchange became monetary, losing its spiritual history.

"The Indigenous Peyote Conservation Initiative formed to reconnect our generations back to the spiritual harvest of the medicine and preserving its spiritual essence," Sandor explained. "Each one that we harvest, we will put

---

* Sandor defined a mature button as "anything with eight to thirteen ribs," which are "little spines of fur on the medicine."

two back. It's a long process, but the process looks generations ahead. I'm not going to be here forever, and I want to leave a sustainable model for peyote."

Being with Sandor, I understood why I had felt a strong desire to visit. He wasn't speaking about theories. He was speaking about what lives inside us and all around. To abstract the "effects of peyote" and the "setting where it's taken" is to isolate variables while missing the full picture. Peyote cannot be understood as a psychedelic plant with unique properties. The medicine is more than the plant. It is the ceremony, the connections, the giving, the preservation, the cultivation, and the honoring of what it reveals through words and actions. It is about as close to the heart of a widespread worldview as a medicine can get. In this worldview, every particle plays an important role, and every fiber of organic life deserves respect and care.

"Life is a ceremony. It's important how you balance that with Western education and what you're going to do, because you're going to leave tracks, and Mother Earth and everybody you care about is going to see them. Is it a good way, or should we not go that way? I say things in the hope that people will be more in tune with themselves and what they're doing to bring harmony to the Earth, to all of us. You are medicine. Are you going to be bad medicine or good medicine? My hope is that the reader will understand, help themselves heal, and be respectful and mindful of everything they do. We're all connected."

He angled his body to speak to me directly. "You are from a different nationality, but you came here to understand about peyote in this rapid movement, to rebalance and reeducate somebody about it within your writing. This movement needs to wake up to get to the point of saying, 'If we engage with this plant medicine, are we infringing on this Indigenous community? We might be doing that. So how are we going to help this community rather than extract it for our own use?' We're trying to heal ourselves, but we're not mindful of what we're doing on a global scale. You have to look at the imbalance of the world. Every Indigenous community was imbalanced in their own way, which in turn affects the natural world. How do we get to harmony? One person at a time. So, stop. Listen."

Ceremony

My conversation with Sandor lasted over two hours. A half hour in, I realized something strange happening within me. I felt moved by his words, but I also felt an inner blankness. I was aware of birdsong and wind, but my thinking mind had all but ceased to function. The questions I'd prepared dissolved into insignificance. Embarrassment took hold, and I feared Sandor would interpret my lack of sharpness as a lack of understanding or care.

He didn't. When I told him what was happening, he nodded. "I could see that," he said. "And that's okay. It's okay."

We took a break and moved to the shade. When he rolled more tobacco, I grabbed one of the American Spirit cigarettes left in my car from a road trip. As I smoked, I focused on the tobacco connecting me to the clouds and trees. Calmness returned. I told Sandor my blankness arose because as I listened to him speak, I felt ignorance and shame in my ancestral and cultural connection to the people who tried to destroy his people's way of life. His clarity about life's spiritual nature made me realize how far I'd slipped from my connection to the spirit, God, the miracle, and mystery. I'd gotten ensnarled in fears and unbalanced habits aimed toward *more productivity* to do *important work*. I was more lost than I had taken the time to admit.

A moment of silence passed. "I'm going to go get something," Sandor said, and he walked to his house. When he returned, he carried a woven pouch. "This is a natural medicine that we use in many ways," he said. "We use it in our ceremonies that come from a grandpa who had the vision of the songs with this medicine. It appeals to us in our Spirit mind. It is for you to think about where you are, to rebalance yourself, and to take that deep breath again when you smell it. When you're done smelling it, you can bless yourself with it."

He poured green powder into my hands. I attuned my senses, brought my hands to my nose, and inhaled the medicine's sharp scent. Sandor stood near me and spoke Lakota words; I didn't need to understand them to feel their power. When he finished speaking, I rubbed the powder on my forehead, focused on an intention, and thanked him.

"You have a purpose," he said. "You have to realign yourself with what you want to do with this book. Rebalance yourself, and nature has its way of keeping us in tune."

Sandor's actions, words, and medicine expressed his values. That, I realized, is the meaning of intention.

"Everybody has a gift," Sandor told me. "You have to find out what your gift is and *cultivate*. Nurture that gift. We're a spirit in a human experience. That spiritual nature keeps us connected."

Take It Slow

Before I left Sandor, I realized I was holding his granddaughter's broken Ninja Turtle. He laughed affectionately when I gave it to him, and he pulled me in for a one-armed hug. "Enjoy your drive home. Remember to take it slow."

I filled up my tank near Deerfield Road. Across the street, large wooden carvings of bears were spread out on a shop's lawn. Amid them stood four life-sized carvings of the Ninja Turtles—strong and confident, all limbs intact.

If the broken action figure Sandor's granddaughter gave me symbolized where I was, these carvings called me toward rebalancing my inner pieces I'd allowed to become fragmented. Recalling the dead buck in the truck in Wyoming, I searched the internet for spiritual meaning. The first blog I found explained that seeing a dead deer "may mean that you need to be careful of your own mortality and learn not to take anything for granted because life can be cut short at any minute."[1]

I thought of my steering-wheel-gripping fear of colliding with the encroaching deer. It wasn't just a fear of totaling my car. It was a fear of death, and it expressed my underlying awareness that I had lost balance. If I had died on the road, I would have died with regret over how distanced I had become from life's spiritual nature. I thought of Sandor and how after he saw the spiritual being and survived the gunshots, he changed his life.

"The experience was a wonderful teacher," he'd told me. "I've been blessed to have another chance to serve, and I'm trying to savor every moment I have. Every moment."

I may not have mentioned the word peyote in a while, but it never left the conversation. The medicine is everywhere, for the cactus points far beyond itself.

To understand peyote, people of Western descent must understand the cactus' complicated history and foster appreciation for the people who preserved its spirit amid violent oppression. Otherwise, we will unconsciously perpetuate a legacy of disregard for their perspective, churning cycles of entitlement brought to North America by Western colonial ancestors. Judgment and disregard harm the cultures being judged, and they harm us as well, blocking us from restoring connection with the natural world, tending to its needs, and healing wounds inflicted by centuries of extraction for personal gain and convenience. Restoring balance starts within, and it was high time I listened to my inner scales calling for attention.

The Trickster Yanks the Rug of Ignorance

I saw no deer on my drive back through Wyoming. The only animal I saw was a coyote, who appeared out of nowhere on the one-lane highway twenty yards ahead. I swerved, and the coyote trotted to the shoulder, observing me each step of the way.

I knew the coyote was significant in numerous Native American mythologies. I knew it was often associated with the "trickster" archetype, which pulls the rug from beneath your feet to shake things up, all but forcing you to see where you've become misaligned. In Lakota mythology the trickster is represented through a character named Iktómi, and the coyote represents something larger and more complex. In "Itkómi and the Coyote," Iktómi believes he has won his battle with the coyote when he throws the animal into the fire. But the coyote comes out unscathed, and with a laugh, he tells a stunned Itkómi, "Another day, my friend, do not take too much for granted."[2]

Like the trickster, psychedelics and plant medicines can shake us up when we need it, presenting a different path. It was clear I'd veered off mine via excessive worry and fear. But when I imagined widening my scope to the vantage point of a hawk, imbalances in the psychedelic revival likewise became apparent, none of which I had adequately investigated.

The branching media arms of the revival have spun a story of miraculous healing medicines bringing little danger when taken in medical settings. In such a positivity palace, less-positive realities are often banished. If I might anthropomorphize psychedelics as trickster beings, these molecular Iktómis and coyotes have begun to resist the intemperate positivity that revival narratives commonly espouse. In response to abundant focus on the light of healing, the dark side has made itself known and must be reckoned with for balance to be restored.

V

THE PSYCHEDELIC
SHADOW

19

Entering the Shadow Realm

"To confront a person with his shadow is to show him his own light."

—Carl Jung, "Good and Evil in Analytical Psychology"

There comes a moment in many psychedelic journeys when a dreaded sensation creeps into the edges of awareness. Amid this, one recognizes the vibes are shifting, and things are about to get darker. This sensation has lurked on the fringes of the previous chapters, and it is now emerging into conscious light.

Folks who prefer a sunshine daydream of psychedelic panacea best buckle in. It can be painful to burst the blissful vision of psychedelic utopia. However, to establish a balanced perspective, certain difficult-to-stomach realities of the revival's shadow need attention.

Shadows, Doppelgängers, and Goosebumps

The concept of "the shadow" was broadly conceptualized in Western psychology by Carl Jung. The idea is that the conscious ego houses one's understanding of personal identity, conceived as a *separate* something distinct from all other autonomous beings. However, ego concepts become limited in their rejection of socially unacceptable realities of the inner world. These realities don't disappear; rather, the psyche's rejected contents live in the exiled realm of the shadow. If the ego is characterized by "I *am*," the shadow is comprised of "I am *not*."

As conceptualized by Erich Neumann, Jung's student: "All those qualities, capacities and tendencies which do not harmonize with the collective values—everything that shuns the light of public opinion, in fact—now come together to form the shadow, that dark region of the personality which is unknown and unrecognized by the ego."[1] Because societal values influence that against which we define ourselves, an indelible relationship exists between each individual's personal shadow and the cultural shadow of thoughts, fantasies, impulses, and behaviors their culture indoctrinates as unacceptable.

If you put a monster in a cage, the monster doesn't cease to exist; all you've done is repress it in a game of "Pretend It's Not There," which you're fated to lose. Jung recognized that the parts of ourselves we banish to the shadow endure, fester, and mutate in barricaded dungeons, continuing to influence our lives whether or not we admit it. Individuation—the process through which the fractured psyche becomes whole—requires integrating the shadow into consciousness.

"No one should deny the danger of the descent," Jung noted. Facing the danger, however, is necessary, for "every descent is followed by an ascent."[2] This is evident in countless narratives. In Haruki Murakami's novel *The Wind-Up Bird Chronicle*, Toru Okada must descend to the bottom of a well to battle his abducted wife's oppressive brother and rescue her from the dreamlike domain where she's imprisoned. In *Toy Story*, Woody must enter the chilling domain of Sid, turning the bully's tarnished toys against him to free Buzz Lightyear and return to the paradise of Andy's room. In *The Shawshank Redemption*, Andy Dufresne must crawl through a "river of shit" to emerge in the glory of freedom and usurp the warden's tyranny. Unless one reconciles with darkness, a limited worldview perpetuates, fragmenting consciousness through indoctrinated avoidance.

The shadow is also represented in stories through the "evil twin," the *doppelgänger*—or "double walker," as the German word is translated—that physically embodies the shadow. Jung wrote, "When the individual remains undivided and does not become conscious of his inner opposite, the world must perforce act out the conflict and be torn into opposing halves."[3] In other words, "When an inner situation is not made conscious, it happens outside, as fate."[4] In Egyptian mythology, it's called a *ka*; in Finnish folklore, it's an *etiäinen*.

The qualities one has determined to constitute their identity form the *persona*. When the shadow is not integrated into the psyche, its contents manifest externally as a doppelgänger with whom the persona engages in a struggle, for the inner opposite threatens the individual's construction of self. Through the doppelgänger's entry into the story, the protagonist (persona) discovers reality to be more complex than they realized. Doppelgängers are found in the works of Dostoyevsky (*The Double*), R. L. Stevenson (*The Strange Case of Dr. Jekyll and Mr. Hyde*), and even R. L. Stine. In Stine's *Goosebumps* universe, it's the bad guy from *I Am Your Evil Twin.**

Did Dostoyevsky, Stevenson, and Stine take psychedelics? I have no idea. But they enjoyed writing about darkness. In this shadow-embracing spirit, let's enter the spectral cave of the psychedelic realm and shine a light on the disturbing markings on the walls, remaining wary of booby traps† on the path to our balanced destination.

Psychedelics and the Shadow

Writing about one of his final meetings with Hofmann before the chemist's death in 2008, Grof noted Hofmann spoke about "the need to embrace creation in its totality, including its shadow side, because without polarity the universe we live in could not have been created."[5] Avoiding the shadow

---

* *Spoiler Alert!* Protagonist Monty's evil twin was actually not his real twin (whom Monty discovers to be his cousin Nan), but a clone made by his Uncle Leo. The plot thickens when Monty and Nan discover there are actually four evil Monty clones! Why would Uncle Leo do such a thing? Well, the plot thickens once again upon revelation that it was not Uncle Leo's doing, but the doing of Uncle Leo's evil clone of himself! Good thing all the clones have little blue dots on them so they can be spotted—until the evil clones put a blue dot on the real Monty! Thrown off, Nan and Uncle Leo's college roommates mistakenly send Monty with the evil clones to South America. Monty tricks them and escapes, leaving Nan to conduct a final test: since Monty is allergic to peanuts, she makes the two Montys eat a peanut-oil-filled donut. Naturally, she puts her faith in the Monty who barfed, sending the protesting second Monty to South America. All is well . . . until later that night, when Monty reveals himself as the evil clone, having switched the donuts when Nan wasn't looking! A baffled Nan asked why evil Monty would do that, and the sinister clone replies, "Nan, I'm your evil twin!" Who could have seen that coming? That's some classic Stine, right there.

† A reference to *The Goonies* (1985), which you might consider watching if you didn't catch that. It features no psychedelic content I'm aware of, but everyone deserves a nostalgic retreat from time to time. For another nostalgia-inducing option, pick up a copy of R. L. Stine's *Say Cheese and Die!*, a literary achievement against which *I Live in Your Basement!* and *The Blob That Ate Everyone* pale in comparison.

of any subject creates a wall of division between the acceptable and the unacceptable, and no wall can withstand the pressure of its opposite over time. When we suggest there are no issues with mainstream adoption of psychedelics, we ignore harmful mainstream trends affecting psychedelics as much as anything. As such perspectives spread, a cultural shadow forms, reinforced by implicit "rules" forbidding certain realities from acknowledgment and dismissing those who voice them as deleterious downers.

Psychedelics can inspire visions of a better world, but they cannot eradicate imperfection. Like the myth of the Garden of Eden, history demonstrates that no matter how pure something is, it is susceptible to corruption once humans become involved. Although the drifter vaping DMT at the music festival may argue otherwise when the bass drops, psychedelics are not *all good*, and they will not "save the world." At a certain point, a dream becomes another means for escaping pain and suffering. All the while, that pain controls us from the shadows, pulling life's strings as we fixate on the marionette shows we desperately want to represent reality.

Psychedelic Research: A White Man's Field

Psychedelic history is interwoven with suppression. The War on Drugs suppressed psychedelic use through harsh punishment, and religious fundamentalism suppressed Indigenous plant medicine use. However, suppressing something doesn't make it vanish. Native Americans continued using peyote in secret, and the Drug War temporarily forced psychedelics underground, from which they reemerged. Rather than eradicating particular histories and perspectives, suppression waters seeds of conflict. As those seeds germinate in the revival, many are calling for recognition of familiar patterns in the roots.

Clinical psychologist Monnica Williams is arguably the most prominent researcher on racial inequality in psychedelic science. In 2018, she co-conducted a methodological research study on the inclusion of people of color in psychedelic therapy. Williams and her team evaluated psychedelic research published between 1993 and 2017, which "utilized a psychedelic substance either alone or in conjunction with psychotherapy in the treatment of a psychological disorder." They looked at sixteen studies from seven countries, focused on five different psychedelics—in the final compilation 82.3% of the 282 participants were non-Hispanic White.[6]

With this statistic in mind, Williams noted that psychedelic science is burdened with a "lack of generalizability of these studies to critical clinical issues for people of color." As promising as results have been, they do not represent the entire population. "In many regards, the psychedelic medicine movement both exemplifies the existing inequities and barriers to mental healthcare treatment inherit in modern psychiatry, while also presenting an enormous opportunity to acknowledge the efficacy and powerful contributions of Indigenous medicine and rectify the injustices of the past," Williams and her team concluded. "However, it will only be successful in doing so to the extent that those with power acknowledge the importance of this issue and consciously make an effort to address the concerns presented herein."[7]

The lack of diversity in the psychedelic field stretches beyond research labs. Psychedelic conferences, which are abundant these days, have been criticized for being whitewashed and featuring a disproportionate number of male presenters. In a conversation with Leia Friedwoman for Lucid News, psychiatrist Julie Holland said, "I'm just exasperated that, at this point, in 2020, there are still so many 'manels' (men only panels) in conferences . . . There's no excuse for it."[8]

I've heard countless people respond to these patterns with a "So what?" Others become angry when it's brought up, scolding the "social justice warriors" for "bringing down the vibes." Perhaps these folks prefer visions of a problem-free world of psychedelic voyagers banging drums and dancing 'round the full-moon fire.

Williams noted that the roots of these issues are complex. An obvious root is the lack of ethnic diversity among psychedelic researchers, while a less obvious one concerns mental health researchers' reliance on the *Diagnostic and Statistical Manual of Mental Health Disorders* (*DSM-5*), which carries a long history of ignoring cultural variations in diagnostic criteria. Another important root is that in many communities of color, scientific research is not regarded as safe, for it has historically been implemented as a means for oppression.

Take, for instance, Georges Vacher de Lapouge, a French anthropologist of the late 1800s who used "craniometry"—the "scientific" measure of the cranium—to "prove" that the "Aryan white race" was biologically superior to all other races.* Then there's the infamous "Tuskegee Study of Untreated Syphilis in the Negro Male," which took place from 1932 to 1972 in Alabama. The US Public Health Service enrolled 600 Black men, nearly 400 of whom had latent syphilis. The men were never informed of their diagnosis, and they were enticed into the research through the promise of "free health care." It turned out their health care denied them the treatment of penicillin, which, after its invention in 1947, became the go-to treatment for syphilis. When the study concluded (after a whistleblower leaked it to the press), over 100 participants had died from syphilis-related complications, and many participants' wives and children were infected.†

A 2016 article in the *Atlantic* stated, "Research has long suggested that the ill effects of the Tuskegee study extend beyond those men and their families to the greater whole of Black culture. Black patients consistently express less trust in their physicians and the medical system than white patients, are more likely to believe medical conspiracies, and are much less likely to have common, positive experiences in health-care settings."[9]

Disparities between White and Black peoples' experiences in health-care settings continue to manifest. In 2020, researchers from George Mason University analyzed data from nearly two million hospital births in Florida from 1992 to 2015. They found Black newborns were about three times more likely than White newborns to die in the hospital when looked after by White doctors. The discrepancy dropped significantly when the doctor was Black, and coauthor Rachel Hardeman called for more research "examining the importance of racial concordance in addressing health care inequities."[10]

The lack of Black participants in psychedelic research is consistent with medical research at large. A 2010 study from Saint Louis University found lower participation among African Americans in "controlled clinical treatment trials, intervention trials, as well as studies on various disease conditions, including AIDS, Alzheimer's disease, prostate cancer and other malignancies, stroke, and cardiovascular disease."[11] Amid the various causes, the researchers

---

* Unsurprisingly, Lapouge's work exerted a strong influence on the development of Nazism.

† For more examples, look at Harriet Washington's *Medical Apartheid*.

asserted, "Mistrust of academic and research institutions and investigators is the most significant attitudinal barrier to research participation reported by African Americans."[12]

Regarding psychedelics, there's also their illegality to consider. Williams and her team wrote, "Minorities fears related to being administer[ed] drugs may be even more intense when the treatment involves controlled substances, given historic and current inequities in the criminal justice system for drug-related offenses."[13] According to a 2015 report by the Drug Policy Alliance, "Black people comprise 13 percent of the U.S. population, and are consistently documented by the U.S. government to use drugs at similar rates to people of other races. But Black people comprise 30 percent of those arrested for drug law violations—and nearly 40 percent of those incarcerated in state or federal prison for drug law violations."[14] As such, research studies on illegal drugs won't spark enthusiasm in populations so heavily afflicted by the War on Drugs.

How much information is missing from psychedelic research due to its lack of diversity? Can we universally apply its procedures and results with so few races and ethnicities represented? Is psychedelic research unconsciously perpetuating ethnocentrism with protocols whose validity for one ethnicity is erroneously applied to all people?

The Need for Diverse Protocols

Camille Barton is neither a therapist nor a scientist, yet they have become a powerful voice bringing attention to numerous underrepresented layers of the revival. When we spoke, Barton described the profound healing they experienced dancing at raves as a teenager.

"I'd find myself in these trance-like states, where thought wasn't really active, and where these amazing energetic currents were running through my body," Barton recalled. Their shift into deeper embodiment helped them heal their trauma-fueled tendency toward dissociation.

Due to the profundity of their experiences, Barton was moved to research their ancestry. They weren't surprised to discover that for their Yoruba ancestors in Nigeria, drumming and dance were integral spiritual practices.

"It feels like remembering a way to connect to wisdom that's beyond me," Barton reflected. "I continue to be curious about precolonial healing traditions in Nigeria, but also how this wisdom can evolve dance therapy by integrating movements common in African diaspora dances. These practices often feel very pleasurable and allow us to start to sense parts of the body that have been numb."

Would Barton have had such a breakthrough while lying on a couch, wearing eyeshades, and listening to ambient music? I doubt it. Why, then, has this become an unquestioned universal standard?

When I interviewed Barton in 2021, they spoke about the MAPS protocol for MDMA therapy. "I don't think that the current protocol will be as effective as it could be for bodies who have an epigenetic legacy or intergenerational memory of healing alongside dance," they said. "I have a strong sense that many African heritage folks, for example, would benefit from being given permission to move their bodies and express using dance during psychedelic therapy sessions, which is currently not possible with the MDMA protocol."[15] While MDMA therapists encourage clients to allow emotions to move and express through their bodies, the rooms are often small, and one's comfort in expressing themselves can be inhibited by the therapist's gaze.

"It is an important practice of cultural humility to understand that what may work for certain communities may not be beneficial for all communities," Barton said. "I hope that as psychedelic-assisted therapies develop, there is more space to weave in dance and different movement practices, and not to medicalize and sanitize all approaches to the point that we're just using a Western psychotherapeutic model where someone has to lie still and be quiet."[16]

Another influential voice on racial disparity in the revival belongs to Joseph McCowan, an MDMA therapist and trainer for MAPS. In an interview in 2021, McCowan told me, "It makes sense that communities who have historically been harmed in research settings—who have not felt seen or heard in mental health settings, or who were disproportionately impacted by the War on Drugs—aren't lining up for this research or these treatments."[17]

These histories and their ongoing impact highlight the limitations of focusing exclusively on the individual. To separate individuals from their history and culture is to operate on the faulty premise that an individual's life unfolds in a vacuum, when really it's broadly influenced by external factors.

"Depression, trauma, addiction . . . are not individual challenges, but challenges occurring in larger sociocultural contexts and environments," McCowan said. "Often, those environments and contexts are creating conditions where more people are actually experiencing trauma, depression, or addiction."[18]

Oppressive sociocultural contexts can manifest as embodied stress for specific populations. "The legacy and the harms of slavery and colonization continue to live on to this day within our bodies, as well as in the experiences we have within the larger systems and structures around us that continue to be traumatizing, even if it looks different than a whip to the back,"[19] McCowan explained.

For those personally affected, these realities are impossible to ignore, even if those who aren't affected scarcely admit their existence. As McCowan noted in an essay, "What I remember most about slavery being covered in my history classes, is the fact that it wasn't."[20]

McCowan explained another element of psychedelic therapy's lack of safety for communities of color. "Most people of color will just imagine, due to implicit bias, that the person they're going to be meeting with is a white therapist. The next thought is going to be, 'Will they understand my experiences, or hear me, or see me?' And they're probably going to think, 'No.' As we move forward, it's really important that we are reorienting how we are working with individuals and communities of color. Supporting these communities requires us to move from the position of expert to the position of learner . . . to move from cultural competency to cultural humility."[21]

McCowan nevertheless advocates for MDMA's potential to heal communities of color. "For people of color with racial trauma, MDMA can provide the opportunity to be with that trauma in a new way: engaging with it, sitting with it, looking at it and feeling it. Just going from patterns of avoidance to acknowledgement and being with what is there provides a pathway to healing."[22]

An important nuance can get overlooked in these kinds of discussions: giving voice to injustices does not equate to victimization. Someone stuck in a victim mentality perceives the injustice of their situation and feels powerless against it, relinquishing the possibility of shifting their circumstances. It's an entirely different thing to voice injustices in an effort to change one's situation for the better, reclaim roots, and mobilize the goodness in others by shining light on inequalities from which they'd previously turned.

"Our collective liberation begins when people of color step out of the colonizer's history and embrace new possibilities," McCowan wrote. "When pushing the limits of the spaces and places we are comfortable, we will begin to transcend the prisons of our outdated patterns, shed our internalized oppression, and heal our individual and collective trauma . . . As we collectively rediscover our roots, we plant our future seeds, helping us emerge from the tangled weeds of our complex histories."[23]

Absence of Sexual and Gender Diversity

I bemoaned the discovery that Timothy Leary, who once inspired my youthful soul in his radical expression, told *Playboy* in 1960 that LSD was a "cure for homosexuality." He cited the "most famous and public of such cases" as Allen Ginsberg, whom Leary claimed "has openly stated that the first time he turned on to women was during an LSD session several years ago."[24] Leary was evidently unaware of Ginsberg's long history of denying his homosexuality before embracing his nature and remaining with his husband, Peter Orlovsky, for the rest of his life.

The point isn't to chastise Leary, but rather to show the subtle ways that marginalization of non-dominant identities happens in plain sight, often going unnoticed by everyone except the people most affected.*

Clinical psychologist and psychedelic researcher Alex Belser speaks on the need for greater representation of queer populations in the revival. In a 2021 interview, he connected Leary's statement with a first-wave trend of using psychedelics for conversion therapy. Such efforts were common practice, even at Canada's Hollywood Hospital, "probably the most famous psychedelic hospital."[25] In the early 1960s, the DSM considered homosexuality a disorder, and the psychedelic research community, enlightened as they presented themselves to be, operated within the manual's pretensions.

---

* Fortunately, Leary's perspective evolved over time, for in 1988 he wrote, "Since homosexuality has always been a part of every society, you have to assume that there is something necessary, correct and valid—genetically *natural*—about it." (Source: James Kingsland, "The shameful history of psychedelic gay conversion therapy," Plastic Brain (blog), May 29, 2019, plasticbrainblog.com/2019/05/29/history-psychedelic-gay-conversion-therapy/)

"The psychedelic clinical psychotherapeutic world is awakening to the way in which, some of the rainbow skeletons of the past are still lurking in the closet," Belser said.[26] He pointed to the skeletons' legacy in many of today's psychedelic studies requiring a male and female co-therapist team for "gender balance."

"First of all, it's incredibly heteronormative," Belser said, "but it doesn't acknowledge gender diversity and trans folks' experience. It centers it in a heteronormative practice and it also essentializes gender stereotypes."[27]

Are the spaces curated in psychedelic therapies safe for people who don't hold specific identities? Will a male and female co-therapist team be helpful for a trans person, or could the binary reinforce the dualistic categories placed on them from an early age from which they have struggled to escape?

Barton broke down the issue. "Generally, the more marginalization you're facing, the harder it is to interface with the Western psychedelic space. Within the space, safety and legitimacy is currently constructed around people with academic or medical credentials, rather than an emphasis on care, embodied ethics and cultural humility, to support people who face marginalization in society. It's difficult for people who don't have these credentials to feel validated and respected for their opinions."

Psychedelics can be powerful tools for exploring identity. When therapeutic models perpetuate norms that inhibit certain individuals' exploration, the tools become rusty, if not obsolete. For psychedelic healing to reach its potential, therapeutic models must create space for all individuals rather than specific people whose backgrounds and appearances mirror those of the facilitators.

How Mushrooms Shifted My Attitude Toward Social Justice

It was not until my early thirties, during my first semester of my master's in transpersonal counseling program, that I confronted the biases I unconsciously held as a result of my upbringing. Without the help of psilocybin mushrooms, I may never have actualized this realization.

During a Social and Multicultural Foundations class, my Latinx teacher spoke about White supremacy. Since my mind conjured images of white-cone-hatted Ku Klux Klan members performing creepy rituals in a wooded glen, I felt shocked when my teacher said, "You are all white supremacists." Fire burned inside my chest. How could she say such a thing? Who was she to compare me, someone she didn't even know, to the KKK? I felt impelled to defend my dignity. I was a good person, *gosh darnit!*

While entwined in the throes of my struggle, I took 3.5 grams of psilocybin mushrooms in my apartment with a trusted sitter. I had no intention of diving into these issues, but I found myself spiraling through the conflict. I heard her accusation on repeat, and I felt my body's resistance as a desperate *fighting* refusing to be overlooked. I breathed with the conflict, and eventually, my identification with the emotions loosened. In the ensuing space, I asked myself, "What are you defending?"

The answers I'd taken as self-evident lacked potency. I was not defending a principle. I was defending my ego. I'd been unwilling to consider certain biases may be indoctrinated into my system, for such consideration threatened my persona.

Revisiting my teacher's words, I no longer heard an accusation. I heard, "Listen to the injustice I've had to endure due to how I look. It's real, and it's important."

The mushrooms revealed the pettiness of my resistance. I had been driven by fear of admitting shameful things about my inner life. It was true that since childhood, when I found myself in a neighborhood of people with different colored skin than mine, fear constricted my gut. It was true that when cops pulled me over, I never felt threatened, the luxury of which was withheld from people who weren't White like me.

These insights shifted my relationship with these issues in a lasting way. When I attended class thereafter, I didn't tense up at the door. I connected with curiosity and humility, aiming to learn from others' experiences of injustices. If I truly cared about human rights, I couldn't overlook these matters without sacrificing integrity.

My point isn't to cast shame but to curate reconsideration of default thought patterns inspired by more dubious sources than commonly acknowledged. Humility opens the heart to compassion, breaking down egoic walls fixated on needing to *prove* something we don't understand. I may not have accessed this humility without the help of mushrooms, and the revival's preponderance of discussions on the potential of psychedelics to bridge cultural divisions suggests I'm not alone in receiving such a boon.

Strong Reactions May Point to the Shadow

My reaction to my teacher's words was powerful because they evoked my shadow. Defending against the perceived onslaught controlled my mind, playing out in class as if I was fated to encounter it. Mushrooms dissolved the barrier separating my ego from my shadow, facilitating descent into parts of my psyche that weren't pleasant to face. It's easier to prop up myself as an open-minded person than to consider the possibility that I might not be as informed as I believed.

Turning away from racial injustice fuels ignorance of important realities for the sake of comfort. This comfort comes at the cost of reinforcing divisions, because it projects a limited worldview onto others in place of listening with compassionate ears. My mushroom journey didn't magically assimilate my full shadow, but it made me aware of important elements inside it. My integration will be a lifelong journey of deepening my understanding and respect for people toward whom contemporary culture is far crueler based on factors they cannot control. But alas, the revival's disparity in racial, ethnic, and gender recognition is but one layer of its shadow. The trip through the underbelly continues.

Debates over the Psychedelic Future

"The Western industrial civilization has so far abused nearly all
its discoveries and there is not much hope that psychedelics
will make an exception, unless we rise as a group to a higher
level of consciousness and emotional maturity."

—Stanislav Grof, foreword to *LSD: My Problem Child*

When I became aware of the revival around 2015, I believed I had stumbled upon something unanimously good. My limited understanding
of the culture of psychedelic research painted a portrait of psychedelic enthusiasts united in their recognition of these substances' value, creating a unified
front organized toward the advancement of a better society. The more I learned,
the more I recognized my portrait depicted a fiction. While there may be a
common belief in the healing potential of these molecules at the core of those
invested in the revival, disagreement populates all sectors of research, policy,
and general perception of what these substances *are*.

Given science's history of regarding religion and spirituality as "unscientific"
and "archaic," it came as little surprise when the Johns Hopkins' mystical
experience conclusion came under scrutiny. Researchers raised questions
on the validity of the Mystical Experience Questionnaire, arguing that the
nature of the questions directs participants toward contemplating mysticism.
The resulting "priming effect" was said to influence participants toward
an intended lens that would not have otherwise framed their perception.
Skeptics maintain that the mystical potential cannot be extrapolated as an

inherent effect of the psychedelic, but rather results from strategically chosen inputs (e.g., spiritual paraphernalia in the office) and suggestibility.

The results of Griffiths' mystical experience study cannot be generalized because each volunteer practiced spirituality or religion in some form. The authors wrote, "It seems plausible that the religious or spiritual interest of the participants may have increased the likelihood that the psilocybin experience would be interpreted as having substantial spiritual significance and personal meaning." The authors acknowledged the possibility "that the novelty of the experience in hallucinogen-naïve individuals enhanced both the intensity and the personal and spiritual significance of the experience,"[1] as the participants had little to no prior experience with psychedelics.

This point on novelty is important. During my early psychedelic journeys, I felt myself connecting directly to a spiritual presence. I perceived an interconnected unity emanating through all things great and small. If I had filled out the Mystical Experience Questionnaire, I'm certain I would have scored high enough to categorize those trips as mystical. It seemed clear that psychedelics produced mystical states, until I took ayahuasca. The foreign, hostile dimension I entered was not the ineffable sense of unity the mystics describe. Everything was not one, and everything was not good.

The experience shook me to my core, crumbling my worldview on what psychedelics were and what existed at the foundation of reality. It was no longer possible for me to abide a viewpoint that God was everything, and everything was God. I had experienced something completely different, and my prior conceptions of mystical unity did not belong.

On that note, plant medicine traditions don't necessarily align with mystical viewpoints either. To argue that a roadman or an ayahuasquero is the same as a mystic would be to lose touch with what either person does. Mystics focus on universality and a sense of identification with all things, eliminating the distinction between the individual self and the Cosmos. An ayahuasquero imbibes ayahuasca to travel through the veil separating this world from another. That other world is home to spirits, and the ayahuasquero communicates and partners with those spirits to bring healing and wisdom to this world. Separation between these two worlds is a fundamental part of their reality. They do not claim that the individual is inherently identical to all spirits, nor do they claim that all spirits have our best intentions in mind. Their journeys are spiritual but not mystical, and yet they catalyze healing that does not depend on a sense of oneness with all things.

I understand now the deeper one travels into psychedelic states, the stranger the states become. Terence McKenna, perhaps the most legendary psychonaut of Western history, took mushrooms on countless occasions for decades, exploring the worlds they revealed with curiosity and boldness that few can match.* For many years, McKenna lectured publicly about his psychedelic exploits, imagining a future that would regard psychedelics with the respect and admiration they deserved. Then, late in his illustrious life, McKenna had a harrowing trip on mushrooms. According to his brother Dennis, the "mushroom turned on him," leaving Terence in "an abyss of utter existential despair."[2]

An all-encompassing mystical explanation for psychedelic healing may be too naïve. Reliance on its objectivity can lead people to imbibe psychedelics with an innocent smile, only to find themselves enmeshed in a foreign reality too frightening to comprehend. To extrapolate such a claim as "psilocybin occasions mystical-type experiences" as scientific fact is to ignore numerous stories of contradiction. Mysticism is a beautiful thing, but it does not encapsulate the full potential of psychedelic states of consciousness.

Psychedelic science ushered the unscientific concept of mysticism into scientific literature, identifying a meeting point between science and spirituality. Before long, science fought back against that science to eliminate such "unscientific" concepts from the literature, lest a mockery be made of psychedelic research before it develops into all it may be. Science and religion can't seem to get along, can they?

---

* An exception is a man named Kilindi Iyi. Before passing away from COVID-related issues in 2020, Iyi became known in the psychedelic world for his "high dose" psilocybin journeys of 20–30 grams, blowing McKenna's 5-gram heroic dose out of the water. Iyi did not speak about mysticism. He spoke about aliens, entities, and all kinds of otherworldly stuff. His reports would not fit into the Johns Hopkins model, and I'd wager a rucksack of shillings that they still wouldn't if he had taken such high doses in a research setting.

External Influences on the Internal

In his paper "Consciousness, Religion, and Gurus: Pitfalls of Psychedelic Medicine," Johns Hopkins' own Matthew Johnson argued that when therapists adorn their offices with religious and spiritual paraphernalia like a Buddha statue or a billowing Ganesh tapestry, they direct their clients' suggestible minds toward religious and mystical conclusions.[3] This brings up an ethical issue: if a client doesn't align with the associated tradition, can a therapist justifiably involve it in the client's psychedelic session? Isn't this work supposed to be non-directive and client-centered?

Things get trickier as these questions dovetail into broader methods of psychedelic therapy. When therapists choose the music, aren't they curating a specific experience for the suggestible client? If the office looks like a jungle with abundant decorative plants, might the client be influenced to see things through an environmental lens? Won't lying on a couch evoke different inner phenomena than lying on the grass?

For a psychedelic session to be truly client-centered, the physical space must extend the client's worldview, rather than the therapist's intentions. Can a therapist offer enough decorative elements to suit diverse worldviews? Or should we admit the impossibility of precisely curating the context of someone's psychedelic session? Might we then consider the possibility that wrapping clients in a mirror of their established worldview may not be ideal?

Plant medicine rites of passage and rituals follow structures and sequences, and the intentionality and meaning of those factors are central to the rituals' effects. They do not reflect initiates' established worldviews but rather call them toward a new and better one. Regardless of whether the Eleusinian *kykeon* was psychedelic, the Mysteries likewise expressed how valuable it is for individuals to move through a structured sequence representative and facilitative of a broader individual and cultural process of transformation.

Might the revival's hyper-focus on the client's worldview be a fresh manifestation of Western society's hyper-individuality, reflecting a late postmodern resistance to establishing a shared value system whose importance extends beyond individual preferences? Perhaps it is, perhaps it's not; psychedelics are, after all, better at raising questions than providing answers. Nevertheless, psychedelic therapy's insistence on framing the setting to mirror the client's belief system puts it at odds with plant medicine traditions, which instill higher echelons of cultural value in ceremonial participants through exposure to novel focal points of archetypal meaning. Reflecting initiates' egos contradicts the point, for the rite is designed to bring death to the identity for the sake of rebirth and evolution.

Healthy Normals and Bad Faith

The revival's focus on psychedelics for treating mental health disorders is generating important breakthroughs, but what about people who don't have a mental health diagnosis? Should they be barred from access? Or can psychedelics help them too?

Psychedelic researchers use a term, attributed to Bob Jesse, to describe folks with no mental health diagnoses. No offense to Jesse, but I find his term quite dumb in its implicit judgment of deviation from "the norm." Nevertheless, it reflects the parlance of our psychedelic times, and so I have no choice but to refer to this broad category with Jesse's term of *healthy normals*.

Although healthy normals haven't been diagnosed with depression or PTSD, plenty face challenges in their lives because, well, they're *human*. Many people with no diagnosed conditions struggle to find purpose, value, and connection. Who among us doesn't carry some inner demons who pester them most days? Who among us couldn't benefit from a shift in perspective time to time?

What defines what it means to be psychologically healthy? In much of America in the 1950s, "healthy" meant being an automaton who drank alcohol, smoked Pall Malls, bought fancy ovens, and probably held racist beliefs. In the late 1960s, being "unhealthy" meant taking LSD in Haight-Ashbury, jamming to Jefferson Airplane, and hopping into Carlos' VW Bus to smoke reefer while cruising the Pacific Coast Highway at sunset—unless, of course, you were one of Carlos' passengers and believed it was the people punching the clock who were unhealthy. Who was correct?

Sometimes, the people who appear the most "healthy" and "normal" on paper are not only suffering deeply but perpetuating collective cycles of suffering and pain, for they've been indoctrinated to believe their lifestyle is the only way to be, and anyone who steps out of line needs an old-fashioned whoopin' or a ten-foot cell. If being a healthy normal means being a close-minded asshole, then such folks undoubtedly qualify.

In the late 1950s, Huxley wrote in *Brave New World Revisited* an illuminating discourse on whether society was moving away from or toward the dystopian vision of his 1932 novel. Huxley wrote, "The real hopeless victims of mental illness are to be found among those who appear to be most normal. Many of them are normal because they are so well adjusted to our mode of existence, because their human voice has been silenced so early in their lives, that they do not even struggle or suffer or develop symptoms as the neurotic does. They are normal not in what may be called the absolute sense of the word; they are normal only in relation to a profoundly abnormal society. Their perfect adjustment to that abnormal society is a measure of their mental sickness."[4]

Many who fit into the healthy normal category are skilled at wearing a socially acceptable mask to conceal their pain. Being "normal" can express less of a positive quality than a practiced suppression of authenticity to conform to cultural norms of acceptable behavior. Perhaps many people with conditions like depression and anxiety are "healthier" in that their condition stems from an honest confrontation with the vices of civilization. Then again, if ignorance is indeed bliss, should anyone be forced to exit a cave where they prefer to reside?

In existential philosophy, the term "bad faith" refers to the psychological phenomenon of giving up your personal freedom in acquiescence to society's values. It's characterized by incongruence and habitual inauthenticity, and it tends to brew what Nietzsche called *ressentiment*, a vicious bitterness toward anyone who lives a life of greater authenticity empowered with freedom from social mechanisms of control.

A culture of adherents to bad faith getting rewarded for sacrificing their dreams plays into why so many people feel deeply dissatisfied. When the values you were taught to revere yield emptiness and longing, where do you turn? The internet? The craps table? The bottles of bourbon and prescription pills?

US culture provides few routes for healthy normals facing such crises to shift their conditions toward alignment. A collective babble-stream shames people who step off the well-worn path and make changes like leaving the job they despise (*Your mortgage! Your 401k! Don't be stupid!*) or traveling the world (*It's dangerous out there! How are you going to pay for it? Think about your children's children!*). As the cycle churns, people continue to confuse bad faith with virtue, denying their hearts and intuition based on a distorted equating of "humility" and "service" with self-sabotage. The result is an unconscious habit of projecting bitterness onto anyone whose presence reminds them that they sacrificed their freedom to languish in an isolated fortress of misaligned being.

A psychedelic journey can disrupt established grooves of perceived identity, reminding such individuals that they are far more than their personas. Seeing new possibilities can be frightening, for they threaten the foundation of one's reality. But with proper care and support, these possibilities can reveal a path toward fulfillment and alignment with one's latent dreams.

The potential for psychedelics to assist self-discovery may be foreign to the research world, but it is well known among users around the world. We are all searching for who we are and where we want to go, and psychedelics can provide unparalleled insight. Regardless of whether the medical model extends its scope past the pages of the *DSM*, healthy normals will continue to benefit in numerous ways from their chosen routes of psychedelic exploration.

Capitalism! Patents! Investors! Oh My!

The time has come to face one of the most formidable white whales of the psychedelic revival: *capitalism*.

As excited as folks have gotten about psychedelics, so too has arisen a trend that would have made the 1960s acidheads freak out amid the grooviest of Dead sets. This trend is the vulture-like swoop of for-profit companies into the world of psychedelics, bringing their shadiest practices with them.

In the 1960s, LSD became the medicine for the counterculture to *wake up* to the ways the system was exploiting them and come together in a spirit of rebellion against personal and collective indoctrination and repression. An ethos of anti-consumerism arose, and the counterculture focused on connection, egalitarianism, and freedom. The psychedelic revolution was in part a reaction against the dominion of financial incentives over human life, prompting an exercise in a new way of living where money was a resource instead of an idol of ultimate value. These days, greed and financial interests have seized upon psychedelic healing, and psychedelics are being adopted by the very systems against which the counterculture rebelled.

Is directing big money toward the research and development of psychedelics a bad thing? Or will it expedite their incorporation into society?

Those who reply "Yes!" to the first option center on a position that capitalism, a system governed by individualism and profit motives, corrupts everything under the sun—perhaps even everything *beyond* the sun, here in the Anthropocene. As Karl "The Beard" Marx argued long ago, capitalism reduces everything to *use value*. That includes human beings, whose capitalistic value is measured not by intrinsic worth but by how much they produce. Once an individual's production value is expended, like when a factory worker named Samson gets his hairy hand mangled by a machine, the person becomes as worthless as a blunt shovel in the eyes of Captain Capital.

Despite the counterculture's best efforts, capitalism emerged victorious, exiling their sunken dreams in the reefer-clouded ruins of Haight-Ashbury. Now, over half a century later, psychedelics are being adopted into the same system. Capitalist nostrils sniffed out a new opportunity, and the greedy sniffers grabbed hold of the psychedelic goldmine wherever they could. This came to public light around 2016, when Compass Pathways arrived on the scene.

Compass Pathways began as a charity, whose stated mission aligned with the not-for-profit ethos of organizations like MAPS. Something changed, and Compass morphed into the biggest for-profit corporation in the psychedelic space, going public in 2020.[5] The company's ambiguous motivations were met with detractors. In 2018, Journalist Olivia Goldhill published a lengthy article on the news website Quartz investigating the possibility that Compass was aiming to create a "magic mushroom monopoly."[6] The thought of making millions off psychedelics struck critics as vile. Edginess entered the psychedelic scene, manifesting as nervous collar-pulling with forced smiles and *everything-will-be-fine!* prophecies presented in a vain attempt to ease the uncertainty. A sense grew of something wicked this way coming to threaten enthusiasts' belief in the goodness of the major players of the revival.

Once they'd become a for-profit company, Compass generated more controversy after receiving significant financial backing from polarizing venture capitalist and PayPal cofounding billionaire Peter Thiel, whose general ideology journalist Max Chafkin described as a conviction "that technological progress should be pursued relentlessly—with little, if any, regard for potential costs or dangers to society."[7] Did Thiel represent the potential of psychedelic medicine, or did he represent its Armani-suit-clad destination?

Because Compass was the first major for-profit psychedelic pharmaceutical research company to emerge, many believed it marked a turning point that would lead psychedelics down the dehumanizing pathways of profit-driven pharmaceutical companies known to champion economic motives over concern for individual well-being. Compass cofounders George Goldsmith and Ekaterina Malievskaia, whose resumes boasted zero history of psychedelic interest before creating Compass, have repeatedly defended the company's integrity and reiterated their commitment to increasing accessibility to psychedelic therapy.

Some of the company's actions haven't appeared to align with such statements. Compass Pathways attracted scrutiny in 2018 for filing a patent on a method of creating synthetic psilocybin. People were concerned that Compass would use their patent to block other manufacturers. Despite the outcry, Compass was granted the patent in 2021.[8] They then made efforts to patent general techniques of psychedelic therapy. If these patents are granted, every provider of psilocybin-assisted therapy will have to pay Compass Pathways to provide their services.

I have no issue with describing these efforts as villainous because these psychedelic therapy techniques were developed and used by a community of healers for more than half a century in the West, and Compass' money-chasing goons had precisely nothing to do with their establishment. Here's how absurd it gets: one of the techniques Compass has tried to patent is the method where "the therapist responds to the subject if the subject initiates conversation." In other words, Compass is trying to patent therapists doing therapy.

Other methods Compass has attempted to patent in psilocybin therapy include soft furniture, high-resolution sound systems, beds or couches in the treatment room, guiding clients through breathing exercises to help them feel calm, and letting clients listen to music.

How are these methods even possible to patent? And how effed up is this capitalist system to empower sketchy businesspeople to make people pay them to care for people in need in a profession centered on caring for people? It would be like business school grads patenting a midwife's use of her hands to deliver a child or a hospice worker's placement of a supportive palm on a dying woman's shoulder.

Moral arguments aside, these psychedelic therapy methods exist as shared knowledge in the public domain. These techniques have been used in psychedelic trials and above-ground practice with ketamine. They stem from first-wave psychedelic therapists, underground therapists who risked their livelihoods to provide this treatment, and countless generations of Indigenous healers who have developed the wisdom to heal with plant medicines.* Once this level of patent-grabbing greed began, people spoke out. There was no denying what was happening and no hoping the criticism and controversy would convince Compass to recalibrate its bearings.

Shayla Love, one of the revival's best journalists, wrote on the subject for VICE in 2021. She quoted Graham Pechenik, the patent and intellectual property lawyer who first sounded the alarms on these claims. "I think if these claims do hold up, it will change the landscape, in the sense that there will be now ownership over these therapy protocols," Pechenik told Love. "Whoever does end up with these patents would be able to really dictate the use of them, either by using them to get revenue through licensing, or by using them to shape what the competition looks like by choosing to license some and not others."[9]

We would then have a monopolistic gatekeeper in the form of tie-choked people making decisions around access according to whatever arbitrary measures they deem most advantageous. For instance, if a therapist who had written a book containing a scathing report of the company's behavior applied to administer psilocybin to clients, Compass could reject him, blocking his ability to practice due to a personal gripe.†

---

*   This stuff doesn't only apply to the States, by the way. The patents Compass Pathways has filed would apply to 153 countries whose signatures can be found on the Patent Cooperation Treaty.

†   I am referring to myself here. If the patent is awarded, I imagine there's a good chance this will happen.

The amount of control over psychedelic therapy Compass or any other company could assume is disturbing at best, terrifying at worst. In Love's wise words, "With a monopoly comes the ability to shape the psychedelic therapy market as a whole: what it will cost, and, therefore, who will have access to it. The granting, negotiating, or rejecting of patents like this one will help define what the future of psychedelic medicine looks like."[10]

I can't say I'm optimistic. As the revival unfolds, more attempts to put access in the hands of people who don't understand psychedelic medicine emerge. Perhaps psychedelic capitalism will fail when the overblown promises of companies and their uninformed methods repeatedly fall short. Perhaps Western society isn't advanced enough to handle psychedelic medicine, and underground treatment is the best option we have.

The Bad Kind of Soma

Many presenters and social media posts claim psychedelic incorporation into the capitalist machine is bound for failure. To these folks, the only way for Western culture to heal is to radically transform political and economic systems, and psychedelics cannot help us accomplish this from within the systems' constructs.

I've heard others relate current models of psychedelic therapy to the drug of *Brave New World*: soma. This bliss-inducing intoxicant is given to all members of Huxley's hierarchical, deterministic dystopia by the elusive rulers controlling from the unseen. The citizens believe they're given the drug because the rulers care about their well-being but fail to see the artificial pleasure it induces stops them from questioning their enslavement.

Robert Forte, a fellow of ambiguous intent who's been close to the heart of psychedelic culture for decades, describes psychedelic therapy as a modern soma. To Forte, recognized for his books on psychedelics and religion and his dissemination of dark theories around sinister underpinnings to the revival, MDMA therapy in particular blisses people out from caring about the world's injustices, leading them to believe all is well because they feel great. Instead of transforming, people stop caring about being manipulated by systems unconcerned with their fulfillment.[11]

Forte has leveraged the same criticism toward microdosing, a trend he unintentionally helped establish when he advised Fadiman to take a tiny dose of LSD to overcome his writer's block. At such small doses, psychedelics don't tend to shed light on global issues, nor do they tend to awaken people to higher levels of responsibility to act in service of creating a better world. It's more like with a pinch of LSD, their desk job for a megalithic corporation doesn't feel so soul-sucking. They feel good again, and so they have less issue with slaving away at the job responsible for draining their vitality in the first place. From this perspective, a microdose is like a sedative taken to numb the pain.

Healing involves feeling better, but this form of feeling better has roots deeper than attachment to impermanent bliss. Feeling better includes responding with increased equanimity to life's inevitable struggles. If healing is equated with pleasure, systemic issues contributing to the negative feelings are never addressed, and widespread transformation is stunted.

I don't know Rick Doblin well, but of the dozens of people I've met and observed in the psychedelic world, there are few, if any, who appear to embody the psychedelic spirit of connection, presence, and joy as much as Doblin. Will his prophesized psychedelic transformation of culture transpire? Is he underestimating the harms that profit-driven motives will cause? I don't know, but the first option is nice to imagine. If it's to manifest, it will be necessary for the world to recognize the less-altruistic companies and individuals purchasing ideological and economic real estate in the psychedelic future. Such recognition will equip people to weed through the false promises being made to fill the piggy banks of people who don't know what they're talking about.

Selling the Miracle Cure

The industry of "self-help" has become massive. According to The NPD Group's market research, the self-help industry grew by 11% between 2013 and 2019, which corresponded to a growth of up to 18 million self-help book sales annually. As of 2020, the industry was worth $10.5 billion.[12*]

---

*   To be honest, I'm not sure what the term "self-help industry" even refers to. Is there an organizational entity connecting all global self-help offerings? Who determines the qualifications something or someone must meet to be included?

At the center of the self-help world are books, courses, and annoying social media accounts that advertise a common claim: *follow my formula and your life will get way better!* These approaches can be helpful. Other times, they reduce well-being to banal platitudes. Sorry, self-help guru, but healing isn't as simple as "letting go," regardless of how many social media followers left emoji-laden comments on your post of the *Tao Te Ching* verse you found on your Google search of "inspiring quotes."

My biggest issue with self-help "healers" isn't their poorly edited e-books or overpriced webinars; it's how they reduce the complexities of human psychology and mental illness to the same cliché axioms found on your neighbor's refrigerator magnets. They'll tell you to change your thinking, and everything else will follow. *Focus on the positive, and low vibes will disappear! It's the law of attraction! Basic physics!*

Self-help charlatans rarely understand that "low vibes" don't "go away." Instead, anti-low-vibe people solidify a thin persona as they accumulate loyal followers, muting the low vibes in themselves and the world. When low vibes reverberate, the persona reinforces the locks and ignores the pounding on the door.

It irks me when charlatan phonies market their services to people who are suffering deeply. They present their programs as if they'll radically improve people's lives with minimal effort required. It's the fad diet of mental health: *10 Easy Recipes to Become Happy and Free!* In other words: *You are Flawed, and If You Pay Me, Your Flaws Will Go Away!*

If this approach helps some folks rediscover happiness, wonderful. No issues there. I'm ranting on behalf of the people it harms. When you sell a package deal of simplified healing to a desperate person living in perpetual pain, what happens when it doesn't work? If you replied, "The desperate person loses even more hope," you answered correctly. They believe something must be horribly wrong with them because the simple program that worked for all the well-adjusted testimonial writers didn't help them one iota. In fact, they feel worse, because their newest hope for a cure—exploited by the program's advertising of false promises—crumbled into despair at their suffering's recurrence. Now, they're beating the hell out of themselves because they couldn't even heal with the *simplest* approach, *guaranteed* to bring results within *days*. It's a cruel thing to sell false hope to people in pain.

Such salespersons have infiltrated the psychedelic revival. They've seen the results of the research, tuned into the excitement, and launched companies that use psychedelic trial results to tell you their new product, service, or program will heal you . . . for a price. They bypass the complexities of healing and ignore the double-digit percentages of folks for whom psychedelic therapy *doesn't* work, instead championing a miracle cure that will transform you into the superhero you've erroneously believed you must become to be happy.

Some of these trends burgeoned via microdosing after *Rolling Stone* published the 2015 article on tech people taking small doses of acid in Silicon Valley. The article quoted one "Ken," a twenty-five-year-old Stanford grad grinding it out in the software world whose "epic time" microdosing was characterized by "making a lot of sales, talking to a lot of people, finding solutions to their technical problems."[13] An unfortunate side effect of the ensuing popularity of microdosing manifested as entrepreneurial hustlers presenting the benefits as scientific facts in order to sell their services alongside the blissful utopia they claimed microdosing would bring.* Suddenly, there emerged microdosing coaches, microdosing schools, and countless microdosing seminars run by business people regurgitating the same claims about an endless array of microdosing benefits, none of which had scientific backing.† I can appreciate people helping others microdose safely, but when the extent of a coach's experience amounts to "I have microdosed and I liked it," I see little more than a charlatan disguised as a healer disguised as a humble servant for the greater good.

The repulsive edges of these trends remind me of a particularly grotesque scene from *Fight Club*, a brutal commentary on capitalist dehumanization.

---

*   I imagine many of these coaches are good-hearted, helpful people. If you seek such services, however, be mindful of the fact that coaching is different from therapy. To become a therapist in the US, one must complete a master's program, which requires hundreds of hours of supervised clinical work. State-specific regulatory bodies preside over therapists with the power to bar them from practice because of an ethical breach. To become a coach in the US, one must decide they are a coach and start calling themselves one. At the time of writing, there is no centralized regulatory agency for coaching and thus no set of rules coaches are required to follow.

†   Perhaps you'll recall Szigeti's "citizen science" study, which concluded microdosing benefits may be attributable to a placebo effect. Unsurprisingly, microdosing coaches were among Szigeti's most vocal critics.

Tyler Durden (Brad Pitt) explains to the Narrator (Edward Norton) that the soap he makes, which sells for top dollar at high-end retail stores, is crafted from a secret ingredient: human fat, stolen from the dumpsters behind a liposuction clinic.

It's a brilliant microcosm of the horrific manifestations of capitalism: people buy food to binge eat because they feel terrible, purchase liposuction to fit the mold of the "perfect" person advertised to symbolize fulfillment, and buy soap to maintain cleanliness and proper appearance in a culture that prizes both. The cycle churns endlessly, and its churners reap the monetary rewards. The system produces the suffering it profits from pretending to cure.*

The self-help crooks swarming the psychedelic space are doing the same thing: profiting off a system that churns cycles of suffering by falsely promising a cure with trivial methods requiring no educational milestones to advertise. Through the shimmering billboard of a rainbow mushroom designed by their unpaid intern, they goad people into the swampy morass of striving for something better. When we exploit cycles of suffering with pretend cures for profit, we are engaging in capitalist dehumanization at its worst.

I fear the revival has succumbed to this trend. In my clinical practice, people frequently contact me to schedule a session as soon as possible. They list their myriad struggles and express their excitement that psychedelic therapy will cure them. They mention neuroplasticity and the default mode network, and they detail specific traumatic histories they intend to "release." The truth is, the treatment does not work for many of them—not in the way they think it will, at least. They have absorbed a simplified narrative due to media coverage of scientific results that filtered out nuance for the sake of mainstream acceptance. I'm left feeling conflicted about the future of psychedelic medicine in the West. If it is to help people as much as I believe it can, the bubble of easy, bliss-inducing healing must pop, and realism must balance the hope for a miracle cure.

---

* If, for instance, I were a doctor who only wanted money, I could prescribe patients a medicine that actually makes them feel worse, so they'll have to come back and pay me for repeated visits without realizing that if they get better, I lose my stream of revenue. Keeping them limping and dependent keeps my pockets bursting at the seams. But no doctor would ever do such a thing! And the pharmaceutical companies who pay them *definitely* want people to get better so they don't need to keep buying the pills they sell. Who *wouldn't* want their livelihood to become obsolete?

21

Psychedelic Stigmatization in Psychedelic Science

"We can evolve no faster than our language allows."

—Terence McKenna, *The Archaic Revival*

After publishing his ergot-Eleusis book *The Immortality Key* in 2020, Brian Muraresku appeared on Joe Rogan's podcast. The ensuing "Rogan Bump" catapulted the book into an overnight bestseller. On the podcast, Muraresku and his wingman, Rogan-favorite Graham Hancock, made one thing clear: Muraresku had never taken psychedelics. They boasted his abstinence meant his research was more legitimate than that of the many psychedelic-taking authors on whose work Muraresku capitalized, implicitly suggesting the prior researchers' words amounted to biased, fallacy-ridden ramblings because they had taken psychedelics.

There's some merit to this approach. In 1978, when Hofmann, Wasson, and Ruck constructed the Eleusinian argument that Muraresku repackaged for a more psychedelic-positive culture, the scientific establishment ignored them. Muraresku didn't want the same fate, so he assumed an "objective" outsider-looking-in persona, which Pollan had proved as journalistically advantageous through the success of *How to Change Your Mind*. Pollan's book, however, hinged on a central "travelogue" wherein he embarked upon three psychedelic journeys to amplify his understanding. Since Pollan's psychedelic use enhanced his legitimacy, why would Muraresku believe the same approach would do the opposite?

Granted, Pollan was exploring how subjective psychedelic effects were yielding breakthroughs in mental health treatment, while Muraresku was wearing the plastic fedora of a cultural anthropologist on a quest to unearth buried archaeological evidence. Nevertheless, I maintain a gripe with Muraresku's self-satisfied stance as a non-user of psychedelics and his pompous suggestion that his abstinence rendered him more legitimate than writers who had taken the substances he claimed lay at the foundation of Western religion. Claiming that enthusiasm drawn from personal psychedelic experiences delegitimizes researching them is like saying enjoyment drawn from reading literature delegitimizes writing a book. And profiting off psychedelic enthusiasm while disowning it is like writing a book while saying you've never read a book, all the while benefiting from the very book-reading enthusiasm you eschew. But alas, Muraresku is but a scapegoat for a broader issue.

Stigmatizing the Subject of Focus

A strange truth of the revival is that prominent psychedelic researchers almost never discuss their personal use. The scientific perception equates personal use with obfuscation of "objectivity," thereby rendering research unscientific. But do we ask nutrition researchers to refrain from putting their conclusions into practice? Of course not. When such researchers don't practice the principles their research suggests, we regard them with skepticism. Would you see a dietician who orders McDonald's four times a day?

Researchers' silence on personal use reflects a psychedelic manifestation of science's fallacious premise that objectivity can only be verified when divorced from emotion. This premise promotes the illusion that people can disengage from subjectivity. Its adherents must have forgotten the "double-slit experiment" of modern physics, which revealed that the observer affects the subject of observation at a molecular level. Ignorance of the observer effect leads to such situations as researchers whose interest in psychedelic healing stems from profound personal experiences being too frightened to speak honestly.

I asked Szigeti, the researcher behind the microdosing-may-be-a-placebo-effect study, about this phenomenon. He felt clear the reasons researchers stay silent about personal experience amounted to reputational risk.

"With scientists, you want to keep some distance from your subject," he said. "People don't want to lose the public perception that they are keeping such distance."

In an interview about her book *Acid Revival*, social scientist Danielle Giffort addressed this trend, noting, "In the popular imagination, we like to think of science as this value-neutral realm that is shielded from the outside world, from the so-called social world specifically. And this image is what grants science a good amount of credibility in the eyes of scientists and the public. But, of course, science is a social endeavor and is impacted by social factors."[1]

Narrative Control

Seeking interviews for this book, I discovered a curious phenomenon: the people most reluctant to be interviewed about psychedelic medicine were often those most involved in the course it's taking. I sent detailed proposals to numerous Johns Hopkins researchers on several occasions, and I didn't receive even an automated reply. Perhaps I was naïve, but I thought leaders of the institution widely recognized as leading the psychedelic science charge would be happy to share their perspective for a book on the subject.

During the scarce interviews I scored with non-Hopkins scientists at the forefront of research, I was often reminded of speaking to the president of the private high school where I used to teach. He was an old Jesuit who'd say calculated things about the direction of the school while tensing up in the presence of major benefactors. With him, as with certain scientists, the vibes felt *political*. These scientists answered with rehearsed responses polished to highlight details determined to bring the most significant advantage and eliminate the specifics determined to risk casting a negative light. It happened too often not to recognize a pattern of narrative control.

There can be a weird tension when prominent psychedelic scientists speak, especially if someone asks a question related to the shadow in the Q&A. This tension is amplified at this precipitous moment, for countless individuals, companies, and academic institutions are banking on the prophesied near-future event of FDA approval of psychedelic-assisted therapies. The backlash of the 1960s likely accounts for a large part of the researchers' reluctance to speak about personal use and shadow content. Basically, they don't want the '60s to happen again, and they fear it might.

One of the ways a backlash could happen is through the media—after all, it was the media that brought widespread attention to the Charles Manson situation, and the images of LSD-taking, forehead-carving hippies outside the courthouse caused fear and mistrust of psychedelic users in the minds of the masses. Fear of another backlash leads researchers to present psychedelics with practiced precision to the mainstream world. Clinical language like "default mode network" and "symptom reduction" are commonplace, but you're unlikely to hear about DMT entities or psychotic breaks on next week's CNN special.

This fear makes sense, especially for those whose careers were upended last time around due to the War on Drugs. Many forefront researchers have labored diligently on the fringes for decades to revive psychedelics from obscurity, chipping away at judicial decrees that seem less likely to change than your eccentric uncle's stance on North Korea. Accomplishing this feat requires an organized effort to present the results in pretty packages to prompt any average brainwashed Joe to consider shifting his Drug-War-induced perspective. It requires a clear and consistent narrative grounded in the enterprise—science—that inspires unquestioned trust. Such narrative precision requires strict adherence to details determined as auspicious for inclusion. Evidently, researchers' personal use doesn't make the cut.

The mainstream narrative glosses over negative psychedelic effects in fear of the sensation-hungry media sinking its ravenous teeth into freaky stories. It doesn't matter how much momentum the movement has accrued. If the media sensationalizes a story like Art Linkletter's daughter Diane jumping out of a window on LSD in 1969, a sea change could occur, and the promise of psychedelic therapy could again crumble beneath Federal fists. And many continue to discover that the deeper they travel into the psychedelic subculture, the stranger things become, spinning a far different story than a cozy room where mystical visions heal the masses.

Then there's the issues around glorification of therapeutic uses while casting stereotypical labels onto "recreational" users. The downstream effect is censorship of discourse. Sure, people have well-grounded fears of being open about personal use: *Will it affect employment opportunities? What will Grandma think?* I'm not talking about these fears. I'm talking about psychedelic leaders shying away from touching the subject of recreational use unless they're referencing it as "irresponsibility." I'm talking about the people most responsible for shepherding psychedelics back into the spotlight shaming people who take psychedelics.

There are irresponsible uses. For example, one should *not*, under any circumstances, take ketamine and operate heavy machinery. But there are beautiful uses of psychedelics outside therapy offices, from dancing with loved ones through the night to marveling at the natural splendor of the mountains and feeling at one with a sky full of stars. Before therapy offices existed, people across the world gathered in communities and journeyed together, gaining insight into themselves and the interconnectedness of the universe. Far more people have taken psychedelics outside a therapy office than inside, but plenty of researchers prefer to focus on the remarkable healing stories of the small percentage who have accessed these therapies than talk about Timothy Leary, the former face of psychedelic research they strive to shed.

"These researchers push away from the pollution of the impure scientist by enacting the sober scientist persona, but at the same time, they still draw on the practices of the impure scientist," Giffort said. "They criticize Leary for failing to follow conventional scientific methods in his psychedelic research, so they actively work to follow the kind of hypothesis-testing methods that grant scientific credibility. But at the same time, they actively incorporate Leary's insights about the psychedelic experience into their therapeutic models. Leary is so central to their stories and to the revival because he is the site of the continuities and divergences between the first and current waves of research."[2]

Although older researchers I interviewed kept their lips sealed on personal use, many younger ones gladly shared personal tales. Among them was Mendel Kaelen, the maestro of music in psychedelic therapy. Young as he may be, Kaelen has made a big name for himself in the research field. If you haven't heard of him, perhaps you've heard a version of his commonly reported, often-misquoted metaphor for psychedelic healing, which he reiterated during our conversation.

"Think of the mind as a hill covered in snow. Sledges are going down this hill and building tracks. When similar information is processed again, we're like sledges attracted to these preexisting trails. That's how our brains evolved—it would be a nightmare if we had to rethink every action again and again. We borrow from previous experiences in an implicit, subconscious way. But that can be disruptive if those trails become patterns of negative thought or addictive behaviors. Psychotherapy aims to change how we perceive the world and our actions, but it can be very hard to change when the rut is deep. Psychedelics temporarily flatten the snow on the hill, so the trails disappear. Then, the question is, when I stand on top of that hill, where can I direct this sledge? What new landscapes and pathways can I explore?"

When I asked him about personal use, Kaelen replied without hesitation. "I had my very first personal experience with mushrooms in 2005. I felt humbled, grateful, and lucky that my first experience was profoundly meaningful. Apart from having resolved inner conflicts and clarifying my attitude toward life, my experience reconnected me with a personal spirituality. Part of that personal spirituality was feeling deeply connected with knowing what I need and want to do."

Here was an established psychedelic researcher explaining how mushrooms helped him become the prominent researcher he is today. Does his admission strip his research of legitimacy? No! Does it compromise the dominant narratives emerging on psychedelic healing? *No!* Is the stigma against scientists talking about personal use rooted in reality? *NO!* It is absolutely an inherited burden from the 1960s insisting academics must remain devoutly silent to avoid being shamed by the scientific establishment and losing everything they've labored to build.

"The case of psychedelic drug research isn't just about the legitimization of psychoactive drugs in medicine but the legitimization of science more broadly," Giffort argued. "One thing that science studies scholars have repeatedly shown is that legitimacy is not automatic and given. It is fragile and can be so easily lost and hard to reestablish. But the ways in which that happens—the ways that we gain and lose legitimacy—aren't based on objective factors; they are very much shaped by the social and historical context."[3]

As an example, Giffort alluded to first-wave psychedelic research using LSD for conversion therapy and to treat "frigid" women. "From today's vantage point, it seems ridiculous and even offensive that the drug was used in this way, but it also reflects the context in which these health professionals were practicing—one in which 'homosexuality' and 'frigidness' were considered valid medical diagnoses . . . In contrast, I have heard presentations in recent years where psychologists have proposed harnessing the self-actualizing potential of psychedelic experiences to facilitate acceptance of one's sexual and gender identity. So, it's a really good example of the social construction of sexuality and medicine."[4]

As psychedelics amplify patterns, the revival amplifies the trends of the academic establishment from which it has emerged. One trend involves people doing one thing (taking psychedelics) and saying another (only *studying psychedelics*). As psychedelic therapy teaches, we cannot shift what we avoid. In our avoidance, the shadow grows in strength.

Pollan, in contrast, promotes discussions of personal use. When he wrote about his psychedelics experiences in *How to Change Your Mind*, he risked his trustworthy reputation with his vast readership, but things played out differently than the risk's forecast. I asked him if he received backlash, and Pollan replied, "No, and I expected that I would. I expected there was some price to pay, reputationally or socially, but there wasn't. What happened is I think it made it more comfortable for many people to tell their stories."

Pollan argues that sharing stories is essential to sway public opinion and eliminate propaganda-fueled stigmas. "It's important for people to come out of the closet," Pollan said. "That is how you normalize something. Look how important that was to the Gay Rights movement. People were willing to tell their stories and come out on television and to their families. It was when everybody realized, 'I know someone who's gay, and they're great,' that suddenly it became socially acceptable, and we could imagine things like gay marriage. I think people coming out of the psychedelic closet helps everybody."

The revival can be viewed as a chess match against the Feds and the unquestioned biases of the culture, where each move aims to curtail a pawn of remaining stigma. Researchers' narrative control benefits the psychedelic medicine field and, to an extent, psychedelics in general. When it stigmatizes people who use psychedelics recreationally, it establishes a hierarchy wherein psychedelic-assisted therapy rules over foolish whippersnappers who take psychedelics at music festivals, scenic parks, and in the comfort of their homes.

Thanks to a new generation of researchers, the supremacy of self-censoring scientists appears to be diminishing. In the meantime, I hope more researchers realize that a movement that stigmatizes its subjects—unless strict and often-inaccessible protocols are followed—seems fated to collapse beneath the hefty weight of its self-denial.

Medical Gatekeepers

The term "gatekeeper" conjures two images in my mind: a cloaked figure holding a scythe at a dark threshold I don't want to find myself approaching, and the old, suited man at the gated entrance of the secret sex cult's palatial manor in *Eyes Wide Shut* who informs Bill Harford (Tom Cruise) he will never be welcome at their mask-clad ritualistic orgies. The second image is more relevant to the current discussion.

Gatekeepers are authorities on accessibility. Who gets to enter the secret club? Who's allowed access to the VIP lounge? The psychedelic gatekeeper of the last five decades has been the Federal Government, whose laws have blocked psychedelic use in all settings.* Ever since Strassman found the narrow path through Federal blockages, those gates have gradually opened. Now, new gatekeepers are forming, and some folks aren't thrilled about how it's shaking out.

The medical research model operates in league with the Federal government. It requires specific settings with specific equipment and staffing, and the individuals dictating who gets approved for treatment are typically doctors holding the power of their prescription pads. Should doctors hold

---

* The exception, ironically, became the Native American Church, whose sacramental use of peyote was granted Federal protection by Bill Clinton's John Hancock two years prior to his *not having sexual relations* with Monica Lewinsky. Fun fact: Clinton's defense during the trial for the perjury he definitely committed included the phrase, "It depends on what the meaning of the word 'is' is . . . if 'is' means is and never has been, that is not—that is one thing. If it means there is none, that was a completely true statement." What might Martin Heidegger say about such complex questions of ontology? Perhaps Slick Willie's *being-toward-deception* would have prompted the German philosopher to add yet another impossibly dense chapter to *Sein und Zeit*.

this power? What if they've never taken psychedelics and have no idea what they're signing people up for? Are they authorities on determining treatment criteria because they graduated from medical schools which, until recently, taught that psychedelics are scientifically verified to be bad?

On this point, psychedelics in the West differ significantly from traditional plant medicine use. In cultures that hold ayahuasca, peyote, and psilocybin mushrooms as sacramental, gatekeepers are the individuals whom Western cultures call shamans. These individuals usually don't attend medical school, but they understand the plants and how to navigate their realms better than anyone.

Then there's the history of underground psychedelic therapy to consider. For decades, practitioners have facilitated psychedelic healing in secret, amassing wisdom along the way. They're not always medically trained, yet many know far more about proper facilitation methods than a doctor who decided to give ketamine to depressed people because he read some statistics in a medical journal.

Some people want to get rid of gatekeepers altogether. These folks advocate for psychedelic legalization, arguing for an inherent human right to take any substance whenever one wants, wherever one wants, and for whatever purpose one desires. Decriminalize Nature is at the forefront, having passed successful measures in several US locations. Decrim fervently resists the medical model, arguing that it supports capitalist agendas and positions medical and pharmaceutical gatekeepers to profit abundantly while controlling access. Carlos Plazola, Decrim's vocal cofounder who appeared on the scene from an ambiguous background around 2019, never misses an opportunity to throw shade at MAPS, Johns Hopkins, and countless other institutions he regards as minions of the medical-industrial complex.

Organizations like Decrim focus on eliminating gatekeepers, suggesting gatekeeping organizations are inevitably infused with capitalistic power dynamics restricting the basic freedom to engage at will with the natural world. It's an appealing argument, and it certainly sounds nice on paper. But as I listened to Decrim's arguments grow louder, I heard a lack of respect for the power of these plants and molecules. Amid Decrim's ethos proclaiming anyone should be able to take psychedelics and plant medicines whenever they want, there's little to no appreciation for the importance of taking them with care and respect in intentional contexts.

Although Decrim's leaders frequently reference the history of Indigenous plant medicine to fortify their libertarian agenda, they appear to forget that Indigenous societies have gatekeepers as well. Plant medicine cultures don't typically have models allowing anyone over eighteen to pick peyote or ayahuasca at will and take it for any purpose they deem fit. The cultures more often regard the medicine with such respect that its consumption is restricted to ceremonial contexts. Their gatekeepers earn the right to serve the medicine after years, if not decades, of disciplined training on navigating the spirit world. Far from the free-for-all model Decrim promotes, this gatekeeping context isn't regarded as a lack of accessibility infringing on human rights but as a necessary condition for honoring the medicine's sacred healing power.

Toward a Meeting Point

I don't think the medicinal approach is the ideal model. But issues of access aren't reducible to a binary between medicalization and legalization. There are important discussion topics in the liminal space between, and potential routes could increase accessibility while establishing intentional contexts of use. Those are the routes I'm most interested in watching develop.

The current wave of psychedelic research has distanced itself from the hippies. While politically advantageous, this approach continues to reinforce stereotypes around personal use. Is this a necessary step for psychedelics to become widely accessible? Or is this the playing out of medico-capitalist initiatives focused on transferring the keys of psychedelic accessibility to the gated community on the hill overlooking the people getting arrested for having the same substances in their pockets?

I hope for future models operating at the intersection of decriminalization and medicalization. If psychedelics become available outside medicalized contexts, I hope their access involves education on harm reduction and intentional use. Just as people gain the privilege of driving a car after undergoing sufficient training, I hope psychedelic use necessitates at least some demonstration of knowledge and care beyond reaching a certain age.

That being said, my beliefs are not emphatic enough to throw stones at those who take psychedelics for non-therapeutic purposes.

If the writers of the revival's narrative continue to shadow widespread non-therapeutic use—not to mention researchers' personal use—seeds of unrest will continue flourishing, and those they wish to write out of existence will rebel. If trends don't shift, these narrators' suppression of "threatening" perspectives will result in the backlash they fear, for things foolishly forced into the shadow inevitably burst through the gimcrack walls built to contain them.

22

Bypassing and Abuses of Power

"The more consciousness gains in clarity, the more monarchic becomes
its content, to which everything contradictory has to submit."

—Carl Jung, *Mysterium Coniunctionis*

The trend that most upsets me about the revival is the ongoing, self-
justified recurrence of *bypassing*. This pattern has more potential than
anything else to destroy the promises of psychedelic medicine.

Psychologist and mindfulness teacher John Welwood invented the term
"spiritual bypassing" to describe a tendency among folks of the spiritual per-
suasion to use techniques like meditation as means for avoidance. Welwood
defined spiritual bypassing as using "spiritual ideas and practices to sidestep
personal, emotional 'unfinished business,' to shore up a shaky sense of self, or
to belittle basic needs, feelings, and developmental tasks."[1] Essentially, one
uses mindfulness tools to tiptoe around challenging personal issues by convincing themselves the issues aren't there.

When we bypass psychological development, we restrict overall growth.
When growth is restricted, we leave parts of ourselves behind, stifling our
capacity to help others. Any number of things can thwart development, such
as experiencing trauma at a young age. As a result of trauma, a part of the
individual becomes frozen in time, and it will remain as such until it gets
the attention and care required to heal from the traumatic incident. Instead
of attending to these developmental needs, spiritual bypassing aims toward
"transcending" the pain and "letting it go," neither of which help the traumatized part become unfrozen.

A tragic example is Christopher McCandless, the young vagabond who died in the Alaskan wilderness and became famous posthumously in Jon Krakauer's book *Into the Wild*. McCandless professed that the only way to achieve Enlightenment was to abandon society and forge transcendental unity with nature. In the end, he realized he had bypassed his need for connection, which he expressed in one of the last things he wrote before dying at age twenty-four: "Happiness only real when shared."[2]

Like meditating alone in the wilderness, psychedelics can be used to access transcendental states and avoid painful realities. As psychedelics can induce ego death, they can paradoxically make the ego denser. They can amplify fears and magnify patterns of avoidance, especially when these patterns are propped up by years of inner work focused on eliminating hardship.

Psychedelic bypassing is a trend of psychedelic users personally and collectively avoiding difficulty and challenge while espousing an ethos of personal and collective healing. Many psychedelic enthusiasts—including therapists and researchers—don't take their potential for harm seriously. Because psychedelics can transform people, many generalize this potential as an inherent quality. When reports of harm arise, such as traumatic trips following unethical facilitation, those prone to psychedelic bypassing shrug them off, ignoring the challenges such stories pose and focusing instead on the psychedelic cure-all story. They sometimes resort to blaming the recipients of harm, citing their unpreparedness without acknowledging psychedelics' potential to harm even those who feel fully prepared.

If psychedelics do nothing but bliss people out in their established worldview, how can they effect healing at a broad scale? The ethos of the 1960s counterculture centered on dismantling and rebelling against the oppressive societal ethos of separation, imperialism, and control; what use are psychedelics if they help us feel better about those realities as we binge-watch the reruns of our personal networks? If we don't use psychedelics to deepen care for ourselves, each other, and the planet, then we will maintain the harmful behaviors, perspectives, and obstructed liberties that generate much of the pain we seek to escape.

Are we creating psychedelic spaces that help us integrate our shadows, or are we elevating approaches that shield us from darkness while calling the resultant pleasure "healing"? What kind of "unity" turns away from the suffering unfolding before our dilated pupils?

IFS, Buddhism, and Bypassing

As discussed earlier, Internal Family Systems calls the inner realities we tend to bypass "exiles." Exiles exist in the shadows behind the thick screen of protective parts, which turn one's attention away from exiles to avoid the pain that accompanies the exiles' expressions.

From this viewpoint, bypassing can be recognized as a protective strategy. Someone who bypasses the pain they cause may be unwilling to acknowledge the pain they feel. It's easy to villainize people who bypass blatant behavioral imbalances, but doing so is unlikely to help them recognize the roots of their behavior. It could end up reinforcing their protective systems, which must defend against the onslaught threatening to expose the exiles they've exerted lifelong effort to keep hidden.

There are clear similarities between IFS and Buddhism. The IFS concept of "Self" parallels the Buddhist notion of the inner "witness," a state of awareness from which one observes one's stream of thoughts, emotions, and desires without gripping on to any of the stream's contents. Buddhism teaches that attachment to those contents—that is, thinking we *are* our thoughts, desires, and emotions—is the source of suffering. In IFS, suffering arises from becoming "blended" with our burdened parts, such as thinking I *am* my inner critic part, or I *am* my reckless thrill-seeker part at my core. In both models, healing relies on relating compassionately to the inner world from an unattached, unblended stance of awareness.*

There's an important difference in Buddhism's and IFS's understanding of that to which we are relating. Buddhism regards the contents of the inner world as illusion. Unattachment involves recognizing that illusory nature, disidentifying with the illusions, and allowing thoughts, emotions, and desires to pass like leaves floating down a river. In recognizing the illusory nature of our identity constructs, and diminishing our attachment to them, we become connected to our "Buddha-nature," a state of pure, unchanging, eternal awareness.

---

* Buddhism teaches that the "self" is an illusion. This Buddhist "self" is not to be confused with the IFS "Self." Through an IFS lens, the Buddhist "self" is an amalgamation of parts that we believe define our identity. It is similar to the psychological construct of the "ego." The IFS "Self" parallels the Buddhist state of pure awareness, for both are always accessible, unchanging, and rooted in our essential identity.

IFS practitioners don't interpret parts as illusions. In Schwartz's eyes, parts are "sacred beings" who desire and deserve the same level of recognition, care, and respect given to our loved ones. Parts are seen as *real*; they are living autonomous lives whether or not we give them attention.

Buddhist meditation can help us disentangle distorted views and thoughts, connecting us with an authentic source of consciousness. By emphasizing the illusory nature of the inner world, these views can promote an ethos of bypassing. IFS can give rise to bypassing if we let our parts that want us to *get somewhere better* run the show. These *get-somewhere-else* parts tend to view other burdened parts as *problems* blocking the intended outcome. An IFS technique of asking parts to "step back" to allow the Self to lead the process can become a crutch pushing away important dynamics of our inner world. For IFS to work, the mind's eye must see clearly enough to recognize when burdened parts are leading us instead of the Self.

If we remain mindful of our inclinations to bypass our strife in effort to feel better, IFS and Buddhism can work symbiotically. Although it may seem counterintuitive, transformation often requires feeling our pain. Few people, if any, have phrased the conundrum better than humanistic psychologist Carl Rogers, when he famously said, "The curious paradox is that when I accept myself just as I am, then I can change."

We Should Not Overemphasize the Negative

In states of desolation and despair, we can direct our attention toward being with the pain, understanding its roots, and feeling compassion for ourselves. At a certain point we may find ourselves wallowing in our suffering. If we focus too much on our struggles, we can embed their reality and block feelings of gratitude and joy. If spiritual bypassing is excessive avoidance, the flip side is overindulgence. Excessive focus on a state constructs a self-fulfilling prophecy that manufactures evidence to support its constructs.

During my psychedelic therapy counseling internship, I worked with a client who'd suffered from depression for decades. Through several ketamine sessions of various doses, I witnessed him remaining stuck in crystallized narratives declaring he was "beyond hope," and the treatment, like everything else, "wasn't helping." The thing is, it was. His wife reflected how much more patient, present, and energized he seemed. His best friend told him he appeared to be exuding light, as if a heavy burden had been lifted. Each session, I listened to him reflect on positive shifts in his daily patterns, and after the medicine peaked, I witnessed him deepening into a calm, restful state. But his habitual emotional patterns took hold again, and by the next session, he'd re-fixated on his inescapable suffering, reconvincing himself he would never get better, even as those closest to him saw significant changes.

Many people remain stuck in negative narratives because the beliefs are serving them, even if they don't realize it. Maybe someone's narrative of powerlessness allows them to refrain from seeking opportunities to avoid rejection. Maybe someone learned to receive love from their caregivers by harshly criticizing themselves. Whatever it may be, fixation on the narrative and its corresponding emotions blocks out the possibility of recognizing anything that threatens the narrative's dominance. If spiritual bypassing ignores the dark for the sake of the light, depression blocks out the light for the sake of the dark.

Focusing on positivity can induce bypassing, but it doesn't necessarily equate to avoidance. It can be transformative to connect to love and bliss amid turmoil. Doing so can also be a slippery slope, for when connecting to the light comes at the expense of acknowledging the dark, the underlying realities fueling the shadow will continue energizing an insatiable conflict between the ego and its inner opposite.

Beware the Ego that Claims No Ego

Perhaps the biggest danger of bypassing is justifying harmful behavior. In the psychedelic world, this shows up in what I call "Guru Syndrome."

Pollan wrote, "It is one of the many paradoxes of psychedelics that these drugs can sponsor an ego-dissolving experience that in some people quickly leads to massive ego inflation. Having been let in on a great secret of the universe, the recipient of this knowledge is bound to feel special, chosen for great things . . . granted sole possession of a key to the universe."[3]

A peculiar and disturbing form of ego can develop through psychedelic use. This takes the form of a master manipulator built on bypassing legitimate concerns through self-aggrandizement. The secret to its endurance is a foundational premise that it is the most humble, nonexistent ego in the known universe. If anyone leverages criticism, Guru Syndrome deflects it, claiming it is the critic's ego projecting its distortions onto the healer, who became a vesicle for eternal truth when psychedelics dissolved their ego long ago. This mentality justifies a remarkable capacity to bypass enormously disturbing behavior.

An example rose to light in 2021, when psychedelic media outlet Psymposia released a video of a man named Martin Ball giving a presentation to the Los Angeles Medicinal Plant Society in 2016. Ball, an influential figure in the psychedelic underground, detailed his experiences administering 5-MeO-DMT. He recounted giving 5-MeO to a seventy-nine-year-old woman, who soon stopped breathing. Ball, who had neither emergency medical training nor medical staff on hand, said, "What happened was I ended up lying down on top of her . . . put my tongue in her mouth . . . pushed against her tongue and there was no push back . . . I just waited with my tongue up against the tip of her tongue, and after a while, she suddenly pushed my tongue out of her mouth, and I was like, 'Okay. She's going to be fine.'"

Ball related a separate incident in which a woman to whom he'd administered Bufo was lying on a mat. "I'm on top of her, and my tongue is on her forehead, and I'm growling," he said. "And then all of a sudden I can feel it . . . and I just *bluargh!* And I threw up all over her head."

As disturbing as the anecdote was, the small gathering he spoke to didn't call him out. They *laughed.*

"I learned, really early on, my job as a facilitator here is simply to follow the energy and to embody it fully, without reservation, without second guessing, without judgment," Ball said. "And if it means I need to throw up on someone, throw up on 'em! Just do it! Because they're going to appreciate it, as odd as it may seem."[4]

This behavior is clearly not okay. How and why does this happen? As far as I can tell, it comes down to a sequence of steps:

1. An individual has a profound psychedelic experience in which their concepts of who they are dissolve.

2. Said person recognizes their *true self* is more expansive than they'd imagined, capable of profound things—in fact, they realize the fundamental religious truth that their essential identity is inseparable from the identity of the Universe and/or God.

3. The individual returns to everyday life, believing their realization translates into baseline consciousness; their issues have been solved, and they can now actualize their role as the healer they've always been.

4. Realities of being human return, including the ego—only now, the individual's ego is structured on the belief that it doesn't exist; by extension, the new ego becomes equated with the Universal/God consciousness to which the individual connected on the psychedelic.

5. Any information or experience that threatens this new ego is either rejected completely or reinterpreted to fit the new schema of faultless self.

6. A tremendous amount of bypassing becomes required to maintain the supremacy of the individual's infallible healing power, pushing their "baser" qualities like anger, lust, and desire for power into the shadow.

7. The individual's shadowed qualities continue influencing them through the shaky walls of bypassing, leading them to perpetuate harms by justifying their behaviors as valid expressions of their inherent divinity.

A cult of personality often surrounds such figures. When controversy is raised, followers cry out in a chorus of support, justifying their leader's ethical breaches on the basis of the healing the leader brought them. There's the American Buddhist teacher Michael Roach, who maintained popularity and influence after numerous controversies of sexual misconduct and harmful teachings. There's also yoga guru Bikram Choudhury, who, after being repeatedly accused of racism, homophobia, and sexual assault, continued to profit from every Bikram Yoga studio whose operators maintained allegiance to their guru. In such cults of personality, a paradigm of victim-blaming shames and shuns the abused individual, deepening their trauma and enhancing its negative ramifications on all facets of life.

Ball represents a dark side of the psychedelic underground, where behaviors like his can proliferate without consequence due to lack of regulatory oversight. Unfortunately, harmful behaviors related to Guru Syndrome are not restricted to the underground. They have manifested in some of the most trusted psychedelic organizations.

Richard Yensen and Donna Dryer

A notorious above-ground instance of facilitator abuse took place during a MAPS-sponsored MDMA-assisted therapy trial in Canada. The co-therapists, Richard Yensen and Donna Dryer, were a married couple who'd been leaders in the psychedelic world for decades. In 2018, a participant submitted complaints to several organizations, including MAPS, explaining that after her treatment concluded in 2015, Yensen engaged in a sexual relationship with her.

MAPS's statement, published in May 2019, read: "At the end of 2015 or early 2016, the relationship between Richard Yensen and the participant became sexual in nature. Donna Dryer reportedly became aware of this and tried to stop the sexual relationship but was unsuccessful. She did not report it to MAPS or any regulatory agencies. Over time, the participant grew uncomfortable with this relationship and eventually moved away in early 2017, breaking ties with both therapists. In January 2018, the participant submitted complaints naming both Richard Yensen and Donna Dryer."[5]

MAPS paid the participant $15,000 Canadian, and Yensen and Dryer "were barred from all MAPS-related activities and from becoming providers of MAPS-affiliated MDMA-assisted therapy if the treatment is approved."[6]

This was a big deal for psychedelic advocates. *A MAPS therapist?* cried the collective voice. *We trusted MAPS! How could this happen?* The unnerving layers grew in 2021, when the media obtained and released videos of Yensen and Dryer's sessions with the participant. The footage included numerous instances of Yensen demonstrating total lack of concern over boundaries in the therapist-client relationship, including a moment when he held her down while she was having a difficult experience.

MAPS denied any knowledge of these behaviors, but given their mandated reviews of session videos, not everyone in the psychedelic world was convinced. While the Yensen-Dryer incident example is the only such controversy to date for MAPS, the same cannot be said for the revival in general.

Françoise Bourzat and Aharon Grossbard

Perhaps the most influential psychedelic book to follow Pollan's *How to Change Your Mind* was Françiose Bourzat's *Consciousness Medicine*, published in 2019. Through her book's success, Bourzat became one of the faces of the psychedelic world, appearing as a keynote-level presenter at countless conferences and webinars in the years following the publication. With her husband Aharon Grossbard and daughter Naama Grossbard, Bourzat cocreated the Center for Consciousness Medicine in 2020, which became one of the world's leading education programs for psychedelic and plant medicine facilitators. Bourzat was lauded for her work with the Mazatec people in Mexico, through whom she claimed to have accumulated ancestral wisdom related to ceremonial psilocybin mushroom use.

Behind the scenes, whispers rose of sketchiness afoot. When I began this book in early 2021, a trusted advisor with deep connections in the psychedelic world instructed me not to interview Bourzat; he was certain the content of these whispers would come to light. He was right.

In September 2021, a man named Will Hall published a detailed article recounting abuses he experienced under Bourzat and Grossbard's care during a lengthy period in which he'd received their underground psychedelic treatment. "The relationship devolved into worse and worse professional boundary violations: staying at Grossbard and Bourzat's home, doing childcare and landscaping work for them, going out to dinner and to a concert, hearing Grossbard's offensive sexual jokes, him greeting me naked in his kitchen one night to tell me to keep the noise down," Hall wrote. "He held my hand in sessions. We hugged and cuddled on the office floor. He and Bourzat told me they loved me and would never leave me and I'd never be alone again. It was wonderful—until it wasn't."[7]

Hall continued, "During one talk therapy session in his office, which was not using psychedelics, Grossbard continued to touch me in ways that felt sexual even after I complained: He embraced me face to face, with my legs wrapped around his waist, sitting genitals-to-genitals in his lap. The touching didn't feel right . . . So I told him, 'This feels sexual.' He dismissed me by stating firmly, 'No, it's not,' and continued."[8]

Hall alluded to Guru Syndrome, writing that Grossbard "did all this presumably because he was convinced his spiritual healing powers entitled him to not play by the rules as a therapist." Then came the requisite gaslighting. "I remembered the many times that Grossbard had called me crazy, sometimes in front of other clients and students," Hall recalled. "When criticized, one of his go-to phrases was 'that's just your crazy ego' to shut down discussion."[9]

Bourzat and Grossbard reached their influential height in the psychedelic world many years after Hall's relationship with them concluded. Seeing their heightened status in the psychedelic world, Hall decided he could not remain silent, especially after learning he was not alone in having received such treatment. His article linked to a lawsuit from 2000, which "alleges sexual battery, fraud, professional negligence, and 12 other violations by a client of Grossbard and Bourzat who said Bourzat had sex with him." The suit was settled out of court, and Hall wrote that a viable source informed him the settlement happened after Grossbard and Bourzat "made a large cash payment."[10]

In the wake of the allegations, the Center for Consciousness Medicine cut ties with Grossbard and suspended Bourzat. Being deeply invested in the psychedelic world as I was, I waited for a proliferation of articles and essays about the revelation, given Bourzat's mighty stature. I was confounded to observe an aftermath of silence. It took weeks, if not months, for large psychedelic organizations to comment. Most denied any connection to Bourzat. Even those who had presented alongside her on numerous occasions washed their hands clean. As a result of this silence, I continually meet people new to this world who fervently recommend *Consciousness Medicine* and speak glowingly of Bourzat, completely unaware of this history.

I do not intend to make any all-inclusive claims about an individual based on one element of their biography. A "witch hunt" mentality can breed extremity. Nevertheless, I feel strongly that folks with such histories should not be in leadership positions in the education of the next wave of psychedelic therapists and guides. To establish such protections, these individuals must be called out, and if their abusive behavior is indicative of a trend, the public should be informed, empowering those seeking treatment to know whom to avoid.

Right Use of Power

While the same standards of practice govern psychedelic and non-psychedelic therapists, adding a substance to the mix changes the ethical dynamics. The power differential between therapist and client expands insofar as the psychedelic amplifies the client's vulnerability and incapacitation. For a client to feel safe, they must trust the therapist's ability to care for them when they cannot care for themselves. Violating this trust is a breach of ethical boundaries and general standards of being a good person.

Psychotherapist Cedar Barstow's book *Right Use of Power: The Heart of Ethics* has influenced the therapy world since its publication in 2005, serving as an ethical guide for people in service professions—therapists, bodyworkers, teachers, clergy, physicians—and helping them navigate the complex power dynamics of their client relationships.

"The power differential is the inherently greater power and influence that helping professionals have as compared to their clients," Barstow wrote. "Consequently, clients are unusually susceptible to harm and confusion through misuses of power and influence."[11]

Caregivers have more "role power" than their clients, for their role inherently exerts more influence over the client than vice versa. Barstow called caregivers to be aware of this and wield their role power with intention. Just as overuse of role power can cause harm, so can underuse, like when a caregiver acts like the client's friend, as if the power differential doesn't exist. Blurred boundaries can yield harmful consequences, as evidenced by Hall's testimony. As much as contemporary culture fears power, power isn't a bad thing. Power is neutral. The good/bad relates to how it is *wielded*.

Barstow named responsibilities for caregivers in a power differential, including:

Setting and maintaining appropriate boundaries

Creating needed safety

Staying in charge

Holding the larger container of wholeness and hope

Keeping your own personal life in the background so that it won't interfere[12]

Barstow was ahead of her time in writing a section on non-ordinary states. She understood such states raise unique concerns, for "the impact of the power differential is heightened and expanded when clients are in a non-ordinary state. Thus, greater sensitivity and skillfulness in understanding and using your increased role power and influence for promoting well-being is needed."[13]

Non-ordinary states bring unique concerns that apply to psychedelic therapy into the dynamic:

Potential for stronger and more complicated transference and counter-transference

Greater suggestibility

Greater need for safety

Increased possibility of triggering the therapist's fears and longings

Greater need to integrate profound experiences[14]

This gets at the impossible-to-overstate importance of psychedelic therapists working with their personal shadows. Without developing a relationship with their desires, fears, and capacity to get triggered into an unconscious response, therapists will likely end up communicating such things nonverbally. This will disorient the client, especially if the therapist denies the reality the client is perceiving. Psychedelics can muddy clarity, but they can also increase it, and clients on empathy-enhancing substances like MDMA may feel an increased ability to peer into the layers underlying the therapist's persona, especially if the therapist is working hard—either consciously or unconsciously—to keep those layers out of sight. Such incongruence obstructs the client's ability to relax into the effects, for human beings, like dogs and horses, can sense inauthenticity and intuit its unsettling effects.

Let Not Psychedelic Bypassing Reign

We cannot deny parts of ourselves or culture out of existence, no matter how skilled we become at bypassing. It can be scary to turn toward the shadow. But as Spielberg demonstrated in *Jaws*, fear of the thing is often bigger than the thing itself. When we let fear run the show, we create barriers to our capacity for compassion and love.

Psychedelic bypassing can be inconsequential when its scope is restricted to an individual's avoidance of unnerving impulses and memories they'd rather not confront. But as the examples of Ball, Yensen and Dryer, and Bourzat and Grossbard evince, excess self-justification and denial can effect sinister manifestations of harming and traumatizing vulnerable people. Psychedelic bypassing has more potential than any other trend to destroy the revival before it takes hold. No enterprise buttressed by its own avoidance can foster widespread healing.

23

Psychedelic Exceptionalism

"Prior to 1907, drug use in western society was viewed as a personal issue rather than a moral one, and drugs like opium and heroin could be purchased with a doctor's prescription from any corner drugstore."

—Jesse Donaldson and Erika Dyck, *The Acid Room*

After the Controlled Substances Act passed in 1970, psychedelics were unequivocally regarded as "drugs." These days, they are commonly referred to as "medicines." This terminological shift reflects cultural revision on the merit of psychedelics. It can also promote excess glorification of their healing potential, as if they occupy the top rung on the ladder of medicinal drugs.

It's somewhat silly to distinguish between drugs and medicines. Western medicines, from Tylenol to morphine, are drugs. Drugs are exogenous substances that, when consumed, affect physiology in discernible ways. Psychedelics fall into this category, as do caffeine, alcohol, and raw cacao.

The cultural distinction between these terms is less categorical than moral. The War on Drugs indoctrinated Western culture with a negativity bias toward the term "drug," morphing it from an inert noun to a politically charged, fear-inducing rhetorical device. In ensuing decades, children received moral messages best summarized by Mr. Mackey's lesson to the kids of *South Park*: "Drugs are bad. You shouldn't do drugs. If you do them, you're bad. Because drugs are bad, *mmkay*?"

As cannabis legalization revealed, the perceived "badness" of a drug doesn't always reflect the substance's objective qualities. What sent people to prison two decades ago is now sold as medicine, and the people profiting the most are doing the same thing—selling it—as thousands of people who are still incarcerated.

While the shift to calling psychedelics "medicines" demonstrates an uptick in their cultural standing, it energizes an elitist trend called *psychedelic exceptionalism*. Adamant enthusiasts, excited to see psychedelics being recognized as powerful medicines, often contrast their "good" drugs with "bad" drugs like stimulants, opiates, and depressants. They cite the cultural shift as "proof" of their righteousness—*I've said it all along, psychedelics are the best*—while reinforcing negative regard for those other drugs—*psychedelics help people, unlike Xanax and cocaine, which are evil.*

Camille Barton summarized this exceptionalism in one of our interviews: "Psychedelics are being removed from the category of 'bad drugs' and elevated into medicine. This stigmatizes people who continue to use 'bad drugs' and paints them as criminals, which perpetuates the war on drugs.

Is this stigmatization what the revival intends? Does its ethos of unity exclude people labeled as criminals?

Carl Hart and Problematic Drug Narratives

Perhaps the most outspoken leader on the subject is Carl Hart, former chair of Columbia University's Department of Psychology. I became aware of Hart's work at the Psychedelic Science Summit in Austin, Texas, in 2019 as he delivered an impassioned lecture demonstrating through abundant scientific research—much of which he conducted—that stigmas around specific drugs are rooted more in misinformation than fact. He wasn't talking about psychedelics. He was talking about cocaine, heroin, and methamphetamine. Hart asserted their "bad drug" label was the perceptual result of War on Drugs propaganda, media bias, and sensationalism of television shows like *Breaking Bad.*[*] In case anyone thought he was just being theoretical, Hart, during a panel discussion, confidently said, "Heroin made me a better person."

---

[*] *Breaking Bad* really is an incredible show, but more so as a character study of power, resentment, and change over time than a factual investigation of methamphetamine.

My gut constricted. Something didn't compute. How could this Ivy League department chair with a PhD in neuropsychopharmacology use a drug that was, according to every perspective I'd ever heard, inarguably evil?

So began a process of dismantling biases I hadn't realized I held. In lieu of my assumptions about heroin, I assumed Hart would have a lot to say about the intended impact of his controversial admissions. I was wrong.

For Hart, such statements—which he made more publicly in his 2021 book, *Drug Use for Grown-Ups*—are not about stirring up controversy. He's troubled that such statements do cause controversy. In his eyes, it's regarded as edgy because people see heroin users through thick veils of stigma rather than as *people*.

In the early 2000s, when psychedelics started gaining mainstream recognition as medicines, Hart recognized a disturbing trend: countless articles, podcasts, and books on psychedelic research positioned them in the "good drug" category while perpetuating "bad drug" stigmas without question. By differentiating their drugs from the "bad drugs," psychedelic users positioned themselves on a moral pedestal and reinforced judgments on "bad drug" users, even though they'd been similarly stigmatized for nearly half a century.

Hart developed a distaste for psychedelics and their users' exceptionalism, yet as he challenges people to question their narratives, so he challenges his own. When he tried 2C-B (a psychedelic phenethylamine growing in popularity) with friends at a festival, he recognized the unique medicinal properties of a powerful drug.

Psychedelics weren't the problem. The problem was the elitism among their staunchest advocates, most of whom were well-educated, upper-middle-class White people.

Hart started speaking at psychedelic conferences to call out what he was seeing. He pissed off a lot of psychonauts, who wondered, "Why's this guy bursting our blissful bubble, telling us psychedelics aren't better than opiates when *obviously* they are?" His message reached many others, and these days, Hart's a leading figure in the revival.

He argues that issues around drug stigmatization come down to breaches of the rights established in the US Constitution.

When Nixon declared a War on Drugs, he effectively declared a war on specific demographics of people.

Unconscious Bias

All drugs have the common factor of altering consciousness. As such, a core tenet of Hart's viewpoint is no drug is morally "better" than another; they are simply different, and judgments on those differences are created by and applied to people. These judgments don't always reflect reality; they express inherited perspectives rooted in misinformation, bias, and oppression of marginalized populations.

A primary example is the crack versus cocaine discrepancy that began in the 1980s. It's well-established that these drugs are identical at the molecular level. However, under President Reagan, the US penalty for crack possession was 100 times more severe than possession of cocaine. The Drug War's media machines fed the population caricatured portraits of crack users as dangerous criminals who must be locked in prison to keep the public safe. Only then could America beat its enemy of the "crack epidemic." The caricatured individuals were usually Black; Hart knows it's no coincidence that the comparatively unstigmatized naughty-but-kind-of-glamorous cocaine was typically associated with wealthy White people. By 1988, Black people were arrested on drug charges at five times the rate of White people, despite no evidence proving they took more drugs.[1] Their drugs were more stigmatized, targeted, and punishable, and their neighborhoods had a higher concentration of drug law enforcement officers.

At the Drug War's inception, its proprietors were less interested in disseminating facts than spinning narratives to serve political agendas. John Ehrlichman, who served as Nixon's domestic affairs advisor until the Watergate scandal landed him in prison, was quoted in a 2016 *Harper's Magazine* article as having said Nixon's two biggest enemies were the "anti-war left and black [*sic*] people."

"We knew we couldn't make it illegal to be either against the war or black [*sic*]," Ehrlichman said, "but by getting the public to associate the hippies with marijuana and blacks [sic] with heroin, and then criminalizing both heavily, we could disrupt those communities. We could arrest their leaders, raid their homes, break up their meetings, and vilify them night after night on the evening news."

In case any doubt remained, Ehrlichman added: "Did we know we were lying about the drugs? Of course we did."[2]

Public safety was not the goal. The goal was to expand control and neutralize communities perceived as threats to "Big" Dick's power by moralizing and criminalizing their drugs of choice.*

Such moralization of drugs generated an excuse to ignore pressing social issues. To scapegoat crack as the problem in specific neighborhoods was to ignore socioeconomic and political factors making prosperity all but impossible for residents to achieve. Low standards of living and lack of opportunity contributed to crack's dissemination, for the economic potential of selling it exceeded most, if not all, economic possibilities available.

"We cannot look at the poor who are addicted to heroin and conclude that heroin is itself a bad drug," wrote Julian Vayne in *Pharmakon*. "Certainly the economic conditions of the world's poor, even in so-called developed nations, are truly terrible, but these are a product of oppressive societies. Our society often uses 'the drug problem' to obscure the problems of homelessness and hopelessness."[3]

As a drug's cultural associations change, associations with its users change. Today's shifting status of psychedelics provides further proof, as does the expansion of criteria determining which drugs belong to the psychedelic category. Although ketamine wasn't as well known as cocaine and methamphetamine, those who had heard of it pre-revival tended to regard it as a dangerous "club" drug of depravity and addiction. As the revival kicked in, ketamine became known as a "miracle" medicine for treating depression. The entire *feel* of the word "ketamine" shifted, especially as it became the first anesthetic to take shelter under the psychedelic-positive umbrella.

But what feelings arise when you think about PCP, a.k.a. "angel dust"? Maybe you think of the scene from *Training Day* when Denzel Washington doses Ethan Hawke with it, leading Hawke to have a bad time that climaxes

---

* It should be noted that the veracity of Ehrlichman's quote has been called into question. It was printed sixteen years after his death, and his family objected to his inability to respond to what they suggested was a fabrication. In a Vox article that followed the *Harper's* publication, journalist German Lopez suggested Ehrlichman's claim was an "oversimplification" of Nixon's drug policy, while at the same time acknowledging the veracity of Nixon's distaste for hippies and Black people. (Source: German Lopez, "Was Nixon's war on drugs a racially motivated crusade? It's a bit more complicated," Vox, March 29, 2016, vox.com/2016/3/29 /11325750/nixon-war-on-drugs.)

with a bad guy shoving a gun into his face as he writhes in a bathtub. Maybe this image contributes to your "knowledge" that PCP is bad.

I'd speculate that PCP's actual history is less widely known than the *Training Day* scene. PCP was developed in 1956 as an anesthetic medication. Due to some undesirable side effects, several analogues were created. One of those was ketamine. As similar as ketamine and PCP are at the molecular level, media-infused cultural associations with these drugs and their users couldn't be more different.

The list continues with Adderall, a stimulant commonly prescribed to treat ADHD. That Adderall is nearly identical to methamphetamine rarely gets acknowledged. Even MDMA is closely related to meth: the "MA" of the acronym stands for "methamphetamine." They aren't identical like crack and cocaine, but important chemical similarities call into question the wide discrepancy between how the general public feels about them. Like ketamine, MDMA was added to the psychedelic category once it was shown to be efficacious for PTSD. At a molecular level, however, MDMA bears more similarities to methamphetamine than to psilocybin or LSD.

If this freaks you out, maybe it shouldn't. After all, in 2021, Hart was elected to MAPS' board of directors.[4] MDMA's similarity to methamphetamine has no negative bearing on the substance for Hart or MAPS' leaders, for its similarity means nothing more than what that sentence says. Moral meaning attributed to the similarity is a human creation, and human creations tend to be more flawed than humans acknowledge. MDMA has unique effects, and so do methamphetamine, LSD, heroin, and all other drugs. When we release our biases and the misinformation they churn, we equip ourselves to understand how specific drugs work and what medicinal applications they have.

As Hart discovered early in his career, neither understanding nor objective truth was the name of the game in academic science. In *Drug Use for Grown-Ups*, he chronicled the significant pushback he received from the scientific establishment after publishing drug research that threatened the establishment's accepted narratives. When superiors discredited his research, trusted colleagues even turned on him, disregarding the validity of his conclusions. Objective truth wasn't the driving force of the establishment. Power, prestige, and security reigned supreme.

Scientific gatekeepers reject research deemed threatening to their conclusions, and their underlings, laboring tirelessly for the Holy Grail of Tenure, must bow to the proverbial gatekeepers lest their shot at the security of a decent salary gets ripped away. I don't care how precise your scientific method is—this context is not conducive to objectivity. Human selfishness tends to prevail when neuroses are activated and basic needs threatened. Hart recognized this pattern, but he didn't submit. In the spirit of his ability to alter neuropsychopharmacological narratives with scientific evidence, he changed narratives proclaiming a bleak fate for dissenters when Columbia University elected him department chair.

How we perceive things doesn't always reflect things as they are. Countless factors influence our narratives, and cultural judgments get wired into our nervous systems, despite their lack of validity.

New Age thinking provides an example. The focus on "trusting intuition" comes with a huge flaw: it champions our biases when they "feel true." Beliefs that are wrong, even downright evil, can "feel" right—that's exactly how propaganda is so effective. When we let our feelings unanimously dictate the rightness or wrongness of a person, thing, or situation, we sacrifice our ability to evaluate those feelings and investigate whatever past experiences caused them to take hold. To the European colonialists who *felt* that Indigenous people were less-than-human, the New Age guru would reply, "Yes. Follow your intuition . . ." without realizing their "intuition" as a physiological expression of dehumanizing indoctrination.

Ivan Pavlov's discoveries in classical conditioning provide grounding. Pavlov found that when he repeatedly paired the neutral stimulus of a bell with the biologically potent stimulus of food set before a hungry dog, he could induce a physiological response (salivation) at the sound of the bell with no food present. He showed that physiological responses—e.g., how we *feel*—to specific associations are programmable. Thus, how we feel is not always the same as intuition or knowledge.

Given the inclinations of politicians and media moguls toward conditioning responses in service of unstated agendas, these points are essential to bear in mind as one evaluates their perceptions of drugs and their users. If one notes a strong physiological response rooted in no personal experience, conditioned biases are likely at play.

Context of Use and Corresponding Effects

Psychedelic exceptionalists sometimes cite Indigenous plant medicine use as evidence of psychedelics' elevated status. Such arguments fail to recognize traditional uses of non-psychedelic plants whose alkaloids led to the synthesis of some of the most notorious "bad drugs."

In the Andean regions of South America, Indigenous cultures chewed *coca* leaves—from which cocaine is derived—to connect to one another and their ancestors in ceremonies and celebrations.[5] They also used coca leaves in medical therapy to relieve pain and sickness.[6] Likewise, heroin was synthesized from morphine, which was first derived from the opium poppy. Opium use has been traced back to 3400 B.C. in Ancient Mesopotamia. In China's Ming dynasty, opium was consumed as an aphrodisiac.

Opium's illegality in Canada arose due to anti-Chinese sentiment. "In the wake of Vancouver's racially motivated anti-Asian riot, in which a white mob destroyed portions of Chinatown," wrote psychedelic historians Jesse Donaldson and Erika Dyck, "future Prime Minister William Lyon Mackenzie King . . . noticed, to his horror, that Chinatown's opium dens were being frequented by both white and Asian customers. Mackenzie King's worry was race-mixing, not addiction, and in his panicked report to the federal government, he recommended an immediate ban on the smoked opium popular with Chinese Canadians (the injectable version preferred by white Canadians remained legal)."[7]

The medicinal value of drugs arises from *how* they are being used. All drugs can be abused. Those abuses manifest differently depending on the drug of choice: you won't overdose on LSD as you might on heroin, but excessive LSD use can catalyze destabilization up to and including psychosis. Don't trust anyone who says LSD-induced psychosis was merely a War on Drugs myth. The Drug War overstated this potential effect, but the risk is real.

Given the essential factors of context and approach, results of clinical psychedelic therapy trials cannot be extrapolated to represent inherent psychedelic properties. Psychedelic research occurs in controlled environments. Trained professionals curate music selections and room decor, monitor doses and vital signs, and provide psychological support to help participants derive enduring value. This context differs radically from a naïve vagabond taking three hits of acid at Coachella and freaking out. The context influences the effects as much as, if not more than, the substance itself.

Strassman arrived at this conclusion after his DMT research. "The spirit molecule is neither good nor bad, beneficial nor harmful, in and of itself," he wrote. "Rather, set and setting establish the context and the quality of the experiences to which DMT leads us. Who we are and what we bring to the sessions and to our lives ultimately mean more than the drug experience itself."[8]

When psychedelics are revered as "good drugs," the harm they can cause is swept under the proverbial rug. Such misinformation prompts many people to imbibe psychedelics in terrible settings to experience healing, leaving them woefully unprepared for the destabilizing outcomes edited out of agenda-driven narratives.

Psychedelics are drugs, and psychedelics are medicines. Like all drugs and medicines, psychedelics can be beneficial and harmful. It's foolish to ignore the latter due to personal or political agendas. Focusing on the harm needn't be detrimental to the incorporation of the molecules into society. Rather, holding an informed and realistic viewpoint on their dangers will help people approach them with care, neutralizing potential harms.

The Courage to Act

One of Hart's core messages is that honesty and integrity are too important to be locked beneath fear. For the Drug War's false narratives to change, people need to speak openly about the benefits they receive from specific drugs, especially when those benefits diverge from stories associated with its users. This openness has been essential in overturning cultural stigmas, but if personal stories continue to glorify psychedelics while stigmatizing users of other substances, they will offer a fractured revision of the Drug War and reinforce harms to communities who, like psychedelic enthusiasts, desire the freedom to change their consciousness as they wish.

Whether or not you align with Hart or continue to believe psychedelics occupy the peak of a moral hierarchy of substances, it's helpful to evaluate your drug-related biases. Important as it is to trust intuition, it's equally important to realize when your "gut reactions" are programmed by influences that don't have everyone's well-being in mind. If nothing else, I hope the psychedelic enthusiasts who plaster "We Are One" stickers on their bumpers while buttressing narratives stigmatizing other drug users make better efforts to practice what they preach.

24

Destabilization and Death

"There are no beautiful surfaces without a terrible depth."

—Friedrich Nietzsche

I used to think bad trips were a myth. My first experiences on mushrooms and LSD brought profound connection, awe, bliss, and confidence. I became somewhat cocky, agreeing with my ego that only fearful people had bad trips, while people like me who meditate and reflect see the true nature of psychedelics. Then, I took ayahuasca.

My first drink had little effect. I saw colors behind my eyelids, and I contemplated my life's new path. Excited to deepen into the tranquility I sensed, I hopped in line for a second dose. Within minutes of lying down, I realized something completely unfamiliar was happening. An African woman lying nearby screamed. She stood, clutching her head, and ran out of the ceremony room into the cold night. Her screams receded into the distance, and the howls of coyotes joined her in a cacophony of chaos.

I sat up and looked around me. The world was no longer the world.

Tendrils and vines materialized, slithering and undulating toward me. I didn't trust them. As my fear grew, they inched closer. They were heading toward my eyes and mouth when the woman's screams stopped. An eerie silence hovered. A blanket rustled, plastic crackled, and another woman vomited into the bag she'd been given. She breathed heavily, then vomited again, and again, each one more guttural than the last. Another person was vomiting now, and another, and another.

This wasn't mere vomiting. This was purging. It was violent release of things too deep to understand. It was the world's chaos and suffering possessing people. I was alone, and I felt more terrified than I could have previously conceived possible. I knew only one thing for certain: this was hell, and I was trapped in it. Abandon hope, all ye who enter. There was no way out.

Bad Trips

You can't possibly understand what a bad trip is like until you have one. Before that, it's only a concept. Nothing can fully prepare you for becoming trapped in a reality more horrifying than your freakiest nightmares. What you must understand is that during a bad trip, the concept plays no role. Every element of your reality—your *physical reality*, all around you—becomes the bad trip. In ways I cannot explain, it becomes more real than anything you've experienced. The darkness takes over, and there's no way back.

Although you can't fully prepare for such an encounter, you can establish supportive structures to help you through it. These must be done in advance, for during a bad trip, you won't be able to explain what's happening. The worst way to experience one is alone. A trusted, sober person can become an anchor, reminding you that the safe place you're used to inhabiting is still there, and you will return to it in time.

As my ayahuasca terror peaked, I found my feet and rushed to the nearest purge bucket. I sent what seemed to be a telepathic distress call, and the Colombian ayahuasquero who spoke little English appeared by my side. He exuded light, and his presence was like a rock. I gripped his shoulder, looked into his eyes, and said, "I don't know . . . what's happening."

He motioned toward the bucket. I looked inside, and I saw life's decay churning, pulling my head like a magnet. I resisted.

He shook his head, leaned in, and whispered, "Surrender."

I faced the bucket. I let the magnet pull me. A force in my stomach collected physical and nonphysical matter accumulated in my body and pushed it up my esophagus. My mouth opened, and I heaved from the bottom of my organs, gagging, spitting, and feeling my soul pulled into a darkness I hadn't prepared to see.

He stood with me, making sure I remained on my feet until my stomach relaxed. He led me to my blanket to lie down. The world was still not the world, but now, I knew I was going to make it back.

Without that compassionate ayahuasquero's powerful act of service, I may never have moved through the terror that strangled my heart. He helped me reconnect to light, and as the medicine began to fade, he handed me a maraca, and I shook it to the rhythm of the sudden burst of music the facilitators conducted. I had found a strength and endurance within that I had not known existed; until then, it hadn't been necessary to access.

I'm still integrating that trip, still working through the terror. Since then, other psychedelics have returned me to that dreadful place, proving how foolish I was to believe bad trips are a myth. They are real and, especially at high doses, always possible.

The revival doesn't talk about bad trips enough. When the subject comes up, a therapist usually revises the story, calling them "challenging experiences which bring the possibility of transformation." Sometimes, that's true. Other times, the trip is just *bad*.

We need to be upfront about bad trips to help people safeguard and either evade them or empower themselves to navigate them. Bad trips can be traumatizing, catalyzing the opposite of healing. If you find yourself in one, do everything you can to remind yourself that you will be okay, and focus on your breath, which can center you even in the deepest circles of the Inferno.

Hallucinogen Persisting Perception Disorder

Bad trips are the most notorious negative psychedelic effects, but they are not the only ones. One psychedelic-induced condition is listed in the *DSM-5*. It's called *hallucinogen persisting perception disorder*, or HPPD, and like bad trips, it is not a myth.

The *DSM* defines HPPD as "the reexperiencing of one or more of the perceptual symptoms that were experienced while intoxicated with the hallucinogen." These symptoms can include "geometric hallucinations, false perceptions of movement in the peripheral visual fields, flashes of color, intensified colors, trails of images of moving objects, positive afterimages, halos around objects, macropsia and micropsia."[1] The symptoms cause distress and/or impairment, aren't attributable to another diagnosed condition, and persist long after the individual is sober.

HPPD commonly corresponds to LSD, but it can arise from other psychedelic and non-psychedelic drugs like cannabis and alcohol. Development is not conditional on heavy use, and the manual references cases following minimal psychedelic exposure. The *DSM* estimates HPPD affects just over 4% of psychedelic users. Symptoms can diminish within weeks, or they can continue for years.[2]

In an episode of the VICE series "My Life Online," Andrew Callaghan, an independent journalist who traveled around the US in an RV interviewing people on the fringes of society, spoke about his HPPD. Callaghan said the more he sits still, "the more I start to feel like I'm living in a simulation, like I'm trapped behind my eyes."[3]

"I have permanent visual damage," he said. "I see visual snow and, like, *tracers*, like, even right now, like, everywhere I look."[4] He took mushrooms regularly when he was thirteen, prompting a pattern of dissociation. Cross-country travel became a way of healing the damage his excessive psilocybin use had caused.

Introduced in a 1954 study about LSD's therapeutic value, HPPD became more widely known in 1969, when psychologist M. J. Horowitz introduced the term "flashbacks" to the medical world. Horowitz described three categories of LSD flashbacks: "*perceptual distortions* (e.g., seeing haloes around objects); *heightened imagery* (e.g., visual experiences as much more vivid and dominant in one's thoughts); and *recurrent unbidden images* (e.g., subjects see objects that are not there.)"[5] Due to the blockage of psychedelic research and the rarity of HPPD, little is known about the condition and how to treat it, although one 2017 study suggested SSRIs and benzodiazepines could alleviate symptoms.[6]

As psychedelic research continues, we will hopefully gain a better understanding of HPPD's causes, risk factors, and treatment methods. For now, we can't do much more than acknowledge its existence and recognize it as an improbable-but-possible psychedelic side effect.

Psychotic Breaks

The healing process ayahuasca potentiates is foreign to Western concepts. In my encounter with it, I saw that as balanced as I believed I was, I'm as vulnerable to destabilization as anyone when powerful non-ordinary states take hold. For some time in the dark space ayahuasca opened, it seemed clear that I would never return to baseline consciousness.

Stories of ayahuasca-induced destabilization are fairly common. The destabilization is usually temporary, but psychotic breaks can occur, especially if facilitators offer the brew alongside other powerful plant medicines. Someone who openly shares his is Ryan Beauregard, a foundational leader of the Zendo Project. Beauregard's experience was fundamental in directing him toward his vocation to help others through challenging trips, but it was no easy road.

After a multi-day ayahuasca retreat in Peru, where he received both ayahuasca and a powerful deliriant called Chiric Sanango, Beauregard returned to the States and found that everything he'd previously believed to be true had collapsed. Reality had no center. His world appeared like a "combination of *The Matrix*, *Groundhog Day*, and *The Truman Show*." Paranoia struck deep, and no one could help him.

Fortunately, his friends and family stayed by his side, and Beauregard eventually returned to reality. His testimony is emblematic of a common crisis people face after taking large doses of psychedelics and plant medicines, especially when integration support is lacking. They are left marooned in a foreign world, forced to navigate unfamiliarity in a culture that provides no adequate maps.

This is a real potential of most psychedelics at high doses, and it must be respected for people to prepare themselves. Practitioners must educate themselves on this possibility and equip themselves to support clients. To administer large doses of psychedelics while underestimating their destabilizing potential is to provide unethical service. If a facilitator isn't prepared to remain calm and compassionate while the client witnesses the collapse of all they had believed to be self-evident, they shouldn't offer psychedelic therapy. Unfortunately, such humility is never guaranteed, and it's far too common to hear stories of tragic consequences, especially in the unregulated underground.

Death and Violence in the Amazon

On April 19, 2018, as psychedelic enthusiasts of the Western world celebrated Bicycle Day through whatever personal rituals they had created, a
violent scene unfolded in the Peruvian Amazon. In the Shipibo-Conibo village of Victoria Gracia, a Canadian man named Sebastian Woodroffe sped
through town on a red motorbike, stopped at a gray wooden house, and
repeatedly yelled the name "Julian." When Julian Arévalo appeared at the
window, Woodroffe pulled out a gun and fired. He missed, and Arévalo ran.
His grandmother, a beloved eighty-one-year-old medicine woman named
Olivia, heard the commotion from her home next door and went outside to
investigate. The villagers chased after Woodroffe, and when he turned toward
his motorbike to flee, he found Olivia blocking the way. He shot her twice
in the chest, killing her.

Woodroffe sped away from the irate villagers, but his escape was thwarted
by a dip in the road. He lost control of the motorbike, and the villagers
surrounded him.[7] They ruthlessly beat him, and when Woodroffe had been
reduced to a moaning, bloody mess, a man wrapped his neck in a seatbelt.
Over a dozen onlookers watched as he dragged Woodroffe into the grass and
strangled him to death.[8]

When a grainy video of the villagers' vengeance on Woodroffe surfaced a
few days later, the story spread through the West. What had caused such a horrific incident? Although much remained a mystery, important pieces coalesced.

Woodroffe had been traveling back and forth from his home on Vancouver
Island to the Peruvian Amazon for three-and-a-half years. He had a nine-year-
old son, but his relationship with the boy's mother hadn't lasted. As he searched
for spiritual meaning in a life of frequent career changes, Woodroffe became
fascinated with Indigenous plant medicine traditions. In 2013, he decided to
become an addiction counselor. He felt called to learn about ayahuasca, which
he saw as superior to any Western medicine. He flew to the ayahuasca hub of
Iquitos, the gateway city to the Peruvian Amazon, to study under Guillermo
Arévalo, a Shipibo medicine man.

As Woodroffe continued traveling to Iquitos and sitting in ayahuasca
ceremonies, a friend on Vancouver Island noticed he appeared distant and
lost. By all appearances, the ayahuasca healing he'd sought had destabilized

him. But Woodroffe remained committed to becoming a healer, and on a trip in 2017, he traveled deeper into the Amazon to the village of Victoria Gracia in hope of doing ayahuasca with Guillermo's cousin, Olivia Arévalo, a respected healer. When Woodroffe arrived in the village, he said he needed Olivia's help because he was "sick" and "crazy."[9] Noting his frantic state, Olivia felt reluctant, but upon learning Guillermo had sent him, she agreed.[10]

Little is known about what happened during Woodroffe's ensuing visits to Victoria Gracia. It's unknown how much ayahuasca Olivia served him. It is known, however, that Woodroffe's primary motivation became connecting with Julian Arévalo, Olivia's son. Woodroffe and Julian may have established a business relationship, planning to open an ayahuasca retreat center together. At some point, the relationship turned for the worse, and in early April 2018, Woodroffe convinced an officer at a police station in the nearby city of Pucallpa to sell him a gun at a high price, claiming he needed protection from animals in the jungle. No one saw the gun on April 18 when Woodroffe showed up in Victoria Gracia looking for Julian, claiming he owed him $4,000. The next day, Woodroffe used the gun to shoot Olivia twice during his vain attempt to escape.

It's impossible to say how prominent a role ayahuasca played in Woodroffe's descent from idealistic seeker to unstable killer. The true nature of the conflict between him and the Arévalo family remains a mystery. But darkness existed in the Arévalo family—nine months later, the BBC published an anonymous woman's report that Guillermo had sexually abused her during an ayahuasca ceremony. When she needed help, Guillermo put his hands down her pants, up her shirt, and around her breasts. A group called Ayahuasca Community Awareness Canada signed and circulated a letter about Guillermo's actions, citing similar complaints of abuse. As the anonymous woman expected, he denied the claims. When she continued seeking ayahuasca healing elsewhere, she underwent even more trauma when she was raped several times "by a [unnamed] healer who is a member of Arévalo's extended family."[11]

These stories are not isolated incidents in an expanse of otherwise unsullied healing. In 2012, an American named Kyle Nolan died during an ayahuasca ceremony, and the shaman subsequently buried him.[12] Three years later, during a retreat in Iquitos, a British man began brandishing a knife and screaming, prompting a Canadian man to grab the knife and stab him to death. Both men were on ayahuasca.[13]

Reports of sexual abuse are more common than murders and deaths, especially as plastic shamans latch onto financial opportunities of the ayahuasca boom. Speaking to *Men's Journal*, Pedro Tangoa López, a Shipibo medicine man with over thirty-four years of experience, said these plastic shamans "often mix the ayahuasca with other, more volatile plants, like toé and floripondio, to create a more explosive trip." He added that "when something goes wrong, they don't know how to help the patient," whereas a "good shaman is capable of snapping a patient out of a dangerous trance in an instant."[14] Grounded as he is in traditional medicine, López rejects the term shaman for himself, instead using maestro.

"It's really sad to see news in the radio, newspaper or other media . . . about huge scams being created by Shipibo masters," López wrote on the dangers of ayahuasca tourism. "There are deaths due to ayahuasca consumption, simply because some of the current young practitioners do not have the training."[15]

Like abusive leaders of major religions, these ill-intentioned people cast a shadow over ayahuasca ceremonies, including those led by the legitimate healers whose primary concerns are protecting their guests. Speaking on behalf of these healers, López wrote, "Our interior is filled with happiness and joy. And that's a really big fortune. It's really valuable. The sacred plants, like ayahuasca, help us strengthen this value. The real masters of ayahuasca are the ones that start to feel this kind of energy inside and then what they do is help, help, help with it. That's our mission, that's our job, that's our responsibility."[16]

As the contrast between Woodroffe's story and López's perspective demonstrates, there is light and shadow in ayahuasca tourism. These dynamics have evolved because cities and villages of the Amazon have been seeing more White people visiting them than ever before, bringing their desires for non-Western healing and their wallets full of money. As the *Men's Journal* article concludes, Nelly Vázquez, Olivia's granddaughter, reminisced about the "peaceful life" her community lived before Woodroffe's arrival. For Vázquez, that peace has left, and she feels haunted by the memory of "the gringo."[17]

The Dark Side of Suggestibility

Psychedelic users can be quite gullible. It's tough to say whether psychedelics make people gullible or gullible people are more drawn to psychedelics. There's at least some truth to the former because psychedelics increase suggestibility. The mind becomes more vulnerable to input, and things that normally seem bonkers can make sense.

Kaelen, who spent years researching the intersection between LSD-induced suggestibility and music, told me, "Suggestibility is primarily defined as the degree to which you follow a suggestion to feel something or behave in a certain way. That suggestion can be explicit, like, 'Stand up, raise your hands,' or it can be more implicit, like with music. Music is not telling you, 'Feel sadness.' It's conveying a process of sadness."

Psychedelic-induced suggestibility can play an important role in healing. Someone locked in a reductionistic worldview may apprehend new perceptions more easily. But the other side of suggestibility, exploited by programs like Project MK-Ultra, is that the mind becomes vulnerable to harmful inputs, and when a compelling narrative takes hold, fact-checking does little to convince the mind of its delusional occupations.

Psychedelic QAnon

QAnon began as a far-right political offshoot and soon came to resemble a cult. Its adherents worshipped Donald Trump as a Christ-like savior and believed liberals were "Satanists" colluding to destroy the American way—by spreading communism and drinking the blood of babies, to be specific. It came as a big surprise when, a few years after QAnon appeared, people deeply involved in spaces typically considered left-wing started spouting QAnon ideas. These spaces were of the "New Age" ilk, and the mentality became known as "conspirituality." One of those spaces was the ayahuasca underground.

As if out of nowhere, many frequent ayahuasca drinkers were claiming Trump had come to save the world and rid international politics of its shadowy overlords. They spoke of a "Great Awakening" approaching, and they deconstructed Trump's tweets to theorize the event's date, believing it would facilitate transcendence for those who saw and fought for "the truth"—namely, themselves. It never came. Nevertheless, no fact could persuade QAnoners against the view, for they dismissed contrarian claims as "fake news" created to enslave them in a mass-media conspiracy. Random QAnon influencers' blogs were cited as facts, and it culminated—at least up to this point in history—in the storming of the US Capitol on January 6, 2021.*

The mascot of the Capitol Storm became known as the "QAnon Shaman," a fellow named Jake Angeli who wore fur and black horns. Angeli, a promoter of far-out, New-Age viewpoints, was a regular psychedelic and plant medicine user, having credited them with his developmental path of becoming a "shaman."[18] Psychedelics did not help him see the lack of foundation to his belief in the vast QAnon conspiracy. He only recognized his delusion when Trump, whom Angeli had perceived as a prophet, did not grant him a Federal pardon, and Angeli was sentenced to forty-one months in prison. Only then did Angeli disavow his QAnon beliefs.

One might think this would convince other QAnon followers of the invalidity of their beliefs. Instead, they decided Angeli was a double agent sent by the political left to try and make them look bad. It didn't matter to them that Angeli insisted this was not true.

Speaking on the subject, Daniel McQueen told me, "I know of multiple ayahuasca communities that have fallen apart because of QAnon. From what I can tell, it's a symptom of delusion. I think psychedelic medicines might make us more susceptible to manipulation and being influenced by our emotions. And I think we also, as a community, are a little questioning of authority. But that can fall into paranoia, delusion, and conspiracy. I'm totally into conspiracy, but I try to stay scientific about it."

Such disregard for facts has roots in postmodern thought. The ramifications of postmodernism linger today, a prominent one of which is the spread of moral relativism, which abolished absolute standards of *right* and *wrong*. While relativism opened the door to cultural humility, making space for diverse cultural and religious perspectives, it eroded collective agreement on moral values and consensus reality.

---

* QAnon adherents were not the only people who stormed the US Capitol. They joined forces with other far-right organizations like the Proud Boys and the Three Percenters.

Our social-media-infused landscape flourishes in echo chambers, where facts that don't align with one's beliefs can be ignored, regardless of whether they're delusional or informed. Conspiracy theories proliferate unchecked as digital communities collectively consolidate their brand of apophenia as "reality." This pattern will likely get worse, for social media megaliths have realized that echo chambers provide economic and political benefit through targeted advertisements for products and viewpoints promoting what individuals already believe.

Many enthusiasts maintain that psychedelics inherently make people more open-minded, compassionate, and morally conscious. To maintain such a view, these enthusiasts must ignore many contradictory examples.

In a 2021 article about "Right-Wing Psychedelia," researchers Brian Pace and Neşe Devenot argued "that any experience which challenges a person's fundamental worldview—including a psychedelic experience—can precipitate shifts in any direction of political belief." Rather than directing people toward a common worldview, psychedelics act as "non-specific amplifiers of the political set and setting."[19]

Pace and Devenot continued, "We believe that the common narratives regarding the effects of psychedelics on political orientation present persistent blind spots within the psychedelic literature . . . Assertions that psychedelics induce a shift in political beliefs will have to address the many historical and contemporary cases of psychedelic users who remained authoritarian in their views after taking a wide variety of psychedelics or became radicalized after extensive experience with them."[20]

Psychedelics do not unilaterally make people "better" and more "aware." Like meditation, they can make you more aware, or they can make you embed your fears, fantasies, and illusions as reality, sealing a perimeter separating your echo chamber from the truth. As described by American Buddhist teacher Jack Kornfield, "Because concentration is a neutral quality, it can be used for both skillful or unskillful, even nefarious purposes. A skilled thief or burglar needs concentration, as does a card shark, a sniper and a terrorist. The power of the concentrated mind can be directed toward the creation of suffering or well-being."[21]

We need to be realistic about the potential of psychedelics to amplify all capacities of the human mind, not solely those deemed virtuous. A new absolutism will further alienate people who don't subscribe to its tenets, but there must be a middle ground, where the best parts of relativity and objectivity can coexist and inform one another. With such an intention, perhaps psychedelics can be tremendously helpful, but if they are used to amplify delusional avoidance of reality, no amount of bypassing can erase the harm they will continue to cause.

Mistaking Visions for Reality

The destabilization that can happen with psychedelics and plant medicines centers on people mistaking their visions for objective reality. People commonly forget that between a vision and its meaning exists *apperception*, the process by which one makes sense of something by assimilating it into an established network of ideas. Psychedelic meaning-making follows a pattern:

Content of Vision → Apperception → Meaning of Vision

In the psychedelic state, the arrows can dissolve, making the separate processes appear one and the same. Unaware of interpretation taking place, people mistake their perception of the vision and their simultaneous interpretation as insight into a "nature of a reality" that extends beyond their ego. Perhaps insight into objective reality is possible, but it's not a guarantee, and there can be some complex trickery at play in a psychedelic state.

At a Colorado music festival I attended in 2019, my partner at the time was volunteering at the medical tent to offer psychological support to people having difficult trips. As the DJ Tipper played his late-night set, I felt a dark shift in the festival's vibes. Sketchiness was afoot. Amid the shift, my partner spent hours working with a guy who'd taken a lot of LSD and thought the apocalypse was happening. He was convinced the only way to stop it was for everyone at the festival to kill themselves—but first, he had to chop off his wang. He repeatedly tried to get naked, and EMTs restrained him as he lunged for scissors.

Before anyone blames LSD, word spread about weird substances floating around the festival sold as LSD. Who knows what this dude took? Even if it was LSD, we can't pin the extent of his delusion on the drug. It may have been a case of an imbalanced individual taking way too much of a powerful substance in a chaotic setting. It may have been related to childhood trauma or any number of factors specific to his background. But no matter what anyone said, this guy was completely convinced his apocalyptic visions expressed absolute truth.

Anecdotal evidence abounds concerning people taking psychedelics repeatedly and embedding their delusions into their reality constructs. Because the psychedelic state leads one to feel what one sees is objectively true, one gradually regards the meaning attributed to their visions as self-evident. Quite often, these "truths" cement previously held beliefs. To the cynical skeptic, a vision of a fiery inferno means, "The world is hopeless!" To the spiritual idealist, it means, "I'm entering the fires of transformation!" To the wide-eyed friend in the corner, it means, "We have to watch *Indiana Jones and the Temple of Doom* right now."* Each interpretation feels equally valid to each person.

Psychedelics probably won't "show you everything" or "reveal the absolute truth." These interpretations are mental constructs applied to an experience and disguised as the experience's inherent qualities. Unfortunately, deluded visions can take hold with Herculean fervor, for they are often symbolic expressions of shadowed fears grown powerful through whatever unconscious resistance has long kept them encaged. Fear is exceptional at convincing us it represents reality, and when it's amplified by a psychedelic, it can become unstoppable.

The Shadow of Ketamine

Bret Michaels once sang, "Every rose has its thorn . . ." In the same way every cowboy sings a sad, sad song, so ketamine has a tragic tale to tell. Amid the myriad ways it helps people heal, uneducated and unethical ketamine use also harms people.

---

* And I highly recommend you do. Rarely has a mainstream Hollywood film been so totally horrific. It was so disturbing that the MPAA created the rating of "PG-13" to prevent children from being traumatized by PG movies like the second *Indiana Jones*, a film for whose creation director Steven Spielberg later apologized to the world.

Ketamine's dark side is arguably darker than any of the classic psyche-delics. More people get addicted to it, and the physical consequences of repeated use are more severe. One of the nastier side effects has been called Ketamine cystitis, or Ketamine Bladder Syndrome. When ketamine enters the bladder, it can damage the cells lining the inner wall. Symptoms can include frequent and urgent urination, pain, and the brutal sense of having to pee but being unable. It can get nastier with blood in the urine, and the bladder can lose its capacity to expand. At the condition's nastiest, the blad-der becomes permanently damaged, and if it's bad enough, the bladder must be surgically removed.

The worst cases of ketamine cystitis appear to be related to heavy ket-amine abuse, like snorting copious amounts every day for years. But everyone is affected differently, and some online reports cite symptoms after minimal use. According to DanceSafe's article on the topic, "The largest-to-date sur-vey of recent ketamine users, for example, found that 26.6% had experienced at least one of the above symptoms, and the majority of these people (70%) said they only used ketamine 1–4 days per month."[22] Since the phenomenon was only discovered in 2007, the best available medical advice for those who notice symptoms is to stop taking ketamine.

Ketamine and Police Brutality

Another dark layer of ketamine involves its use by first responders who don't understand it. Ketamine is powerful enough to knock out a rhino, so it can be helpful to sedate an agitated individual who poses a threat to others. Police officers have thus used ketamine to apprehend suspects in states of "excited delirium," a term law enforcement and first responders use for what they describe as a state of superhuman strength and aggression catalyzed by a stimulant like methamphetamine or cocaine.

The thing is, excited delirium has been used to justify hundreds of deaths at the hands of law enforcement personnel, a large percentage of whom were Black men. This issue came to light in 2019 when officers in Aurora, Colorado accosted twenty-three-year-old Elijah McClain, an unarmed Black man, on his walk home from a store. The officers physically restrained McClain, and when paramedics arrived on the scene, they injected him with a seismic dose of 500 milligrams of ketamine, claiming McClain was in a state of excited delirium.

Their justification was bogus. McClain had no stimulants in his system. Secondly, he was 5'6, 140 pounds, and there were several officers on the scene—did he really pose a physical threat? Finally, a video was released of the incident, which showed three officers aggressively wrestling McClain to the ground and holding him submissive as he cried out, "Why are you attacking me?" McClain pleaded, "I don't even kill flies."

Minutes after the EMTs jacked him up with 500 milligrams of ketamine, McClain had no pulse. The paramedics resuscitated him and brought him to the hospital, but the damage had been done. Three days later, he was declared braindead, and three days after that, Elijah McClain died.

The coroner initially reported the death could not be attributed to anything during the arrest. Once the video surfaced, this report struck many people as total bullshit. The hold with which the officers restrained McClain put pressure on his carotid arteries, cutting off blood flow to his brain. When such a hold is combined with a massive dose of ketamine, there's a damn good chance of an adverse reaction.

It took three years for a cause of death to be released. In September 2022, McClain's death was attributed to "complications of ketamine administration following forcible restraint." Stephen Cina, the author of the amended autopsy report, wrote, "Simply put, this dosage of ketamine was too much for this individual and it resulted in an overdose, even though his blood ketamine level was consistent with a 'therapeutic' blood concentration. I believe that Mr. McClain would most likely be alive but for the administration of ketamine."

The officers justified their ketamine administration on the pretense of excited delirium. In late 2020, the Board of the American Psychological Association (APA) declared that the condition was an invalid diagnosis. The APA maintained that this term should no longer be allowed to justify administration of ketamine, citing it as "too non-specific." A study published by doctors at Harvard, the University of Michigan, Massachusetts General Hospital, and a team of civil rights lawyers described excited delirium as a "scientifically meaningless" term which has "come to be used as a catch-all for deaths occurring in the context of law enforcement restraint, often coinciding with substance use or mental illness, and disproportionately used to explain the deaths of young Black men in police encounters."[23]

This discussion is not meant to rebuke all first responders' uses of ketamine. It is safe in specific dose ranges and can be incredibly helpful to treat someone in severe pain. This discussion concerns specific instances of first responders tranquilizing people with ketamine based on a made-up condition. Such usage is about as far from therapeutic uses of ketamine as taking Advil is from injecting morphine into your eyeball. The dose given to McClain was about five times more than what he would have received at a ketamine therapy clinic, where he'd be greeted with a comfortable sofa instead of an artery-constricting chokehold.

The World Health Organization included ketamine on its list of essential medicines because of its numerous positive applications. Ketamine administration during the unjustified arrest and ensuing death of a young Black man does not qualify. I hope the unfolding rescinding of the fabricated condition called "excited delirium" will promote reform in whichever training systems justify wrongful use of a powerful psychedelic. This change is essential, and for it to happen, the death of Elijah McClain was far too great a price to pay.

Where Is It Heading?

I sometimes wonder what the moment felt like in the 1960s when the hippies first realized their dream was dying. I imagine that in 1968, after the Summer of Love, the realization trickled in slowly: more arrests, more violence, more Nixon and J. Edgar Hoover. Surely the shifting vibes prompted abundant denial.

"Nah, man, that's just the *fear* talking," said the aimless drifter hanging around Haight-Ashbury. "It's all good! Acid! Freedom!"

Eventually, the scale tipped, and the people realizing the dream was dying outnumbered those clinging on. Altamont and Family Manson didn't "end the '60s" out of nowhere. They confirmed what the culture had all but realized: reality had defeated the utopian dream.

One of the biggest fears among the older generation of second-wave researchers is that history will repeat itself. The biggest mistakes of the '60s counterculture, they say, was over-exuberance. Unfortunately, people have been doing that again, including psychedelic researchers. Rosalind Watts, a forefront researcher from Imperial College London, came to regret her overenthusiasm in her 2017 TEDx talk on psilocybin's potential at Oxford. "I can't help but feel as if I unknowingly contributed to a simplistic and potentially dangerous narrative around psychedelics; a narrative I'm trying to correct," she wrote.[24]

Watts defined that new narrative as "a tidal wave of hype, over promising, magical thinking, marketing, sugar-coating, simplistic sound bytes, hopeful shareholders, gold rushing, territory-claiming," which has also brought a "sidelining of critical voices, like those of the victims of sexual assault in psychedelic contexts turned away by countless respected professionals in the field lest they tarnish the shine." Watts asserted that the revival narrative feels "like a PR campaign for a celebrity that was wrongfully imprisoned and now needs to be shown to be utterly beyond reproach, sunshine personified."[25]

Psychedelics have been subjected to Disneyfication, a fantabulous term referring to a sanitization of a place or thing in order for it to appear simple, safe, and of course, *marketable*. Public perception has shifted, but to what end? In 2023, numerous psychedelic businesses have gone bankrupt, including forefront training centers like the Synthesis Institute, which promised to lead training of psilocybin facilitators.[26] Has the second wave crested? If so, is it destined for a crash or a smooth roll to shore?

I don't know. What I do know is I never anticipated the psychedelic world would stage so much drama. I suppose people love conflict at some level, and large-scale collaboration across the movement is more fantasy than possibility. It was a real bummer when I caught wind of this conflict, for it prompted the erosion of my conviction that the psychedelic revival was an undeniably *good thing*. But perhaps excessive focus on the drama expresses an addiction to reinforcing our sense of self-importance.

I hope the Western world reconciles with its shadow. Perhaps its linear, scientific models are too limited to lay the groundwork for psychedelic healing. Maybe the dream of the revival, like that of the 1960s, cannot escape its inevitable termination.

Or perhaps Doblin is on to something by focusing on the good in every-thing, including the for-profit sectors many see as bad. I don't want to bypass legitimate concerns, but obsessing over them distances my perception of the revival from the profundity that garnered such enthusiasm when I first took mushrooms in that Australian sculpture park, long ago. Doblin has main-tained his steadfast belief in the healing power of psychedelics through nearly four decades of rigorous work. If nothing else, he's living testimony that hope can endure, and perhaps a microdose of naïveté can be a helpful ally as one navigates a labyrinthine world.

Epilogue

Speculative Synthesis of the Philosopher's Stone

"When I sitting heard the astronomer where he lectured
with much applause in the lecture-room,
How soon unaccountable I became tired and sick,
Till rising and gliding out I wander'd off by myself,
In the mystical moist night-air, and from time to time,
Look'd up in perfect silence at the stars."

—Walt Whitman, "When I Heard the Learn'd Astronomer"

It's common for the end of a psychedelic journey to bring disappointment. The vast illumination of its magical spell fades, and no matter how much the journeyer felt certain they had connected to the essence of reality, the ego's familiar stories return. In such disappointment, the journeyer is left wondering, "What now?"

These pages have constituted a semantic journey through scientific, recreational, spiritual, ancestral, and shadow realms of a variety of topics related to psychedelics and plant medicines. And here we are, right where we began, breathing and perceiving the present moment. I recall Lao Tzu's words that began the book: *The further one goes, the less one knows.*

I suppose I could take a swing at prophecy, visualizing how this might play out. Inevitably I would miss plenty of pitches and probably strike out.

In these pages, I've used models and theories to help make sense of psychedelic states and their content. As far out as some of these models go, they are as limited as the human mind at grasping the totality of existence.

Science builds upon frameworks and explanations. The more widely applicable the framework, the more important it becomes. To apply an existing framework to non-ordinary experiences is to eliminate space for discovery. It is to double down on tightly held models of the psyche and the Universe, no matter how significantly these states threaten the models' premises. It is to limit possibilities in fear of what those possibilities suggest.

Human beings have a primordial desire to make sense out of reality. Doing so affords us the ability to find—or perhaps fabricate—stability and security in a destabilizing world. This desire is at the core of the ongoing tension in academic science around new generations of researchers calling into question not only the results but the very premises upon which a previous generation's results depended. Even Einstein resisted the onset of quantum mechanics, scoffing at the implications of Heisenberg's Uncertainty Principle with the assertion, "God does not play dice with the Universe."[1]

The mysteries of the universe are not grasped through rational discourse. It is more fruitful to contemplate mystery, for the irrational directions these contemplations travel can unlock layers of truth rooted deeper than anything the rational mind can comprehend. I think again of Isaac Newton, who considered his esoteric studies of the occult to be at least as important as his mathematical inquiries into the physical world.

From the Indigenous people of North America to the hippies of the 1960s, psychedelics and plant medicines have inspired resistance against structures, especially when those structures restrict thought, behavior, and identity. These substances and plants break down structures not out of an anarchistic, nihilistic drive toward chaos but to resuscitate inherent freedoms limited by oppressive structures. To custodians of oppressive structures, this freedom is threatening, for the imposition of structure yields the power to control.

If these molecules have a fundamental purpose, it may be to dismantle the mechanisms of ideological dominance. This can manifest at a personal level, such as a psychedelic user becoming more aware of how their default mode network restricts expression through repressive imperatives, and it can manifest at a cultural level, as demonstrated through the hippies of the 1960s who rebelled against indoctrination into a flawed and dehumanizing system. Perhaps the revival is a fresh playing out of this psychedelic agenda: unwilling to be repressed and controlled, psychedelics have tricked their way back into the forefront of medicine and culture after half a century of imprisonment.

As valid as some of these speculations may be, they will never encapsulate the whole. The mystery at the heart of these inquiries will continue burning explanations in their eternal fires, and those who grip explanations too tightly will continue regarding these fires as threats to their illusory concepts of reality.

As complicated as psychedelics and their contexts get, the core of healing may be quite simple. Through the tangled traumas, sunken dreams, violent fantasies, and desperate yearnings psychedelics evoke, a common thread in the many stories of transformation is their capacity to restore a sense of profound peace amid life's chaos. Healing need not involve meditating like a hermit or taking a pilgrimage to the other side of the world in hope to recover some lost fragment of the soul. Healing can be as simple as reawakening to a sense of bounty in the here and now, intuited through a fire of gratitude burning brightly in the chest.

Perhaps healing is as simple as getting out of our own way and seeing the world through eyes of wonder again. It might be complicated to get there, or it might be simpler than you imagine.

My most beneficial psychedelic experiences cut through life's complexity, revealing how much chaos I create by fueling desires for some outcome I've deluded myself into mistaking as a final arrival. There's no getting *there*; there's only getting *here*, where everything is.

These concluding contemplations on simplicity have arisen through a personal need. I got so twisted up and tangled in pulling this book together that I found myself further from my heart than any previous point in my life. Stress consumed me. I thought a psychedelic might heal me, and perhaps it could have helped, but deep down, I knew I'd already received the answers I needed. I'd simply been too afraid to hang up the phone, for the answers required shifts I didn't want to make. Still, my heart provided the same clarity again and again in the words the great Ram Dass evoked in the title of his most famous book: *Be here now.*

Be here now . . . and follow what brings you energy instead of that which drains it. A collective burden instructs us to do things we don't want to do. Yes, we must do unpleasant things at times, and virtue can be found in the self-sacrifice of doing essential tasks so others don't have to. But a lifestyle of self-sacrifice paves the road to self-annihilation, of saying "No" to life's possibilities because that's what we were taught is noble. It's time to drop this burden.

In his famous conversation with Bill Moyers, Joseph Campbell said, "Follow your bliss and don't be afraid, and doors will open where you didn't know they were going to be."[2] The bliss to which he referred is more than fleeting pleasure. Bliss is the energy of life, and it fills one's cup with an endless stream that was always here and shall remain. When we fill our cups, we serve the world, offering our gifts and feeling rejuvenated in the giving.

As I approached my final deadline, I found myself drawn by a peculiar presentiment toward an essay I hadn't read in years called "Albert Hofmann and the Quest for the Alchemical Philosopher's Stone," written by Ralph Metzner and published in the invaluable *Hofmann's Elixir: LSD and the New Eleusis*. I reread Metzner's words over several weeks, receiving them one page at a time to properly digest their beauty and profundity. Each sentence filled my cup a little more, and I found it to be the most inspiring and evocative piece of psychedelic-inspired writing I'd chanced upon reading.

Throughout the essay, Metzner charted the history of alchemy, drawing parallels between alchemy and the wisdom traditions commonly called shamanism. These traditions share a common aim of *spiritual transformation*. Metzner argued alchemy broke off from shamanism, thereby rendering it the Western world's deepest connection to the elemental roots of healing perceived in numerous plant medicine traditions.

Like shamanism, practitioners of alchemy were met with social and political resistance and oppression. The rituals and practices of alchemists came to be regarded as the work of the devil, forcing them to carry on their ancient lineage in secret. They wrote in complex codes and symbols to protect themselves and to ensure their discoveries did not end up in the hands of those who would use such transformative powers for dark purposes.

The aim of alchemy was the discovery of the *lapis philosophorum*, the philosopher's stone. Contrary to popular belief, the stone was not merely a material object synthesized from raw metal, the boons of which would allow one to live forever. Metzner dug through alchemy's history to establish that the philosopher's stone resides *within*. Only through this realization can one contact its powers.

The stone's central power is to dissolve the density of the inner world and create a new solution infused with the spiritual substance at the foundation of matter. This spirit can transform anything it touches, and one who brings it forth from within will be granted eternal life. Eternal life is not life everlasting. Eternal life is the fulfillment of self-realization in eternal connection to life's essence in the present moment.

To Metzner, psychedelics—when used with the right intention, set, and setting—catalyze a similar process. They dissolve calcified ego structures and broaden awareness of the Spirit for reconstitution into a more highly developed embodiment of authentic being. As alchemy was concerned with the intersection of physical and spiritual matter, psychedelics come in physical form to catalyze a spiritual process of renewal.

Hofmann once said, "Any scientist who is not a mystic, is no scientist."[3] Nevertheless, the Western scientific establishment has long been skeptical of the Spirit as a living, tangible reality. The Johns Hopkins research helped bridge the Spirit back into scientific awareness, but backlash resulted, prompting Johns Hopkins' own Matthew Johnson to argue that terms like "mystical" and "consciousness" should be reevaluated in scientific literature. Maybe he's right. Maybe we should let scientists do their scientist thing. But if we do, it is essential to release our cultural attachment to inherited dogmas prizing science as the ultimate guide to reality and its constituent parts. Science is concerned with the physical, and alchemists and shamans have known for eons that the physical world is but one plane of reality. The mental, emotional, and spiritual planes are equally real, even if microscopes and telescopes fail to observe them.

I don't know how the psychedelic revival will play out, but I hope it refrains from succumbing to the inherent limitations of science. My wish is for psychedelics to reconnect the Western world with the immediacy of the

Spirit by way of any form of symbolic language and imagery through which it presents itself. My hope is that in this reconnection, the Western world revives the elements of the soul that its architects cut off through persecution of ancestral practices built around maintaining connection with the Spirit as it lives and breathes in all molecules constituting the planet and the ever-expanding universe. These hopes may point toward a new paradigm of healing, because this paradigm transcends and includes the many essential medicinal developments that have come before. This new paradigm rediscovers the philosopher's stone, the key to redeeming the widespread desolation and fragmentation so many of us feel every day.

Transformation is not waiting in the wings for some molecule to get approved by the FDA. Transformation is waiting for us right here, calling for us to change how we see ourselves, the world, and the unseen realities permeating all things and connecting us all far more than Descartes and others led us to believe. Regardless of the revival's fate, I hope psychedelics and plant medicines continue to wash our windshields so we may clearly see routes both ancient and new, evoking the shadowed Spirit and saying *sayonara* to the myriad ways scientific materialism keeps it locked away.

"Whereof we cannot speak, thereof we must remain silent," wrote Wittgenstein. May the release of a reductionistic, linear worldview revive a depth of Truth no words can possibly define.

Acknowledgments

Writing a book is very much an isolated endeavor, but far less so than I had believed. Without the help of the people I hope to honor here, this book would exist as a formless assemblage of ideas overwritten in the many journals stored in my closet.

First, I sincerely thank all the people who gave their time to be interviewed. Regardless of whether your words appear in the final draft, you informed the content and helped me immeasurably in reaching this point of completion. I'm beyond grateful for your generosity.

Jennifer Brown: thank you for trusting me to write this book and giving me the space to explore this material authentically. Anastasia Pellouchoud: thank you for helping me carve a disorganized mass into a coherent whole, and thank you for holding this complex process with care every step of the way. Tami Simon: thank you for supporting me since the random day I met you and for being an unparalleled example of an authentic visionary guided by a caring heart. Thank you also to Joe Sweeney, Ivory Fields, Emily Stewart, Chloe Prusiewicz, and all the other people at Sounds True who helped make this book a real thing.

Alice Peck: how did I get so lucky to have you as an editor? Your immense wisdom and editorial alchemy are matched by your enormous compassion. Thank you for helping me form this book into its final shape, pointing me toward its heart, and keeping everything grounded when I got lost in the weeds.

Thank you to my great teachers through the years, especially Dennis Clausen, Peter Gratton, Mike Callahan, Sherrie Flick, Marc Nieson, Sheryl St. Germain, Heather McNaugher, Uri Talmor, and Clarissa Cigrand.

To those who helped without asking anything in return: Rob Colbert, for your mentorship as I entered the psychedelic world; Rolf Potts, for always answering emails, offering advice, and embodying humility and generosity; Sam Jones, for teaching me how to get paid as a writer when it seemed impossible; Rafaelle Lancelotta, for sitting for several interviews in the early days; Dori Lewis, for trusting me to offer ketamine-assisted therapy under your license; Jason Sienknecht and Bri Bendixsen, for your friendship and encouragement through the years; and Scott Shannon, for your generous mentorship, support, and kindness. Thank you all.

Thank you to all the editors who developed and published my work, especially Brian Frederick, Simon Berger, Wesley Thoricatha, Pat Smith, Lorna Liana, and Bia Labate. Special thanks go to Joe Moore for your encouragement, trust, and genuine goodness in the center of the psychedelic world.

To all my friends who have supported my writing, thank you. Special thanks go to Will Erker, my oldest friend, for being an architect of your unique vision and always showing how much more is possible than we realize.

Thank you to the countless artists who have inspired me, especially Haruki Murakami, David Foster Wallace, David Lynch, Stanley Kubrick, and the musicians of Pink Floyd and the Beatles, whose explorations of strangeness have helped me feel more at home in it.

To BK Loren: this book never would have happened without you. Your magical, inspired vision planted its seeds, and I'm eternally grateful. I'm beyond blessed for your guidance, your care, and most of all, your friendship. I'm so glad I bumped into you that rainy day in Pittsburgh, for you have bettered my life in immeasurable ways.

Thank you, Mom and Dad, for giving me a great home and childhood, supporting my detouring decisions, and always loving me for who I am.

To my brothers: Mike, for your unending goodness and joviality; Kevin, for your honesty, bravery, and resilience; and Conor, for your curiosity, rebelliousness, and reliability to be there when I need to talk with someone who understands how weird things can get. I love you guys more than I can say.

Most of all, I want to thank Alex Warren for always being there to celebrate the highs, navigate the lows, talk out the confusion, laugh at the absurdity, and remind me that all is well. I love you so much, and I'm so glad you have been with me since the day I received my contract.

Finally, thank you, reader, for taking this journey with me. I don't expect you to agree with everything I wrote, but I hope my words prompted fruitful contemplations on your unique vision of this wild trip we're all on. May many blessings meet you on the road ahead.

Notes

Introduction

1   Marc B. Stone et al., "Response to Acute Monotherapy for Major Depressive Disorder in Randomized, Placebo Controlled Trials Submitted to the US Food and Drug Administration: Individual Participant Data Analysis," *BMJ* 378 (August 2, 2022): e067606, doi.org/10.1136/bmj-2021-067606.

2   Charles S. Grob and Jim Grigsby, eds., *Handbook of Medical Hallucinogens* (New York: Guilford Press, 2022), 176.

Chapter 1: Setting the Stage

1   Stanislav Grof, *Realms of the Human Unconscious: Observations from LSD Research* (London: Souvenir Press, 2016).

2   Lauren Johansen et al., "The Psychological Processes of Classic Psychedelics in the Treatment of Depression: A Systematic Review Protocol," *Systematic Reviews* 11, no. 85 (2022), doi.org/10.1186/s13643-022-01930-7.

3   Jack Kornfield, *Bringing Home the Dharma: Awakening Right Where You Are* (Boulder: Shambhala, 2012), 240.

Chapter 2: Foundations of Psychedelic-Assisted Therapy

1   Shayla Love, "It's Time to Start Studying the Downside of Psychedelics," Vice, March 3, 2022, vice.com/en/article/m7vxm8/its-time-to-start-studying-the-downside-of-psychedelics.

2   Carl Rogers, "The Necessary and Sufficient Conditions of Therapeutic Personality Change," *Journal of Consulting Psychology* 21, no. 2 (1957): 95–103, doi.org/10.1037/h0045357.

3   Rogers, "Therapeutic Personality Change."

4   "Sensorimotor Psychotherapy," GoodTherapy, last updated August 24, 2015, goodtherapy.org/learn-about-therapy/types/sensorimotor-psychology.

5   Suzannah Weiss, "How to Set an Intention for Your Drug Trip," Vice, August 19, 2021, vice.com/en/article/akg8ap/how-to-set-an-intention-for-your-drug-trip.

6   Sean Lawlor, "Buddhist University Partners with MAPS to Offer MDMA-Assisted Psychotherapy Training," Lucid News, August 19, 2020, lucid.news /naropa-maps-offer-mdma-assisted-psychotherapy-training/.

Chapter 3: Psilocybin: The Bridge
Between Science and Mysticism

1   José Manuel Rodríguez Arce and Michael James Winkelman, "Psychedelics, Sociality, and Human Evolution," *Frontiers in Psychology* 12 (2021): 729425, ncbi.nlm.nih.gov/pmc/articles/PMC8514078/.

2   Colin Marshall, "Algerian Cave Paintings Suggest Humans Did Magic Mushrooms 9,000 Years Ago," Open Culture, January 27, 2021, openculture.com/2021/01/algerian-cave-paintings-suggest-humans-did -magic-mushrooms-9000-years-ago.html.

3   María Sabina, *María Sabina: Selections*, ed. Jerome Rothenberg (Berkeley, CA: University of California Press, 2003), 28.

4   R. Gordon Wasson, "Seeking the Magic Mushroom," *LIFE*, May 13, 1957, at Trippingly Peak Experiences, accessed January 21, 2024, trippingly.net /lsd/2018/5/14/seeking-the-magic-mushroom.

5   Sabina, *Selections*, 56.

6   Stanislav Grof, "Stanislav Grof Interviews Dr. Albert Hofmann" (Esalen Institute, Big Sur, CA, 1984), MAPS, accessed December 9, 2023, maps.org /news-letters/v11n2/11222gro.html.

7   R. R Griffiths et al., "Psilocybin Can Occasion Mystical-Type Experiences Having Substantial and Sustained Personal Meaning and Spiritual Significance," *Psychopharmacology* 187, no. 3 (2006): 268–83, doi.org/10 .1007/s00213-006-0457-5.

8   Albert Garcia-Romeu et al., "Optimal Dosing for Psilocybin Pharmacotherapy: Considering Weight-Adjusted and Fixed Dosing Approaches," *Journal of Psychopharmacology* 35, no. 4 (2021): 353–61, doi .org/10.1177/0269881121991822.

9   "Hallucinogenic Drug Psilocybin Eases Existential Anxiety in People With Life-Threatening Cancer - 12/02/2016," Johns Hopkins Medicine, December 2, 2016, hopkinsmedicine.org/news/media/releases /hallucinogenic_drug_psilocybin_eases_existential_anxiety_in_people_with _life_threatening_cancer.

10 Alan K. Davis et al., "Effects of Psilocybin-Assisted Therapy on Major Depressive Disorder: A Randomized Clinical Trial," *JAMA Psychiatry* 78, no. 5 (2021): 481–89, doi.org/10.1001/jamapsychiatry.2020.3285.

11 Matthew W. Johnson, Albert Garcia-Romeu, and Roland R. Griffiths, "Long-Term Follow-up of Psilocybin-Facilitated Smoking Cessation," *The American Journal of Drug and Alcohol Abuse* 43, no. 1 (2017): 55–60, doi.org/10.3109/00952990.2016.1170135.

12 Matthew W. Johnson et al., "Pilot Study of the 5-HT2AR Agonist Psilocybin in the Treatment of Tobacco Addiction," *Journal of Psychopharmacology* 28, no. 11 (2014): 983–92, doi.org/10.1177/0269881114548296.

13 William James, *The Varieties of Religious Experience: A Study in Human Nature; Being the Gifford Lectures on Natural Religion Delivered at Edinburgh in 1901-1902* (New York: Penguin, 1985), 388.

14 Griffiths et al, "Psilocybin Can Occasion Mystical-Type Experiences."

15 Rick Doblin, "Pahnke's 'Good Friday Experiment' A Long-Term Follow-Up And Methodological Critique," *Journal of Transpersonal Psychology* 23, no. 1 (1991): 1–28.

16 Huston Smith, *Cleansing the Doors of Perception: The Religious Significance of Entheogenic Plants and Chemicals* (New York: Tarcher, 2000), 101.

17 W.N. Pahnke, "Drugs and Mysticism: An Analysis of the Relationship Between Psychedelic Drugs and the Mystical Consciousness," (unpublished thesis, Harvard, 1963).

18 Kwonmok Ko et al., "Psychedelics, Mystical Experience, and Therapeutic Efficacy: A Systematic Review," *Frontiers in Psychiatry* 13 (2022): 917199, doi.org/10.3389/fpsyt.2022.917199.

19 Aldous Huxley, *The Doors of Perception and Heaven and Hell* (New York: HarperCollins, 2009), 53–54.

20 Robin L. Carhart-Harris et al., "The Entropic Brain: A Theory of Conscious States Informed by Neuroimaging Research with Psychedelic Drugs," *Frontiers in Human Neuroscience* 8 (2014): 20, doi.org/10.3389/fnhum.2014.00020.

21 Carhart-Harris et al., "The Entropic Brain."

22 "The Entropic Brain."

23 "The Entropic Brain."

24 "The Entropic Brain."

25 "Breakthrough Therapy," US Food and Drug Administration, updated January 4, 2018, fda.gov/patients/fast-track-breakthrough-therapy-accelerated-approval-priority-review/breakthrough-therapy.

26 James Kent, "Compass Pathways Phase 2 Psilocybin Results Far from Spectacular," Psychedelic Spotlight, November 2, 2022, psychedelicspotlight.com/compass-pathways-phase-2-psilocybin-results-far-from-spectacular/.

27 "Usona Institute PSIL201 Study Site Now Recruiting Patients with Depression," Businesswire, press release, October 24, 2019, businesswire.com/news/home/20191024005233/en/Usona-Institute-PSIL201-Study-Site-Now-Recruiting-Patients-with-Depression

28 Usona Institute website, accessed December 9, 2023, usonainstitute.org/campus.

29 Benjamin Kelmendi et al., "Single-dose psilocybin for treatment-resistant obsessive-compulsive disorder: A case report," *Heliyon* 8, no. 12 (December 2022): E12135, doi.org/10.1016/j.heliyon.2022.e12135.

30 "Repeat Dosing of Psilocybin in Migraine Headache," clinicaltrials.gov, accessed December 9, 2023, clinicaltrials.gov/ct2/show/NCT04218539.

31 "Psilocybin for the Treatment of Cluster Headache," clinicaltrials.gov, accessed December 9, 2023, clinicaltrials.gov/ct2/show/NCT02981173.

32 Scott LaFee, "New Grant Funds Clinical Trial to Assess Psychedelic as Treatment for Phantom Limb Pain," UC San Diego Today, February 17, 2021, today.ucsd.edu/story/new-grant-funds-clinical-trial-to-assess-psychedelic-as-treatment-for-phantom-limb-pain.

33 LaFee, "New Grant Funds Clinical Trial."

34 "New Grant Funds Clinical Trial."

35 Hub Staff report, "'60 Minutes' segment explores psychedelics research at Johns Hopkins," Hub, Johns Hopkins University, October 14, 2019, hub.jhu.edu/2019/10/14/60-minutes-anderson-cooper-psychedelics/.

36 Angela Chen, "Magic mushrooms help cancer patients cope with fear and depression," The Verge, December 1, 2016, theverge.com/2016/12/1/13799142/magic-mushrooms-psilocybin-cancer-nyu-johns-hopkins-palliative-care.

37 Tyler Fyfe, "Aldous Huxley's wife wrote this letter about injecting him with LSD right before he died," The Plaid Zebra, June 7, 2015, theplaidzebra.com/aldous-huxleys-wife-wrote-this-letter-about-injecting-him-with-lsd-right-before-he-died/.

38 Fyfe, "Aldous Huxley's wife."

39 Steve Paulson, "How a pioneering psychedelic researcher 'leaned in' to his terminal cancer diagnosis," Wisconsin Public Radio, April 8, 2023, wpr .org/how-pioneering-psychedelic-researcher-leaned-his-terminal-cancer -diagnosis.

40 Paulson, "Pioneering psychedelic researcher."

41 "Pioneering psychedelic researcher."

42 David Marchese, "A Psychedelics Pioneer Takes the Ultimate Trip," *New York Times*, April 7, 2023, nytimes.com/interactive/2023/04/03/magazine /roland-griffiths-interview.html

43 "Pioneering psychedelic researcher."

44 Marchese, "A Psychedelics Pioneer."

Chapter 4: LSD: Transformation in Death and Rebirth

1 Albert Hofmann, *LSD: My Problem Child* (Santa Cruz, CA: MAPS, 2009), 36.

2 Hofmann, *LSD: My Problem Child.*

3 *LSD: My Problem Child,* 47.

4 *LSD: My Problem Child.*

5 *LSD: My Problem Child,* 48.

6 *LSD: My Problem Child,* 49.

7 *LSD: My Problem Child.*

8 *LSD: My Problem Child,* 50.

9 *LSD: My Problem Child.*

10 *LSD: My Problem Child,* 50-51

11 *LSD: My Problem Child.*

12 John Lennon, *The Beatles Anthology* (San Francisco: Chronicle Books, 2000), 179, libquotes.com/john-lennon/quote/lba5r0w.

13 Terry Gross, "The CIA's Secret Quest For Mind Control: Torture, LSD And A 'Poisoner In Chief,'" NPR, September 9, 2019, npr.org/2019/09 /09/758989641/the-cias-secret-quest-for-mind-control-torture-lsd-and-a -poisoner-in-chief.

14 Brianna Nofil, "The CIA's Appalling Human Experiments with Mind Control," History, accessed January 21, 2024, history.com/mkultra -operation-midnight-climax-cia-lsd-experiments.

15 Dylan Cahn, "The Acid Tests," Origins: Current Events in Historical Perspective, Ohio State University, December 2015, origins.osu.edu /milestones/december-2015-acid-tests?language_content_entity=en.

16 S. Rufus, "The Acid Wars," Psychology Today, January 26, 2010, psychologytoday.com/us/blog/stuck/201001/the-acid-wars.

17 Alexander Trope et al., "Psychedelic-Assisted Group Therapy: A Systematic Review," *Journal of Psychoactive Drugs* 51, no. 2 (2019): 174–88, doi.org/10.1080/02791072.2019.1593559.

18 Stanislav Grof, *LSD Psychotherapy*, 4th ed. (Santa Cruz, CA: MAPS, 2008), 141.

19 Frederick Streeter Barrett, "The Neuroscience of Psychedelic Drugs, Music, and Nostalgia," filmed at TEDMED 2020, March 2020, video, 14:01, ted.com/talks/frederick_streeter_barrett_the_neuroscience_of_psychedelic_drugs_music_and_nostalgia?language=en.

20 Grof, *LSD Psychotherapy*, 141.

21 "Our Story," wavepaths.com, accessed December 10, 2023, wavepaths.com/story.

22 Robin L. Carhart-Harris et al., "The Entropic Brain: A Theory of Conscious States Informed by Neuroimaging Research with Psychedelic Drugs," *Frontiers in Human Neuroscience* 8 (2014): 20, doi.org/10.3389/fnhum.2014.00020.

23 Timothy Leary, Ralph Metzner, and Richard Alpert, *The Psychedelic Experience* (New York: Citadel Press, 2007), 23.

24 Thomas Taylor, *The Elusinian and Bacchic Mysteries: A Dissertation*, ed. Alexander Wilder (New York: J.W. Bouton, 1891), via Internet Archive, uploaded December 5, 2014 archive.org/details/EleusinianBacchicMysteriesADissertation.

25 Cicero, *De Legibus*, 2.31, via Loeb Classical Library, Harvard University Press, accessed January 24, 2024, loebclassics.com/view/marcus_tullius_cicero-de_legibus/1928/pb_LCL213.415.xml?readMode=recto.

26 Simon Andrew Vann Jones and Allison O'Kelly, "Psychedelics as a Treatment for Alzheimer's Disease Dementia," *Frontiers in Synaptic Neuroscience* 12 (2020): 34, doi.org/10.3389/fnsyn.2020.00034.

27 Johannes G. Ramaekers et al., "A low dose of lysergic acid diethylamide decreases pain perception in healthy volunteers," *Journal of Psychopharmacology* 35, no. 4 (2021): 398–405, doi.org/10.1177/0269881120940937.

28 Albert Hofmann, *Hofmann's Elixir: LSD and the New Eleusis*, ed. Amanda Feilding (London: Strange Attractor Press, 2010), 34.

Chapter 5: MDMA and Nonlinearity

1   Alexander T. Shulgin and David E. Nichols, "Characterization of Three New Psychotomimetics," in *The Psychopharmacology of Hallucinogens*, ed. Richard C. Stillman and Robert E. Willette (New York: Pergamon Press, 1978), 74–83.

2   Michael C. Mithoefer et al., "MDMA-assisted psychotherapy for treatment of PTSD: study design and rationale for phase 3 trials based on pooled analysis of six phase 2 randomized controlled trials," *Psychopharmacology* 236 (2019): 2735–45, link.springer.com/article/10.1007/s00213-019-05249-5.

3   Michael C. Mithoefer, *A Manual for MDMA-Assisted Psychotherapy in the Treatment of Posttraumatic Stress Disorder*, version 7 (Santa Cruz, CA: MAPS, 2015), 27, maps.org/research-archive/mdma/MDMA-Assisted -Psychotherapy-Treatment-Manual-Version7-19Aug15-FINAL.pdf.

4   Julie Holland, *Good Chemistry: The Science of Connection, from Soul to Psychedelics* (New York: HarperCollins, 2020), 92.

5   MAPS, "MAPS-Sponsored Pilot Study: MDMA-Assisted Therapy for PTSD in Couples May Reduce PTSD Symptoms, Improve Couples' Happiness," news release, December 7, 2020, maps.org/news/media/press-release-maps -sponsored-pilot-study-mdma-assisted-psychotherapy-for-ptsd-in-couples -may-reduce-ptsd-symptoms-improve-couples-happiness/.

6   MAPS, "MAPS-Sponsored Pilot Study."

7   Holland, *Good Chemistry*, 93.

8   Mithoefer, *A Manual for MDMA-Assisted Psychotherapy*.

9   Jane Alison, *Meander, Spiral, Explode: Design and Pattern in Narrative* (New York: Catapult, 2019).

10 Steve Paulson, "Isaac Newton's Secret Alchemy," Wisconsin Public Radio, September 19, 2020, wpr.org/isaac-newtons-secret-alchemy.

11 Steve Paulson, "Isaac Newton's Secret Alchemy."

12 John Maynard Keynes, "Newton, the Man" (lecture, given by Geoffrey Keynes, Royal Society of London, July 1946), mathshistory.st-andrews.ac.uk /Extras/Keynes_Newton/.

13 Keynes, "Newton, the Man."

14 Pema Chödrön, *When Things Fall Apart: Heart Advice for Difficult Times* (Boston: Shambhala, 2005), 10.

Chapter 6: Ketamine and Connection

1   Phil Wolfson, *The Ketamine Papers: Science, Therapy, and Transformation* (Santa Cruz, CA: MAPS, 2016), 129–30.

2   Wolfson, *Ketamine Papers*, 12.

3   *Ketamine Papers*, 9.

4   *Ketamine Papers*, 9.

5   Katie MacBride, "I am certain that the LSD experience has helped me very much: 66 years ago, the founder of Alcoholics Anonymous tried LSD — and ignited a controversy still raging today," Inverse, February 9, 2022, inverse.com/mind-body/alcoholics-anonymous-lsd-bill-wilson.

6   Johann Hari, *Chasing the Scream: The First and Last Days of the War on Drugs* (New York: Bloomsbury, 2015), 172.

7   Robert Beverley, The History and Present State of Virginia, in Four Parts (London: Printed for R. Parker, 1705), docsouth.unc.edu/southlit/beverley /beverley.html.

8   Aldous Huxley, *Island: A Novel,* (New York: Harper, 1962), 197.

9   Albert Hofmann, "LSD: Completely Personal" (lecture, Worlds of Consciousness Conference, Heidelberg, Germany, 1996), maps.org/news -letters/v06n3/06346hof.html.

10   *Ketamine Papers.*

11   *Ketamine Papers.*

12   *Ketamine Papers.*

13   *Ketamine Papers.*

Chapter 7: Recreational Use

1   Roland R. Griffiths et al., Psilocybin can occasion mystical-type experiences having substantial and sustained personal meaning and spiritual significance," *Psychopharmacology* 187, no. 3 (August 2006): 268–83, www .hopkinsmedicine.org/press_releases/2006/griffithspsilocybin.pdf.

2   Michael Pollan, *How to Change Your Mind* (New York: Penguin Press, 2018), 38, 228.

3   "Who We Are: What Is Harm Reduction?" Harm Reduction International, accessed December 10, 2023, hri.global/what-is-harm-reduction.

4   "What Is Harm Reduction?"

5 Kristen Philipkoski, "Ecstasy Study Botched, Retracted," Wired News, September 5, 2003, web.archive.org/web/20061231144742/http://www .wired.com/news/business/0,1367,60328,00.html

6 Philipkoski, "Ecstasy Study."

7 Philipkoski, "Ecstasy Study."

8 Robert Colbert and Shannon Hughes, "Evenings with Molly: Adult Couples' Use of MDMA for Relationship Enhancement," *Culture, Medicine, and Psychiatry* 47 (2023): 252–70, doi.org/10.1007/s11013-021-09764-z.

9 Colbert and Hughes, "Evenings with Molly."

Chapter 8: Microdosing

1 Andrew Leonard, "How LSD Microdosing Became the Hot New Business Trip," *Rolling Stone*, November 20, 2015, rollingstone.com/culture/culture -news/how-lsd-microdosing-became-the-hot-new-business-trip-64961/.

2 Balázs Szigeti et al., "Self-blinding citizen science to explore psychedelic microdosing," *eLife* 10 (2021): e62878, elifesciences.org/articles/62878.

3 Joseph M. Rootman et al., "Adults who microdose psychedelics report health related motivations and lower levels of anxiety and depression compared to non-microdosers," *Scientific Reports* 11 (2021): 22479, doi.org /10.1038/s41598-021-01811-4.

4 Joseph M. Rootman et al., "Psilocybin microdosers demonstrate greater observed improvements in mood and mental health at one month relative to non-microdosing controls," *Scientific Reports* 12 (2022): 11091, doi.org/10 .1038/s41598-022-14512-3.

Chapter 9: Creativity and Imagination

1 James Fadiman, *The Psychedelic Explorer's Guide: Safe, Therapeutic, and Sacred Journeys* (Rochester, VT: Park Street Press, 2011).

2 Fadiman, *The Psychedelic Explorer's Guide,* 116.

3 *The Psychedelic Explorer's Guide,* 4.

4 Drake Baer, "How Steve Jobs' Acid-Fueled Quest For Enlightenment Made Him The Greatest Product Visionary In History," Business Insider, January 29, 2015, businessinsider.com/steve-jobs-lsd-meditation-zen-quest-2015-1.

5 Tim Adams, "Amanda Feilding: 'LSD can get deep down and reset the brain – like shaking up a snow globe,'" *The Guardian*, February 10, 2019,

theguardian.com/politics/2019/feb/10/amanda-feilding-lsd-can-reset-the
-brain-interview.

6   Sian Boyle, "Now that is mindblowing! She's the way-out aristocrat
    who drilled a hole in her own head and spent years dabbling in every
    psychedelic drug imaginable. But Lady Amanda Feilding has turned it all
    into a healthcare revolution worth £58million," *Daily Mail*, August 26,
    2021, dailymail.co.uk/news/article-9931169/Way-artistocrat-drilled-hole
    -head-started-healthcare-revolution-worth-58M.html.

7   Joe Moore, "Amanda Feilding – The Beckley Foundation: Changing Minds
    through Psychedelic Research," April 28, 2020, in *Psychedelics Today*,
    podcast, MP3 audio, 60:17, psychedelicstoday.com/2020/04/28/amanda
    -fielding-the-beckley-foundation-changing-minds-through-psychedelic
    -research/.

8   Moore, "Amanda Feilding."

9   Isabel Wießner et al., "LSD and creativity: Increased novelty and
    symbolic thinking, decreased utility and convergent thinking," *Journal
    of Psychopharmacology* 36, no. 3 (2022): 348–59, doi.org/10.1177
    /02698811211069113.

10 N.L. Mason et al., "Spontaneous and deliberate creative cognition during
    and after psilocybin exposure," *Translational Psychiatry* 11, no. 209 (2021),
    doi.org/10.1038/s41398-021-01335-5.

11 Mikal Gilmore, "Beatles' Acid Test: How LSD Opened the Door to
    'Revolver,'" *Rolling Stone*, August 25, 2016, rollingstone.com/feature/beatles
    -acid-test-how-lsd-opened-the-door-to-revolver-251417/.

12 "Paul McCartney takes LSD for the First Time," The Beatles Bible, accessed
    December 11, 2023, beatlesbible.com/1965/12/13/paul-mccartney-takes-lsd
    -first-time/.

13 "Imagination Is More Important Than Knowledge," Quote Investigator,
    January 1, 2013, quoteinvestigator.com/2013/01/01/einstein-imagination/.

14 World Health Organization, *Guidelines for the Management of Conditions
    Specifically Related to Stress* (Geneva: WHO, 2013), web.archive.org/web
    /20131027071552/http://apps.who.int/iris/bitstream/10665/85119/1
    /9789241505406_eng.pdf.

15 "The Beatles and Drugs: LSD (Part Four)," The Beatles Bible, accessed
    December 11, 2023, beatlesbible.com/features/drugs/6/.

16 "The Beatles and Drugs."

17 "The Beatles and Drugs."

18   George Harrison (direct quotation), Harrison Archive, posted April 26, 2022, harrisonarchive.tumblr.com/post/682608490228875264/scan-george -harrison-in-greece-summer-of-1967.

19   Kory Grow, "Brian Wilson Talks Mental Illness, Drugs and Life After Beach Boys," *Rolling Stone*, October 11, 2016, rollingstone.com/music/music -features/brian-wilson-talks-mental-illness-drugs-and-life-after-beach-boys -103541/.

20   Nick Mason, *Inside Out: A Personal History of Pink Floyd* (San Francisco: Chronicle, 2017), 207.

Chapter 10: Mescaline and the Garden of Eden

1   Aldous Huxley, *The Doors of Perception and Heaven and Hell* (New York: HarperCollins, 2009).

2   Rick Strassman, *DMT: The Spirit Molecule: A Doctor's Revolutionary Research into the Biology of Near-Death and Mystical Experiences*, (Rochester, VT: Park Street Press, 2001), 23.

3   Gabrielle Agin-Liebes et al., "Naturalistic Use of Mescaline Is Associated with Self-Reported Psychiatric Improvements and Enduring Positive Life Changes," *ACS Pharmacology and Translational Science* 4, no. 2 (2021): 543–52, doi.org/10.1021/acsptsci.1c00018.

4   Eric Bender, "Finding Medical Value in Mescaline," *Nature*, updated October 4, 2022, nature.com/articles/d41586-022-02873-8.

5   "Our Research," Journey Colab, accessed January 22, 2024, journeycolab .com/our-research.

6   Huxley, *The Doors of Perception*.

7   *Waking Life*, directed by Richard Linklater (Century City, CA: Searchlight Pictures, 2001), 1 hour, 39 minutes.

8   Joe Rogan, "#1661- Rick Doblin," June 2021, in *The Joe Rogan Experience*, podcast, MP3 audio, 3:15:32, open.spotify.com/episode /1Z8lzhvHCMv0c8qZWXbzzK.

9   Marguerite Uhlmann-Bower, "Embracing Deer Medicine - The Flower of Kindness," Plant Pioneers, December 20, 2019, plantpioneers.org/blog /2023/6/24/embracing-deer-medicine-the-flower-of-kindness.

10   Bill Richards, "Flight Instructions for Psychedelic Journeys," Maps of the Mind, accessed January 13, 2024, mapsofthemind.com/2020/08/26 /psilocybin-sessions-instructions/.

11 Janis Phelps, "Developing Guidelines and Competencies for the Training of Psychedelic Therapists," *Journal of Humanistic Psychology* 57, no. 5 (2017): 450–87, kodu.ut.ee/~hellex/aya/kirjandus/ps%C3%BChhoioogia /Developing_Guidelines_and_Competencies_f.pdf.

12 Anthony de Mello, *Awareness: The Perils and Opportunities of Reality* (New York: Image, 1992), 104.

13 David Foster Wallace, "This Is Water," Kenyon College commencement speech, 2005, Gambier, Ohio, fs.blog/david-foster-wallace-this-is-water/.

14 Foster Wallace, "This Is Water."

15 Ludwig Wittgenstein, *Tractatus Logico-Philosophicus* (New York: Harcourt, Brace & Co, 1922; Project Gutenberg, 2021), gutenberg.org/files/5740 /5740-pdf.pdf.

Chapter 11: Ibogaine and Practical Integration

1 John Martin Corkery, "Chapter 8 - Ibogaine as a treatment for substance misuse: Potential benefits and practical dangers," *Progress in Brain Research* 242 (2018): 217–57, doi.org/10.1016/bs.pbr.2018.08.005.

2 Jessica A. Meisner, Susan R. Wilcox, and Jeremy B. Richards, "Ibogaine-associated cardiac arrest and death: case report and review of the literature," *Therapeutic Advances in Psychopharmacology* 6, no. 2 (April 2016): 95–98, doi.org/10.1177/2045125315626073.

3 Jeffrey E. Noller, Chris M. Frampton, and Berra Yazar-Klosinski, "Ibogaine treatment outcomes for opioid dependence from a twelve-month follow-up observational study," *American Journal of Drug and Alcohol Abuse* 44, no. 1 (2018): 37–46, doi.org/10.1080/00952990.2017.1310218.

4 Sherman Peabody, "Ibogaine and Parkinson's Disease," Brain Talk Communities forum, September 22, 2017, braintalkcommunities.org/forum /neurological-disorders-and-injury/parkinson-s-disease/7619-ibogaine-and -parkinson-s-disease.

5 Alan Watts, *The Joyous Cosmology: Adventures in the Chemistry of Consciousness*, rev. 1st ed. (New York: Vintage, 1965), 26. Author's note: for some reason, this quote has been removed from subsequent editions of the book. It is only present in this particular version.

6 Christopher Germer, Ronald D. Siegel, and Paul R. Fulton, eds., *Mindfulness and Psychotherapy* (New York: Guilford Press, 2005), 7.

Chapter 12: 5-MeO-DMT and Nonduality

1 See Dr. Octavio Rettig Hinojosa's webpage, octaviorettig.com/.

2 Albert Most, *Bufo Alvarius: The Psychedelic Toad of the Sonora Desert* (1983), via Internet Archive, uploaded June 28, 2020, archive.org/details /bufoalvariusbooklet_202006/page/3/mode/2up.

3 Alan K. Davis et al., "The epidemiology of 5-Methoxy-N,N-Dimethyltryptamine (5-MeO-DMT) use: Benefits, consequences, patterns of use, subjective effects, and reasons for consumption," *Journal of Psychopharmacology* 32, no. 7 (2018): 779–92, doi.org/10.1177 /0269881118769063.

4 Psychedelic Times Staff, "5-MeO-DMT: Light and Shadow in the Psychedelic Toad," Psychedelic Times, November 20, 2019, psychedelictimes.com/5-meo-dmt-psychedelic-toad/.

5 Alan K. Davis et al., "5-methoxy-N,N-dimethyltryptamine (5-MeO-DMT) used in a naturalistic group setting is associated with unintended improvements in depression and anxiety," *American Journal of Drug and Alcohol Abuse* 45, no. 2 (2019): 161–69, doi.org/10.1080/00952990.2018 .1545024.

6 Johannes Reckweg et al., "A Phase 1, Dose-Ranging Study to Assess Safety and Psychoactive Effects of a Vaporized 5-Methoxy-N, N-Dimethyltryptamine Formulation (GH001) in Healthy Volunteers," *Frontiers in Pharmacology* 12 (2021), doi.org/10.3389/fphar.2021.760671.

7 JL, "Healing Trip Tales: One Vet's Ibogaine & 5-MeO-DMT Experience for PTSD and TBI," Psychedelics Today, August 28, 2020, psychedelicstoday .com/2021/05/26/healing-trip-tales-one-vets-ibogaine-5-meo-dmt -experience-for-ptsd-and-tbi/.

8 JL, "Healing Trip Tales."

9 Albert Hofmann, *LSD: My Problem Child* (Santa Cruz, CA: MAPS, 2009), 17–18.

10 *LSD: My Problem Child*, 13.

11 *LSD: My Problem Child*, 13.

12 *LSD: My Problem Child*.

13 Albert Hofmann, *Hofmann's Elixir: LSD and the New Eleusis*, ed. Amanda Feilding (London: Strange Attractor Press, 2010), 98.

14   Israel Regardie, *Philosopher's Stone: Spiritual Alchemy, Psychology, and Ritual Magic*, ed. Chic Cicero and Sandra Tabatha Cicero (Woodbury, MN: Llewellyn Publications, 2013), 26.

15   Regardie, *Philosopher's Stone*, 26.

16   *Philosopher's Stone*, 26.

17   *Philosopher's Stone*, 26.

18   C. G. Jung, *The Collected Works of C. G. Jung*, vol. 14, *Mysterium Coniunctionis*, trans. Gerhard Adler and R. F. C. Hull (Princeton, NJ: Princeton University Press, 1970).

19   *Philosopher's Stone*, 27.

Chapter 13: DMT: Beholding the Mystery

1   Alan K. Davis et al., "Survey of entity encounter experiences occasioned by inhaled N,N-dimethyltryptamine: Phenomenology, interpretation, and enduring effects," *Journal of Psychopharmacology* 34, no. 9 (2020): 1008–20, doi.org/10.1177/0269881120916143.

2   Sergio A. Mota-Rolim et al., "The Dream of God: How Do Religion and Science See Lucid Dreaming and Other Conscious States During Sleep?" *Frontiers in Psychology* 11 (2020): 555731, doi.org/10.3389/fpsyg.2020.555731.

3   David Foster Wallace, "This Is Water," Kenyon College commencement speech, 2005, Gambier, Ohio, fs.blog/david-foster-wallace-this-is-water/.

4   Foster Wallace, "This Is Water."

5   Kendra Cherry, "What Are the Jungian Archetypes?" VeryWell Mind, updated March 11, 2023, verywellmind.com/what-are-jungs-4-major-archetypes-2795439.

6   Ralph Metzner, *The Unfolding Self: Varieties of Transformative Experience* (Ross, CA: Pioneer Imprints, 2010).

7   Davis et al., "Survey of entity encounter experiences."

8   "Small Pharma Successfully Completes Phase I Clinical Trial of DMT in Combination with Supportive Psychotherapy," GlobeNewswire, press release, September 21, 2021, globenewswire.com/news-release/2021/09/21/2300464/0/en/Small-Pharma-Successfully-Completes-Phase-I-Clinical-Trial-of-DMT-in-Combination-with-Supportive-Psychotherapy.html.

Chapter 14: Deconstructing Shamanism down the Amanita Rabbit Hole

1   Editorial Staff, "Salvia vs. DMT: Effects & Differences," American Addiction Centers Oxford Treatment Center, updated July 19, 2023, oxfordtreatment.com/substance-abuse/hallucinogens/salvia-vs-dmt/.

2   Julian Vayne, *Pharmakon: Drugs and the Imagination* (Oxford, UK: Mandrake of Oxford, 2006), 45.

3   *Pharmakon*, 45.

4   Shelly Beth Braun, "Neo-Shamanism as a Healing System: Enchanted Healing in a Modern World" (PhD diss., University of Utah, 2010), 29, collections.lib.utah.edu/dl_files/6f/4b/6f4b3fa9de4747bc4ca6f9568b9e8544ce250f0a.pdf.

5   Piers Vitebsky, *The Shaman: Voyages of the Soul: Trance, Ecstasy and Healing from Siberia to the Amazon* (New York: Little, Brown, 1995).

6   Vitebsky, *The Shaman*, 11.

7   Ibid. p. 46

8   Vitebsky, *The Shaman*, 8.

9   *The Shaman*, 10

10 Lewis Carroll, *Alice's Adventures in Wonderland* (New York: T.Y. Crowell & Co., 1863; Auckland, NZ: The Floating Press, 2009).

11 Mike Jay, "Mushrooms in Wonderland," Mikejay.net, accessed December 12, 2023, mikejay.net/mushrooms-in-wonderland/.

12 Matthew Byrd, "How Super Mario's Most Iconic Power-Up Was Inspired by Magic Mushrooms," Den of Geek, April 20, 2022, denofgeek.com/games/is-super-marios-most-iconic-power-up-really-based-on-magic-mushrooms/.

13 Amanita Dreamer, "Pt. 2 My Story Panic Anxiety and Healing," Amanita Dreamer, September 10, 2019, YouTube video, 7:37, youtube.com/watch?v=E0AVZwWWJIM.

14 See Amanita Dreamer's blog, amanitadreamer.net/blog.

15 Maria Voynova et al., "Toxicological and pharmacological profile of Amanita muscaria (L.) Lam. – a new rising opportunity for biomedicine," *Pharmacia* 67, no. 4 (2020): 317–23, pharmacia.pensoft.net/article/56112/.

16 Voynova et al., "Amanita muscaria."

17 "A brief cultural history of the mushroom," Deutsche Welle, October 17, 2022, dw.com/en/a-brief-cultural-history-of-the-mushroom/a-63461380.

18 "A brief cultural history of the mushroom."

19 *Rig Veda*, 8.48.3, www.sacred-texts.com/hin/rigveda/rv08048.htm.
20 *Bhagavad Gita* 9, 20.
21 R. Gordon Wasson, *Soma: Divine Mushroom of Immortality* (San Diego: Harcourt Brace Jovanovich, 1972).
22 Sofie Mikhaylova, "A Cultural History Of The Amanita Muscaria Mushroom," Psychedelic Spotlight, October 25, 2022, psychedelicspotlight.com/a-cultural-history-of-the-amanita-muscaria-mushroom/.
23 Mikhaylova, "A Cultural History."
24 Justin Mullis, "Santa's Reindeer and Psychedelic Urine," AIPT, December 22, 2022, aiptcomics.com/2022/12/22/santa-reindeer-shaman-urine-folklore/.

Chapter 15: Iboga and the Single Story

1 Rachel Nuwer, "This psychoactive plant could save lives—and everyone wants to cash in," *National Geographic*, March 8, 2023, nationalgeographic.com/animals/article/ibogaine-pschedelic-drug-root-fair-trade-gabon.
2 Charles Eugène Aubry-Lecomte, "Note sur quelque poisons de la côte occidentale d'Afrique," *Revue Maritime et Coloniale*, vol. XII, 1864.
3 Nuwer, "This psychoactive plant."
4 "The Bwiti Tradition: All Things Bwiti and Its Relation to Iboga," Bwiti Life website, accessed December 12, 2023, bwitilife.com/bwiti-tradition.
5 Uwe Maas and Süster Strubelt, "Music in the Iboga initiation ceremony in Gabon: Polyrhythms supporting a pharmacotherapy," *Music Therapy Today* 4, no. 3 (June 2003), s3.amazonaws.com/arena-attachments/2150825/90b79d90b39e553a1d99e9f0211866bf.pdf?1525805022.
6 Maas and Strubelt, "Music in the Iboga initiation ceremony."
7 "Music in the Iboga initiation ceremony."
8 "Music in the Iboga initiation ceremony."
9 "Music in the Iboga initiation ceremony."
10 "Music in the Iboga initiation ceremony."
11 "Music in the Iboga initiation ceremony."
12 "Music in the Iboga initiation ceremony."
13 "Music in the Iboga initiation ceremony."
14 "Music in the Iboga initiation ceremony."
15 "Music in the Iboga initiation ceremony."
16 "Music in the Iboga initiation ceremony."
17 "Music in the Iboga initiation ceremony."

18 "Music in the Iboga initiation ceremony."

19 Stephanie Hegarty, "Can a hallucinogen from Africa cure addiction?" BBC News, April 13, 2012, bbc.com/news/magazine-17666589.

20 Dan Engle, "Dr. Dan's Journey," DrDanEngle.com, accessed January 14, 2024, drdanengle.com/dr-dans-journey/.

21 Teafaerie, "Hard Reset," The Vaults of Erowid, December 18, 2014, erowid .org/columns/teafaerie/2014/12/18/hard-reset/.

22 Dunja Hersak, "Power Objects: On the Transient Nature of Classifications, with Examples from the Kwilu Region in Congo-Brazzaville," *African Arts* 55, no. 2 (2022): 26–35, doi.org/10.1162/afar_a_00654.

23 Hersak, "Power Objects."

24 "Power Objects" (emphasis mine).

25 "Power Objects."

26 "Power Objects."

27 "Power Objects."

28 Chimamanda Ngozi Adichie, "The Danger Of A Single Story," filmed at TEDGLOBAL 2009, July 2009, video, 18:33, ted.com/talks/chimamanda _ngozi_adichie_the_danger_of_a_single_story?language=en.

29 Juan Scuro and Robin Rodd, "Neo-Shamanism," in Henri Gooren, ed., *Encyclopedia of Latin American Religions* (Switzerland: Springer, 2015): 1–6.

30 Shelly Beth Braun, "Neo-Shamanism as a Healing System: Enchanted Healing in a Modern World" (PhD diss., University of Utah, 2010), 29, collections.lib.utah.edu/dl_files/6f/4b /6f4b3fa9de4747bc4ca6f9568b9e8544ce250f0a.pdf.

31 See the Foundation for Shamanic Studies website on their workshops page, shamanism.org/workshops/ index.php.

Chapter 16: Ayahuasca and the Spirit World

1 Daiara Tukano, "The First Indigenous Ayahuasca Conference (Yubaka Hayrá) in Acre Demonstrates Political, Cultural and Spiritual Resistance," Chacruna, February 14, 2019, chacruna.net/the-first-indigenous-ayahuasca -conference-yubaka-hayra-in-acre-demonstrates-political-cultural-and -spiritual-resistance/.

2 Mark Hay, "The Colonization of the Ayahuasca Experience," JSTOR Daily, November 4, 2020, daily.jstor.org/the-colonization-of-the-ayahuasca -experience/.

3   Bernd Brabec de Mori, "Is Ayahuasca Possibly Less than Five Hundred Years Old?" Chacruna, June 18, 2020, chacruna.net/is-ayahuasca-possibly-less -than-five-hundred-years-old/.

4   Dennis J. McKenna, "Ayahuasca: An Ethnopharmacologic History" (2003), semanticscholar.org/paper/1-Ayahuasca-%3A-An-Ethnopharmacologic -History-Mckenna/6f48aadc69f805030e385ca630f01f0337cf2375.

5   McKenna, "Ayahuasca."

6   Denyse O'Leary, "Yes, Plants May Be Conscious Too, Says Researcher," Mind Matters, August 29, 2022, mindmatters.ai/2022/08/yes-plants-may -be-conscious-too-says-researcher/.

7   Robert Macfarlane, "The Secrets of the Wood Wide Web," New Yorker, August 7, 2016, newyorker.com/tech/annals-of-technology/the-secrets-of -the-wood-wide-web.

8   Gemini Adams, "How Ayahuasca Retreats Gamble with Your Life: 13 Ways to Protect Yourself," Medium, March 3, 2020, geminiadams.medium.com /ayahuasca-how-to-not-die-while-getting-high-e44f40adf306.

9   Isaiah 14:12-14 (New International Version).

10   Revelation 12:7-9 (New International Version).

11   Job 1:6-7 (New International Version).

12   2 Corinthians 11:14 (New International Version).

13   Maria Mohsin, "Legend of the Wendigo," Business Standard, February 14, 2020, tbsnews.net/splash/legend-wendigo-44773.

14   "Sluagh," Emerald Isle, accessed December 12, 2023, emeraldisle.ie/sluagh.

15   Kim McNamara-Wilson, "Irish Faerie Folk of Yore and Yesterday: The Sluagh," GotIreland.com, accessed December 12, 2023, gotireland.com /2012/10/24/irish-faerie-folk-of-yore-and-yesterday-the-sluagh/.

16   "Sluagh."

17   "Funayūrei," Yokai.com, accessed January 15, 2024, yokai.com/funayuurei/.

18   "Mogwai," Monster Wiki, accessed January 15, 2024, monster.fandom.com /wiki/Mogwai.

19   Lion's Roar Staff, "What Are Hungry Ghosts?" Lion's Roar, August 27, 2020, lionsroar.com/what-are-hungry-ghosts/.

20   Gabor Maté, In the Realm of Hungry Ghosts: Close Encounters with Addiction (Berkeley, CA: North Atlantic Books, 2010), 1.

21   Piers Vitebsky, The Shaman: Voyages of the Soul: Trance, Ecstasy and Healing from Siberia to the Amazon (New York: Little, Brown, 1995), 74.

Chapter 17: Peyote and Reciprocity

1 Michael Pollan, *This Is Your Mind on Plants* (New York: Penguin, 2021), 170.

2 Sean Lawlor, "Blessings of Life and Peyote with Debi Roan," Chacruna, February 11, 2021, chacruna.net/debi_roan_blessings_life_and_peyote/.

3 Lawlor, "Blessings of Life."

4 "Blessings of Life."

5 Karol Liver, "Kené – The Visual Language of Nature," Pangea, August 8, 2018, pangeanpath.com/2018/08/08/kene-the-visual-language-of-nature/.

6 John G. Neihardt, ed., *Black Elk Speaks: The Complete Edition* (Lincoln, NE: Bison Books, 2014), 53.

7 Shelly Beth Braun, "Neo-Shamanism as a Healing System: Enchanted Healing in a Modern World" (PhD diss., University of Utah, 2010), 29, collections.lib.utah.edu/dl_files/6f/4b /6f4b3fa9de4747bc4ca6f9568b9e8544ce250f0a.pdf.

8 Carolina Ivanescu and Sterre Berentzen, "Becoming a Shaman: Narratives of Apprenticeship and Initiation in Contemporary Shamanism," *Religions* 11, no. 7 (2020): 362, doi.org/10.3390/rel11070362.

9 Piers Vitebsky, *The Shaman: Voyages of the Soul: Trance, Ecstasy and Healing from Siberia to the Amazon* (New York: Little, Brown, 1995), 10-11.

10 Vitebsky, *The Shaman*, 11.

11 Charles Duits, *Peyote Dreams*, trans. Zara de Yazd (Rochester, VT: Park Street Press, 2013), 17.

12 Duits, *Peyote Dreams*.

13 Brian P. Akers, "Peyote and Peyotism" (master's thesis, Western Michigan University, 1986), scholarworks.wmich.edu/cgi/viewcontent.cgi?article= 2298&context=masters_theses.

14 Pollan, *This Is Your Mind on Plants*, 189.

15 Richard Evans Schultes and Albert Hofmann, "The Tracks of the Little Deer," from *Plants of the Gods: Their Sacred, Healing, and Hallucinogenic Powers* (Rochester, VT: Healing Arts Press, 1992), peyote.org/.

16 Keeper Trout, "Inquisition law: peyote use," *Trout's Notes* (blog), December 5, 2014, sacredcacti.com/blog/inquisition/

17 Keeper Trout, "Inquisition law."

18 Dianna Everett, "The Encyclopedia of Oklahoma History and Culture: Indian Territory," Oklahoma Historical Society, accessed December

12, 2023, okhistory.org/publications/enc/entry?entryname=INDIAN
%20TERRITORY.

19   James Mooney, "The Ghost Dance Religion and the Sioux Outbreak
      of 1890," in J.W. Powell, *Fourteenth Annual Report of the US Bureau
      of Ethnology to the Secretary of the Smithsonian Institution 1892–93*
      (Washington, DC: GPO, 1896), 771, via Internet Archive, last updated
      May 11 2008, archive.org/details/ghostdancerelig01moongoog/page/770
      /mode/2up

20   Mooney, "The Ghost Dance Religion," 772.

21   "The Ghost Dance Religion," 772.

21   Author's interview with Sandor Iron Rope

22   *This Is Your Mind on Plants,* 197.

23   Decriminalize Nature website, accessed January 16, 2024,
      decriminalizenature.org/contribute/volunteer.

24   Psychable Team, "Peyote Pilgrimage of the Wixárika," Psychable, last
      updated October 25, 2022, psychable.com/mescaline/peyote-pilgrimage-of
      -the-wixarika.

25   Psychable Team, "Peyote Pilgrimage."

26   Students for Sensible Drug Policy, "National Decriminalization Advocacy
      Groups Launch Community Healing Alliance to Decriminalize Entheogens
      and Repair the Damage Done by the War on Drugs," press release, January
      27, 2022, ssdp.org/blog/ssdp-decrim-nature-become-partners/.

27   Bia Labate and Kevin Feeney, "Decriminalize Nature Targets Peyote: Drug
      Reform or Settler Colonialism?" Chacruna, July 1, 2022, chacruna.net
      /decriminalize_nature_drug_reform_settler_colonialism/.

Chapter 18: Crossing the Threshold

1   Bryan Samoy, "Dead Deer Symbolism – A Number Of Implied Meanings,"
     RichardAlois Blog for Spirituality & Symbolism, May 9, 2021, richardalois
     .com/symbolism/dead-deer-symbolism.

2   "Iktomi and the Coyote," Aktá Lakota Museum & Cultural Center, accessed
     January 16, 2024, aktalakota.stjo.org/lakota-legends/iktomi-and-coyote/.

Chapter 19: Entering the Shadow Realm

1   Erich Neumann, *Depth Psychology and a New Ethic* (UK: Harper
     Torchbooks, 1973).

2   C.G. Jung, *The Collected Works*, ed. Herbert Read, Michael Fordham, and
    Gerhard Adler, trans. R.F.C. Hull (London: Taylor & Francis, 2023), 357.

3   Jung, *The Collected Works*.

4   C. G. Jung, *The Collected Works of C. G. Jung*, vol. 9, part 2, *Aion: Researches
    into the Phenomenology of the Self*, ed. Herbert Read, Michael Fordham,
    Gerhard Adler, and William McGuire, trans. R.F.C. Hull (Princeton, NJ:
    Princeton University Press, 1953), 71.

5   Albert Hofmann, *LSD: My Problem Child* (Santa Cruz, CA: MAPS, 2009),
    20–21.

6   Timothy I. Michaels et al., "Inclusion of people of color in psychedelic-
    assisted psychotherapy: a review of the literature," *BMC Psychiatry* 18
    (2018): 245, doi.org/10.1186/s12888-018-1824-6.

7   Michaels et al., "Inclusion of people of color."

8   Leia Friedwoman, "It's 2020 and White Men Still Dominate Psychedelic
    Conferences," Lucid News, July 15, 2020, lucid.news/men-still-dominate
    -psychedelic-conferences/.

9   Vann R. Newkirk II, "A Generation of Bad Blood," *Atlantic*, June 17, 2016,
    theatlantic.com/politics/archive/2016/06/tuskegee-study-medical-distrust
    -research/487439/.

10 Rob Picheta, "Black newborns more likely to die when looked after by
    White doctors," CNN, August 20, 2020, cnn.com/2020/08/18/health/black
    -babies-mortality-rate-doctors-study-wellness-scli-intl/index.html.

11 Darcell P. Scharff et al., "More than Tuskegee: Understanding Mistrust
    about Research Participation," *Journal of Health Care for the Poor and
    Underserved* 21, no. 3 (August 2010): 879–97, ncbi.nlm.nih.gov/pmc
    /articles/PMC4354806/.

12 Scharff et al., "More than Tuskegee."

13 "Inclusion of people of color."

14 Drug Policy Alliance, "The Drug War, Mass Incarceration and Race,"
    June 2015, unodc.org/documents/ungass2016/Contributions/Civil
    /DrugPolicyAlliance/DPA_Fact_Sheet_Drug_War_Mass_Incarceration_and
    _Race_June2015.pdf.

15 Sean Lawlor, "Decolonizing Psychedelics and Embodied Social Change with
    Camille Barton," Chacruna, March 11, 2021, chacruna.net/camille_barton
    _embodied_social_change/.

16 Lawlor, "Decolonizing Psychedelics."

17 Sean Lawlor, "Using Psychedelic Therapy to Heal Intergenerational Racial Trauma with Dr. Joseph McCowan," Chacruna, February 4, 2021, chacruna .net/joseph_mccowan_healing_racial_trauma_psychedelics/.

18 Lawlor, "Using Psychedelic Therapy."

19 "Using Psychedelic Therapy."

20 Joseph McCowan, "Rediscovering Our Ancestral Roots of Exploration," Chacruna, August 8, 2022, chacruna.net/rediscovering-ancestral-roots/.

21 "Using Psychedelic Therapy."

22 "Using Psychedelic Therapy."

23 McCowan, "Rediscovering Our Ancestral Roots."

24 "Playboy Interview: Timothy Leary," *Playboy*, September 1966, via Internet Archive, uploaded November 29, 2007, archive.org/stream /playboylearyinte00playrich/playboylearyinte00playrich_djvu.txt.

25 Sherry Walling, "Queering Psychedelic Research: A Pride Special," June 28, 2021, in *MIND CURIOUS*, podcast transcript, archived March 24, 2023, at the Wayback Machine, web.archive.org/web/20230324052439/www .mindcure.com/podcast/celebrating-pride-with-dr-alex-belser.

26 Walling, "Queering Psychedelic Research."

27 "Queering Psychedelic Research."

Chapter 20: Debates over the Psychedelic Future

1 R. R Griffiths et al., "Psilocybin Can Occasion Mystical-Type Experiences Having Substantial and Sustained Personal Meaning and Spiritual Significance," *Psychopharmacology* 187, no. 3 (2006): 268–83, doi.org/10 .1007/s00213-006-0457-5.

2 Peter Bergmann, "All You Ever Wanted to Know About McKenna's Bad Trip," McKennite, June 13, 2016, mckennite.com/articles/badtrip.

3 Matthew W. Johnson, "Consciousness, Religion, and Gurus: Pitfalls of Psychedelic Medicine," *ACS Pharmacology and Translational Science* 4, no. 2 (2021): 578–81, doi.org/10.1021/acsptsci.0c00198.

4 Aldous Huxley, *Brave New World Revisited* (London: Chatto & Windus, 1972), 35–36.

5 Kimberly Chew, Edward Gamson, and Andrew Landsman, "Patent Controversies in Psychedelics," Psychedelic Spotlight, October 21, 2022, psychedelicspotlight.com/patent-controversies-in-psychedelics/.

6   Olivia Goldhill, "A millionaire couple is threatening to create a magic mushroom monopoly," Quartz, November 8, 2018, qz.com/1454785/a -millionaire-couple-is-threatening-to-create-a-magic-mushroom-monopoly.

7   Anna Wiener, "What Is It About Peter Thiel?" *New Yorker*, October 27, 2021, newyorker.com/news/letter-from-silicon-valley/what-is-it-about-peter -thiel.

8   Compass Pathways, "Compass Pathways granted fifth US patent for crystalline psilocybin," press release, November 23, 2021, compasspathways .com/fifth-us-patent-crystalline-psilocybin/.

9   Shayla Love, "Can a Company Patent the Basic Components of Psychedelic Therapy?" Vice, February 9, 2021, vice.com/en/article/93wmxv/can-a -company-patent-the-basic-components-of-psychedelic-therapy.

10   Love, "Can a Company Patent?"

11   Joe Moore and Kyle Buller, "Robert Forte – The Hidden History of Psychedelics," August 7, 2018, in *Psychedelics Today*, podcast, MP3 audio, 1:50:53, psychedelicstoday.com/2018/08/07/robert-forte/.

12   Dimitrije Curcic, "Self-Help Books Statistics," WordsRated, December 16, 2022, wordsrated.com/self-help-books-statistics/.

13   Andrew Leonard, "How LSD Microdosing Became the Hot New Business Trip," *Rolling Stone*, November 20, 2015, rollingstone.com/culture/features /how-lsd-microdosing-became-the-hot-new-business-trip-20151120.

Chapter 21: Psychedelic Stigmatization in Psychedelic Science

1   Emily Dufton, "The Points Interview: Danielle Giffort," *Points* (blog), updated January 26, 2022, archived February 4, 2023, at the Wayback Machine, web.archive.org/web/20230204120433/pointshistory.com/2020 /08/25/the-points-interview-danielle-giffort/.

2   Dufton, "The Points Interview."

3   "The Points Interview."

4   "The Points Interview."

Chapter 22: Bypassing and Abuses of Power

1   John Welwood, *Toward a Psychology of Awakening: Buddhism, Psychotherapy, and the Path of Personal and Spiritual Transformation* (Boston: Shambhala, 2002).

2   Jon Krakauer, *Into the Wild* (New York: Knopf Doubleday, 2009).

3   Michael Pollan, *How to Change Your Mind* (New York: Penguin Press, 2018), 193.

4   Martin Ball, "Excerpts from Dr. Martin Ball's 2016 LAMPS Lecture (Reupload)," Psymposia, YouTube video, 9:56, youtube.com/watch?v= PzcpGtFs7SQ&t.

5   "Statement: Public Announcement of Ethical Violation by Former MAPS-Sponsored Investigators," MAPS, updated March 25, 2022, maps.org/2019 /05/24/statement-public-announcement-of-ethical-violation-by-former -maps-sponsored-investigators/.

6   "Public Announcement of Ethical Violation."

7   Will Hall, "Ending The Silence Around Psychedelic Therapy Abuse," Mad in America, September 25, 2021, madinamerica.com/2021/09/ending-silence -psychedelic-therapy-abuse/.

8   Will Hall, "Psychedelic Therapy Abuse: My Experience with Aharon Grossard, Francoise Bourzat … And Their Laywers," Medium, September 18, 2021, medium.com/@willhall/psychedelic-therapy-abuse-my-experience -with-aharon-grossbard-francoise-bourzat-and-their-a1f0f6d06d64.

9   Hall, "Psychedelic Therapy Abuse."

10 Hall, "Ending The Silence."

11 Cedar Barstow, *Right Use of Power: The Heart of Ethics*, 10th anniv. ed. (Boulder, CO: Many Realms Publishing, 2015), 23.

12 Barstow, *Right Use of Power*, 27.

13 *Right Use of Power*, 129.

14 *Right Use of Power*, 131.

Chapter 23: Psychedelic Exceptionalism

1   Michael Tonry, *Malign Neglect: Race, Crime, and Punishment in America* (New York: Oxford University Press, 1995).

2   John Ehrlichman, "Drug War Confessional," Vera, accessed December 13, 2023, vera.org/reimagining-prison-webumentary/the-past-is-never-dead /drug-war-confessional.

3   Julian Vayne, *Pharmakon: Drugs and the Imagination* (Oxford, UK: Mandrake of Oxford, 2006), 43.

4   "MAPS Announces Appointment of Carl L. Hart, Ph.D., to the Board of Directors," MAPS, press release, November 3, 2021, maps.org/news

/media/maps-announces-appointment-of-carl-l-hart-ph-d-to-the-board-of
-directors/.

5   "The Ancient Ritual of Coca Leaf Reading in the Andes," Inkaterra, January
    25, 2019, www.inkaterra.com/blog/coca-leaf-reading/.

6   "Buried deep – the medical benefits of an ancient herbal plant," University
    of Sydney Faculty of Science, January 22, 2021, sydney.edu.au/science/news
    -and-events/2021/01/22/ancient-herbal-plant.html.

7   Jesse Donaldson and Erica Dyck, *The Acid Room: The Psychedelic Trials and
    Tribulations of Hollywood Hospital* (Vancouver, BC: Anvil Press, 2022).

8   Rick Strassman, *DMT: The Spirit Molecule: A Doctor's Revolutionary Research
    into the Biology of Near-Death and Mystical Experiences*, (Rochester, VT: Park
    Street Press, 2001), 327.

Chapter 24: Destabilization and Death

1   American Psychiatric Association, *Diagnostic and Statistical Manual of
    Mental Disorders*, 5th ed. (Arlington, VA: American Psychiatric Association,
    2013), 531.

2   APA, *DSM-5*.

3   Andrew Callaghan, "Andrew Callaghan: Documenting America's
    Underbelly," Vice, January 21, 2021, YouTube video, 23:14, youtube.com
    /watch?v=zUbod5t_2oM#t=1256.

4   Andrew Callaghan, "Documenting America's Underbelly."

5   Laura Orsolini et al., "The 'Endless Trip' among the NPS Users:
    Psychopathology and Psychopharmacology in the Hallucinogen-Persisting
    Perception Disorder. A Systematic Review," Frontiers in Psychology 8
    (2017): 240, doi.org/10.3389/fpsyt.2017.00240.

6   Orsolini et al., "The 'Endless Trip.'"

7   Matthew Bremner, "The True, Complicated Story of the Ayahuasca
    Murders," *Men's Journal*, January 9, 2020, mensjournal.com/adventure
    /blurred-vision-a-shamans-murder-uncovers-the-dark-side-of-ayahuasca/.

8   Scott Anderson, "Descent into Darkness," CBC News, October 28, 2018,
    newsinteractives.cbc.ca/longform/sebastian-woodroffe-death-ayahuasca-peru.

9   Bremner, "The True, Complicated Story."

10 "The True, Complicated Story."

11 Simon Maybin and Josephine Casserly, "'I was sexually abused by a shaman at an ayahuasca retreat,'" BBC, January 15, 2020, bbc.com/news/stories-51053580.

12 Tricia Escobedo, "Teen's quest for Amazon 'medicine' ends in tragedy," CNN, October 27, 2014, cnn.com/2014/10/24/justice/ayahuasca-death-kyle-nolan-mother/index.html.

13 "Briton Unais Gomes killed in Peru 'during shamanic ceremony,'" BBC, December 18, 2015, bbc.com/news/uk-35133580.

14 Maestro Pedro Tangoa López, "The Dangers of the Ayahuasca Tourism Boom," Kahpi: The Ayahuasca Hub, January 22, 2020, kahpi.net/ayahuasca-tourism-boom-pedro-tangoa-lopez/.

15 Tangoa López, "The Dangers of the Ayahuasca Tourism Boom."

16 "The Dangers of the Ayahuasca Tourism Boom."

17 "The True, Complicated Story."

18 Emma Parry, "HE'S A RIOT: QAnon 'shaman' Jake Angeli first got high aged 11, takes psychedelic cactus & used to go to school dressed as Brad Pitt," U.S. Sun, January 9, 2021, the-sun.com/news/2104357/qanon-horned-shaman-jake-angeli-high-psychedelic-brad-pitt/.

19 Brian A. Pace and Neşe Devenot, "Right-Wing Psychedelia: Case Studies in Cultural Plasticity and Political Pluripotency," Frontiers in Psychology 12 (2021): 733185, doi.org/10.3389/fpsyg.2021.733185.

20 Pace and Devenot, "Right-Wing Psychedelia."

21 Jack Kornfield, "How Concentration Works," jackkornfield.com, June 10, 2015, jackkornfield.com/how-concentration-works/.

22 Emanuel Sferios, "Ketamine Bladder Damage – What You Need to Know," DanceSafe, September 9, 2020, dancesafe.org/ketamine-bladder-damage-what-you-need-to-know/.

23 Brianna da Silva Bhatia et al., "'Excited Delirium' and Deaths in Police Custody," Physicians for Human Rights, March 2, 2022, phr.org/our-work/resources/excited-delirium/?CID=701f40000018pCHAAY&ms=FY20_SEM_GoogleAd&gclid=CjwKCAiAg6yRBhBNEiwAeVyL0MLe0cfsU9OOQ2h3yxBloHm8vQxxSa5IeE5YWqTx6rS4avOGK2F0UhoCtpwQAvD_BwE.

24 Rosalind Watts, "Can magic mushrooms unlock depression? What I've learned in the five years since my TEDx talk," Medium, February 28, 2022, medium.com/@DrRosalindWatts/can-magic-mushrooms-unlock-depression-what-ive-learned-in-the-5-years-since-my-tedx-talk-767c83963134.

25 Watts, "Can magic mushrooms unlock depression?"

26 Ryan Haas, "Major trainer for Oregon's psilocybin program runs out of funding," Oregon Public Broadcasting, March 6, 2023, opb.org/article /2023/03/06/oregon-psilocybin-mushroom-psychedelic-therapy-synthesis -institute/.

Epilogue: Speculative Synthesis of the Philosopher's Stone

1 Kelly Dickerson, "One of Einstein's most famous quotes is often completely misinterpreted," Business Insider, November 19, 2015, businessinsider.com /god-does-not-play-dice-quote-meaning-2015-11.

2 Joseph Campbell, "Follow Your Bliss," Joseph Campbell Foundations, accessed December 13, 2023, jcf.org/about-joseph-campbell/follow-your -bliss/.

3 Mona Sobhani, "'A scientist who is not a mystic, is no scientist:' The value of non-ordinary states of consciousness for science," *The Brave New World of Psychedelic Science* (Substack), June 30, 2022, psychedelicrenaissance.substack .com/p/a-scientist-who-is-not-a-mystic-is.